D1616053

PHARMACOKINETICS
Principles and Applications

Notice

Medicine is an ever-changing science. As new research and clinical experience broaden our knowledge, changes in treatment and drug therapy are required. The authors and the publisher of this work have checked with sources believed to be reliable in their efforts to provide information that is complete and generally in accord with the standards accepted at the time of publication. However, in view of the possibility of human error or changes in medical sciences, neither the authors nor the publisher nor any other party who has been involved in the preparation or publication of this work warrants that the information contained herein is in every respect accurate or complete, and they disclaim all responsibility for any errors or omissions or for the results obtained from use of the information contained in this work. Readers are encouraged to confirm the information contained herein with other sources. For example and in particular, readers are advised to check the product information sheet included in the package of each drug they plan to administer to be certain that the information contained in this work is accurate and that changes have not been made in the recommended dose or in the contraindications for administration. This recommendation is of particular importance in connection with new or infrequently used drugs.

PHARMACOKINETICS
Principles and Applications

Mehdi Boroujerdi, Ph.D.
Professor of Pharmaceutics
Department of Pharmaceutical Sciences
School of Pharmacy
Bouve College of Health Sciences
Northeastern University
Boston, Massachusetts

McGRAW-Hill
Medical Publishing Division

New York   Chicago   San Francisco   Lisbon   London   Madrid
Mexico City   Milan   New Delhi   San Juan   Seoul
Singapore   Sydney   Toronto

McGraw-Hill

A Division of The McGraw-Hill Companies

Pharmacokinetics: Principles and Applications

Copyright © 2002 by The **McGraw-Hill Companies,** Inc. All rights reserved. Printed in the United States of America. Except as permitted under the United States Copyright Act of 1976, no part of this publication may be reproduced or distributed in any form or by any means, or stored in a data base or retrieval system, without the prior written permission of the publisher.

1 2 3 4 5 6 7 8 9 0   DOC/DOC   0 9 8 7 6 5 4 3 2 1

ISBN: 0-07-135164-7

This book was set in Times New Roman by Matrix Publishing Services.
The editors were Stephen Zollo and Barbara Holton.
The production supervisor was Richard Ruzycka.
The cover designer was Mary McKeon.
The index was prepared by Katherine Pitcoff.
The illustrator was Mehdi Boroujerdi

R. R. Donnelley & Sons, Inc. was the printer and binder.

This book is printed on acid-free paper.

Library of Congress Cataloging-in-Publication Data
Boroujerdi, Mehdi.
    Pharmacokinetics : principles and applications / author, Mehdi Boroujerdi.
       p. ; cm.
    Includes bibliographical references and index.
    ISBN 0-07-135164-7
    1. Pharmacokinetics.   I. Title.
    [DNLM: 1. Pharmacokinetics. QV 38 B736p 2001]
  RM301.5 .B66 2001
  615'.7—dc21

All quotes from ancient Greek philosophers in this textbook are from the following book:

Readings in Ancient Greek Philosophy
From Thales to Aristotle
Edited by S. Marc Cohen, Patricia Curd, and C. D. C. Reeve
Indianapolis/Cambridge: Hackett Publishing Company, Inc., 1995

Dedicated to my wife, Parvin, and my sons,
Mazy and Bob

CONTENTS

CHAPTER 11: Multicompartment Models: Linear Two-compartment Model with Instantaneous Input and First-order Disposition 233

CHAPTER 12: Multiple-dosing Kinetics: Two-compartment Model 255

PREFACE

This book is intended to serve as a text for the course in pharmacokinetics that is usually taken by upper-level undergraduates in pharmacy or by first-year graduate students in pharmaceutical sciences. In the preparation of this text the author maintained two main objectives: first, to present the mathematical principles underlying the concepts and theories of pharmacokinetics; second, to present the practical utility of the principles. The mathematical techniques used have been kept as elementary as possible and are mostly standard results in matrix algebra and calculus, including the elementary theory of Laplace transforms. For this reason the author did not delve deeply into such areas as nonlinear pharmacokinetics and population pharmacokinetics. This textbook provides a judicious introductory-level overview of pharmacokinetics. Emphasis is placed on the basic principles that form the foundation for more advanced courses or more applied courses such as therapeutic drug monitoring.

Each chapter is written as self-contained as possible with application examples and assignments of varied difficulty. If the book is used as a basis for course lectures, it will be necessary to select the assignments based on the expectations of students, students' interest, and students' mathematical ability. The extra-credit (EC) assignments are included mainly for students who wish to be challenged, honor students, and graduate students, or as a case study topic for small groups of students who are expected to work together on the assignment and present their findings to the class. The assignments with numerical data provide the opportunity for computer simulation. Obviously the choice of software and the emphasis of the simulation are the instructor's prerogative. Thus, the text is designed as a teaching instrument. It can be used to introduce novices to pharmacokinetics and guide them until they understand the fundamentals well enough to read both articles in the literature and more advanced texts with understanding. The instructor of the course, obviously, can flesh out this framework by providing additional assignments and delving into the wealth of published scientific and clinical articles.

Notices of errors and suggestions for improvement of the text will be greatly appreciated by the author.

Mehdi Boroujerdi

All teaching and all intellectual learning result from previous cognition. This is clear if we examine all the cases; for this is how mathematical sciences and all crafts arise. This is also true of both deductive and inductive arguments, since they both succeed in teaching because they rely on previous cognition: deductive arguments begin with premises we are assumed to understand, and inductive arguments prove the universal by relying on the fact that the particular is already clear. Rhetorical arguments also persuade in the same way, since they rely either on examples (and hence on induction) or on argumentations (and hence deduction).

Aristotle (Posterior Analytics—Book I)

PHARMACOKINETICS
Principles and Applications

CHAPTER 1

GROUNDWORK

Education is not implanted in the soul unless one reaches a greater depth.
PLUTARCH (ON PRACTICE, STOBAEUS SELECTIONS 178.25)

OBJECTIVES

■ To sharpen mathematical skills of students.

■ To review the relevant topics from algebra, calculus, and differential equations that are useful in developing mathematical relationships of pharmacokinetics.

1.1 INTRODUCTION

The indispensable aids to pharmacokinetic analysis are some selected concepts and principles of mathematics. The contribution made by mathematics to the field of pharmacokinetics is not limited to the use of arithmetic, calculus or differential equations. It also encompasses statistical analysis, numerical analysis, and concepts related to probability and stochastic processes. The goal of this chapter is to review briefly the mathematics most useful to students in their understanding of pharmacokinetics. Emphasis is placed on problem solving rather than on the theory of the mathematical concepts.

1.2 DEPENDENT AND INDEPENDENT VARIABLES

The study of kinetics of any process is the evaluation of its time dependency. Pharmacokinetics is the study of the time dependency of physiological processes such as absorption, distribution, metabolism, and excretion (usually abbreviated as ADME) and the pharmacologic response of a drug. Therefore, time is the independent variable in the study of these physiologic processes and the way a drug is handled in the body. The variable that is measured with respect to time is the dependent variable. The dependent variables in pharmacokinetics are drug-related parameters such as plasma concentration of drug, amount excreted in urine and bile, or therapeutic outcome. There are cases, however, when time is not the independent variable and it is difficult to differentiate between the two variables. In this type of situation the variable that is measured more reproducibly would be the independent variable.

A set of two-variable measurements is usually reported as a table with two columns or rows of numbers, or it may be presented as a graph. Plotting the data as a graph, by hand or computer, enables us to interpret the relationship between the two variables, draw conclusions, and arrive at a mathematical relationship describing the behavior of one variable with respect to the other. The most convenient relationship that provides useful information about two-variable measurements is the straight-line relationship.

1.3 STRAIGHT-LINE RELATIONSHIPS

The following are various forms of straight-line relationships and each defines a different relationship between the two variables.

■ The equation of $y = b$, where b is the y intercept and a constant. This equation signifies that changes in the dependent variable, y, are independent of changes of independent variable, x. The line $y = b$ is horizontal and parallel to the x axis (Figure 1.1). We may also have a vertical line when the equation of the line is $x = C$, where C is the x intercept.

■ The relationship $y = \pm mx$, where the slope of the line, m, is the ratio of the two variables. Therefore, the slope is the proportionality constant for conversion of one variable to the other. It can be negative or positive. A positive slope identifies a positive and direct relationship between the two variables (Figure 1.1); that is, the magnitude of y increases or decreases as x increases or decreases. A negative slope, on the other hand, indicates that the magnitude of y decreases as x increases and vice versa. According to equation $y = \pm mx$ the line with negative or positive slope passes through the origin where both variables are zero and therefore the y intercept is equal to zero. When the data set is ideal, the slope is determined by estimating the equivalent ratio between corresponding data (i.e., $y_1/x_1 = y_2/x_2 = y_n/x_n = m$). The equivalent ratio can be used to predict an unknown value of the dependent variable. For example, assume y_n is the unknown. As $y_1/x_1 = y_n/x_n$, and $y_1 \cdot x_n = y_n \cdot x_1$, then the unknown value would be

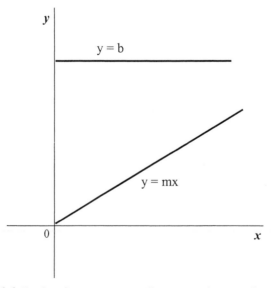

FIGURE 1.1 Graphs of y versus x according to equations $y = b$ and $y = mx$.

$y_n = y_1(x_n/x_1)$. When the data are scattered (i.e., data with random errors), the slope must be determined by regression analysis, which is discussed in Section 1.5.

■ The equation $y = \pm mx + b$, where b is the y intercept and m is the slope. Both the slope and y intercept can be positive or negative. When m is positive, the relationship between x and y is a direct positive proportion and the equivalent ratio for the ideal data is expressed in terms of the difference between the corresponding data:

$$\frac{y_2 - y_1}{x_2 - x_1} = \frac{y_3 - y_2}{x_3 - x_2} = \cdots \frac{y_n - y_{n-1}}{x_n - x_{n-1}} = m \qquad (1.1)$$

When m is negative the relationship between the two variables is negative direct proportion and the calculation of slope is the same as Equation 1.1 (Figure 1.2). The equivalent ratio or slope, positive or negative, remains constant for a reproducible process and should not vary significantly from experiment to experiment. The y intercept, however, may change from one experiment to the next. If multiple sets of data generate a family of parallel straight lines it would indicate that the slopes are the same and y intercepts are different (Figure 1.3). If the lines radiate from the same y intercept it would be a sign of the same y intercepts and different slopes (Figure 1.4).

For a line with a known slope of m, a known coordinate of (x_1, y_1) and an unknown coordinate (x, y), the following point–slope relationship can be developed:

$$\frac{y - y_1}{x - x_1} = m$$

Therefore

$$y = y_1 + m(x - x_1) \qquad (1.2)$$

This equation represents a line with slope of m that passes through (x_1, y_1).

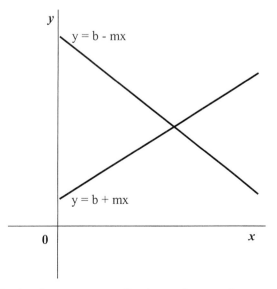

FIGURE 1.2 Graphs of y versus x according to equations $y = b - mx$ and $y = b + mx$.

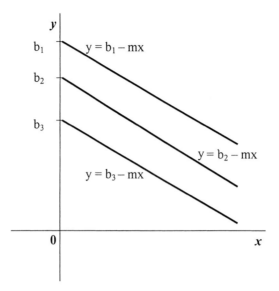

FIGURE 1.3 By keeping slope the same and changing y-intercept, a series of parallel lines can be generated. An analogy would be when different doses of a drug are administered to a patient, plasma concentration is determined at different time after each dose and log plasma concentration is plotted versus time. The lines would be parallel and the y-intercepts, which are dependent on dose, would be different.

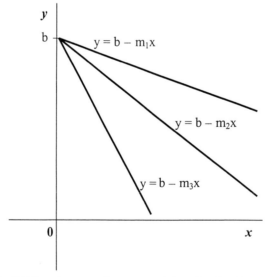

FIGURE 1.4 By keeping the y-intercept the same and changing the slope, a series of lines radiated from one intercept can be generated. An analogy would be when the same dose of a drug is given to different patients with different renal functions and log plasma concentration at different time after the dose is plotted versus time for each patient.

1.4 GRAPHIC ANALYSIS

1.4.1 Numerical Data

A first step in analysis of a set of data when little is known about the relationship between y and x is to plot y against x on a linear graph. Obviously, the simplest approach would be to analyze the data according to one of the straight-line relationships. If the graph of y versus x did not yield a straight-line pattern attempts should be made to acquire a linear relationship from the data. This may well be achieved by plotting different adaptations of y, such as log y, y^2, and $1/y$, against x or different alterations of x such as log x, x^2, and $1/x$.

1.4.2 Numerical Data with an Equation

At times a set of data are presented in conjunction with an equation that at first glance may or may not represent a straight-line relationship. If the equation resembles one of the straight-line relationships, then plotting the data by knowing the y and x of the straight-line would be straightforward. However, if the equation does not look like a straight-line relationship we may modify it to achieve a relationship of the types discussed in Section 1.3. Then, according to the modified linear relationship the variables are plotted to give us the straight line. Some examples of identifying the variables of straight-line relationships and modification of equations are given in Table 1.1.

In addition to linear graph, the data can be plotted on either a semilogarithmic or a log–log graph. The grid lines of the semilog and log-log graph are so distributed that the raw data take up the positions they would have if the log y versus x (for semilog plot) or log y versus log x (for log–log plot) had been plotted on a linear scale. A semilog plot is used in conjunction with common logarithms. Each cycle corresponds to a placement number within the data, that is, to a factor of 10. Therefore, it would be necessary first to decide how many cycles are required on the y axis for the data to be well spread across the graph. One cycle is required for each factor of 10. For instance, if the plasma concentrations ranged from 6 to 735 mg/L, then a three-cycle semilog graph would be adequate. The first cycle would be between 1 and 10 mg/L where 6 mg/L is located, the second cycle between 10 and 100 mg/L, and the third cycle between 100 and 1000 mg/L. It follows that a range of concentrations between 0.17 to 735 would require a four-cycle graph.

1.5 REGRESSION ANALYSIS

In real-life situations due to the presence of experimental error, assuming that it is confined only to the measurement of dependent variable such as the variability of measurement of drug concentration in biological fluid, the data are most often scattered. To fit a set of such data to a straight line does not necessarily mean that one is justified in drawing an arbitrary line through the scattered data points. There is only one straight line that

TABLE 1.1 Examples of Linear Conversions

Relationship	Linear Conversion	x	y	m	b
1. $Ax + By = C$	$y = (C/B) - (A/B)x$	x	y	A/B	C/B
2. $(x/m) = kC^n$[a]	$\log(x/m) = \log k + n \log C$[a]	$\log C$	$\log(x/m)$	n	$\log K$
3. $A = A_0 e^{-kt}$	$\log A = \log A_0 - (kt/2.303)$[b]	t	$\log A$	$-k/2.303$	$\log A_0$
4. $xy = K$	$y = K/x$	x^{-1}	y	K	0
5. $v = (V_{max}C)/(K_m + C)$[c]	$v^{-1} = (K_m/V_{max}\ C) + (1/V_{max})$	C^{-1}	v^{-1}	(K_m/V_{max})	V_{max}^{-1}
6. $dy/dx = -KA$	$dy/dx = -KA^b$	A	dy/dx	$-K$	0
7. $dy/dx = R_0$	$dy/dx = R_0^d$	—	dy/dx	0	R_0
8. $A - A_0 = R_0 t$	$(A - A_0) = R_0 t^d$	t	$A - A_0$	R_0	0
9. $A - A_0 = R_0 t$	$A = A_0 + R_0 t^d$	t	A	R_0	A_0
10. $\ln(A/A_0) = -kt$	$\ln(A/A_0) = -kt^b$	t	$\ln(A/A_0)$	$-k$	0
11. $\ln(A/A_0) = -kt$	$\log A = \log A_0 - (kt/2.303)$[b]	t	$\log A$	$-k/2.303$	$\log A_0$
12. $y = x^2$	$y = x^2$	x^2	y	1	0
13. $y = x^2$	$\log y = 2 \log x$	$\log x$	$\log y$	2	0
14. $x - y = 1$	$y = x - 1$	x	y	1	-1

[a] Freundlich equation.
[b] First-order kinetics.
[c] Michaelis–Menten equation.
[d] Zero-order kinetics.

6

lies near all points. The line is called the regression line (or least-squares line) and is the "best" straight line through a set of scattered points on the graph.

To draw the regression line by hand on graph paper, we need only two coordinates. The straight line can then be drawn between and beyond these two coordinates. The first coordinates are the mean values of x and y,

$$\bar{x} = \left(\sum x\right)/n \tag{1.3}$$

$$\bar{y} = \left(\sum y\right)/n \tag{1.4}$$

where n is the number of observations. The following calculations are needed to establish the second coordinate:

$$\sum d^2x = (\bar{x} - x_1)^2 + (\bar{x} - x_2)^2 + (\bar{x} - x_3)^2 + \cdots$$

$$\sum dxdy = (\bar{x} - x_1)(\bar{y} - y_1) + (\bar{x} - x_2)(\bar{y} - y_2) + (\bar{x} - x_3)(\bar{y} - y_3) + \cdots$$

$$m = \frac{\sum dxdy}{\sum d^2x} \tag{1.5}$$

Here, dx is the deviation of the independent variable and dy is the deviation of the dependent variable from their corresponding mean values. The square of deviation in x is d^2x, the product of deviation in x and y is $dxdy$, and m is the slope of the regression line. For Equation 11 in Table 1.1, dx is dt, dy is $d \log A$, and the slope is

$$m = \frac{\sum d \log Adt}{\sum d^2t}$$

The next step is substituting the calculated values of slope and averages of x and y in the point–slope equation of the straight line:

$$y = \bar{y} + m(\bar{x} - x) \tag{1.6}$$

After multiplication and addition of known values, the equation takes the form

$$y = b \pm mx$$

If the plot were on graph paper then the coordinates of the straight line would be:

$$\text{first coordinate:} \quad x = \bar{x} \quad \text{and} \quad y = \bar{y}$$

$$\text{second coordinate:} \quad x = 0 \quad \text{and} \quad y = b$$

The y intercept can be used as the second coordinates of the regression line, but we may also use and calculate other coordinates by substituting different x values and calculating the corresponding y values.

TABLE 1.2 Serum Concentrations of the Aminoglycoside after the First Dose

Time (h)	Serum Concentration (mg/L)	Log Concentration
0.50	10.10	1.004
0.75	8.20	0.914
1.00	6.40	0.806
1.50	6.20	0.793
2.00	5.60	0.748
3.00	5.30	0.724
4.00	3.50	0.544
6.00	2.90	0.462
8.00	2.00	0.301
12.00	0.91	−0.041
16.00	0.72	−0.142
24.00	0.40	−0.398

APPLICATION

An 80-year-old man with a urinary tract infection receives 60 mg of an aminoglycoside intravenously on a multiple dosing regimen. He receives no other antimicrobial agents and no diuretics during the treatment. The concentration of free drug in serum was determined at different time (t) after the first dose (Table 1.2). Using regression analysis, determine the slope, y intercept, and equation of the line.

The stepwise solution of this problem is as follows:

■ The plot of serum concentration versus time on a linear graph (Figure 1.5) is not a straight line.
■ The plot of log concentration versus time (Figure 1.6) yields scatter data that are linear. Therefore, y = log serum concentration and x = time.

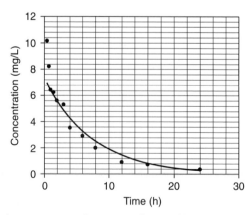

FIGURE 1.5 Plot of plasma concentration versus time on linear graph paper. The curve has the profile of exponential decline.

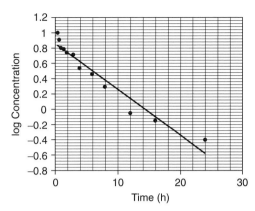

FIGURE 1.6 Plot of log concentration versus time on linear gradation of x and y axes (log concentration $= -0.0601t + 0.871$, $r^2 = 0.946$).

■ The first coordinates of the line, namely, the mean values of x and y are:

$$\bar{t} = \frac{\sum t}{n} = \frac{78.75}{12} = 6.56 \text{ h}$$

$$\bar{y} = \frac{\overset{n}{\sum} \log C}{n} = \frac{5.71}{12} = 0.476$$

■ Determine the slope of the line:

$$\text{slope} = \frac{\sum dydx}{\sum dx^2} = \frac{\sum d \log Cdt}{\sum dt^2} = \frac{-35.62}{592.22} = -0.06 \text{ h}^{-1}$$

■ Determine the equation and the second coordinates of the line (ie, the y intercept).

$$y = \bar{y} + m(x - \bar{x})$$

Therefore,

$$\log C = 0.476 - 0.06(t - 6.56)$$

$$\log C = 0.870 - 0.06t$$

Therefore, if the data set is plotted on linear graph paper with log concentration on the y axis and time on the x axis, the coordinates of the line would be $\{t = 0, y = 0.87\}$ and $\{t = 6.57 \text{ h}, y = 0.476\}$. If the data set is plotted on semilog graph paper with concentration on the y axis and t on the x axis, the coordinates of the line would be $\{t = 0 \text{ h}, y = \text{antilog } 0.87 = 7.43 \text{ mg/L}\}$ and $\{t = 6.57 \text{ h}, y = \text{antilog } 0.476 = 2.992 \text{ mg/L}\}$ (Figure 1.7).

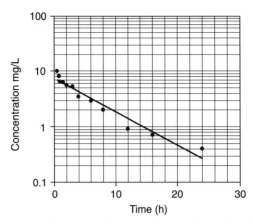

FIGURE 1.7 Plot of concentration versus time on a three-cycle semilogarithmic gradation (concentration = $7.4291e^{-0.1385\,(t)}$, $r^2 = 0.946$).

NOTE

■ The real data set presented in this Application has two distinct linear phases: an initial sharp decline (the first three or four points) followed by a slower decline of the terminal phase. This type of graph is called biphasic and because it is logarithmic and can be converted to exponential, it is also known as a biexponential graph. Because the data are fitted to one straight line only, which represents one exponential, the y intercept of the equation is less than the initial values of the data set. This characteristic of the data set that requires more than one exponential is discussed in Chapter 11.

■ As it will be discussed in the next section, since $\ln x = 2.303 \log x$ and $e^{\ln x} = x$, where x is the independent variable, the equation of the line may also be presented as $\ln C = 2 - 0.138t$ or monoexponential equation of $C = 7.41$ (mg/L)$e^{-0.138(h^{-1})t}$

■ Log values have no units.

1.6 EXPONENTIAL AND LOGARITHMIC FUNCTIONS

Consider the algebraic function $y = x^2$ (Equation 12 from Table 1.1). If the places of x and 2 are switched, the equation changes to a new function that is no longer algebraic, the magnitude of its dependent variable is not the same as y, and the exponent is the independent variable. This new function $Y = 2^x$ is called exponential function and is defined by the general equation $Y = m^x$, where m, called the base, is a constant and can be any number greater than zero. The exponent is the independent variable, x. Different numbers for the base may be convenient choices for some; however, an irrational number, denoted by e, is by far the most popular and frequently used exponential function. The general equation would then take the form $Y = e^x$. The actual value of e is approximated by the equation $e \approx (1 + (1/n))^n$, where n is an integer. For very large values of n, the value of e would be approximately 2.718 281 83. This number is named after Leonhard Euler (1707–1783), who calculated this value up to 25 decimal places. The properties of exponential functions are presented in Table 1.3.

TABLE 1.3 Properties of Exponential Functions

$$e^0 = 1$$
$$e^\infty = 0$$
$$e^{-x} = 1/e^x$$
$$e^x = 1/e^{-x}$$
$$e^x e^z = e^{x+z}$$
$$(e^x)^z = e^{xz}$$
$$e^x/e^z = e^{x-z} = 1/e^{z-x}$$
$$e^x = e^z \text{ if and only if } x = z$$
$$e^{x/z} = (e^{1/z})^x = (e^x)^{1/z}$$

If the variables of equation $Y = m^x$ are interchanged, a new function is formed called the logarithmic function with base m, that is, $x = m^Y$. This means that the logarithm of x to base m, when m is greater than zero, is the exponent Y to which m is raised, or $Y = \log_m x$ if and only if $x = m^Y$. Among all possible logarithmic bases that can be chosen for m, only base 10 and base e are used in science. Therefore, $\log x$ should be interpreted as $\log_{10} x$, and $\ln x$ as $\log_e x$. Logarithms to base 10 are also known as *common logarithms* and logarithms to base e as *natural logarithms*. The properties of logarithmic functions are presented in Table 1.4.

By the use of logarithmic properties, multiplication can be converted to addition, division can be changed to subtraction, and power can be transformed to multiplication (properties 3–5, Table 1.4). Furthermore, the conversion factor between common logarithm and natural logarithm can be estimated from properties 1 and 2. For example, for $x = 10$, the Y value according to the first property is 1, and according to the second property, it is ≈ 2.303; that is, $10^1 = e^{2.303}$, or $\log 10 = 1$ and $\ln 10 = 2.303$. Therefore, $\ln x = 2.303 \log x$, where x is any positive value.

Exponential and logarithmic functions are commonly encountered in pharmacokinetics. The following assignment will sharpen your skills in using the basic properties of these functions.

ASSIGNMENT

Using exponential properties, simplify the following equations.

1.1 $Y = (20e^3)(0.2e^4)$

1.2 $Y = (5e^{-0.5})(2e^{0.9})$

TABLE 1.4 Properties of Logarithmic Functions

1. $\log x = Y$ is comparable to $x = 10^Y$
2. $\ln x = Y$ is comparable to $x = e^Y$
3. $\log xz = \log x + \log z$
4. $\log x/z = \log x - \log z$
5. $\log x^z = z \log x$
6. $\log x = \log z$ if and only if $x = z$
7. $\log 1 = 0$
8. $\log 1/x = -\log x$
9. $\log \sqrt{x} = (1/2)\log x$

1.3 $Y = e^5/e^7$
1.4 $Y = (e^{-5}/e^{-3})^{-2}$
1.5 $Y = e^2 e^{-6}$
1.6 $Y = (2e^{-3}e^3)^{-3}$
1.7 $Y = (15e^{0.2})(0.2e^{0.1})$
1.8 $Y = (e^{-0.6}/e^{-0.2})^{-1}$
1.9 $Y = e^{2/3}$
1.10 $Y = e^{-0.2}(1 - e^{-0.2})/2e^{-0.2}$

Change the following from logarithmic form to exponential form and find x.

1.11 $\log_4 16 = 4$
1.12 $\log_4 2 = \frac{1}{2}$
1.13 $\log_3(1/9) = -2$
1.14 $\log x = 3$
1.15 $\log x = 6$
1.16 $\ln x = 0.2$
1.17 $\ln x = -0.3$
1.18 $\log x = -0.2$
1.19 $\log(x + 1) = 0.2$
1.20 $\ln(x + 2) = 0.6$

Change the following from exponential form to common logarithmic form.

1.21 $64 = 4^3$
1.22 $1/8 = 2^{-3}$
1.23 $Y = 10^5$
1.24 $Y = 10^{-2}$
1.25 $Y = e^{-0.5}$
1.26 $Y = 10e^{-0.1}$
1.27 $Y = 100e^{-5}/20e^{-0.5}$
1.28 $Y = e^5/e^7$
1.29 $Y = (20e^{-0.2})(10e^{-2})$
1.30 $Y = 50(e^{-0.4}/e^{-2})$

1.7 DERIVATIVES OF EXPONENTIAL AND LOGARITHMIC FUNCTIONS

This section offers only a brief review of some of the principles of the first derivative that will be used in future chapters.

Taking the first derivative of a function provides the rate of change of dependent variable, y, with respect to change of independent variable, x. When the equation of first derivative is based on two or more coordinates (i.e., more than two pairs of x and y), the rate equation gives an average rate of change. When the rate is based on one coordinate it is considered the instantaneous rate. The slope of the straight-line equations is the first derivative of the related function beween x and y and provides the average rate of change of y with respect to x. The instantaneous rate of functions with concave or convex, determines the direction of the curves. For example, when the rate is positive it indicates that the curve is rising, when it is negative the curve is falling and when it is equal to zero it identifies the maximum or minimum of the curve and the corresponding x value.

TABLE 1.5 First Derivatives of Selected Functions

Function	Derivative
1. $y = $ constant	$dy/dx = 0$
2. $y = x^n$	$dy/dx = nx^{n-1}$
3. $y = cu$	$dy/dx = c\,(du/dx)^a$
4. $y = cx^n$	$dy/dx = cnx^{n-1}$
5. $y = u(x) \pm v(x)$	$dy/dx = (du/dx) \pm (dv/dx)$
6. $y = u(x)v(x)$	$dy/dx = u(dv/dx) + v(du/dx)$
7. $y = u(x)/v(x)$	$dy/dx = (v(du/dx) - u(dv/dx))/v^2$
8. $y = f(u) = f[g(x)]$	$dy/dx = (dy/du)(du/dx)$
9. $y = [g(x)]^n$	$dy/dx = n[g(x)]^{n-1}(dg/dx)$
10. $y = \ln x$	$dy/dx = 1/x$
11. $y = \ln u(x)$	$dy/dx = (1/u(x))(du/dx)$
12. $y = \log_b x$	$dy/dx = (1/x)(\log_b e)$
13. $y = \log_b u$	$dy/dx = (1/u)\log_b e\, du/dx$
14. $y = e^x$	$dy/dx = e^x$
15. $y = e^{u(x)}$	$dy/dx = e^u\, du/dx$
16. $y = b^x$	$dy/dx = b^x \ln b^b$
17. $y = b^{u(x)}$	$dy/dx = b^u \ln b\, du/dx^b$

^{a}Where c is a constant and $u = f(x)$.
^{b}Where $b > 0$ and $\neq 1$.

The general rules of taking first derivatives that are useful in pharmacokinetics are presented in Table 1.5.

ASSIGNMENT
Find the first derivative of each function.
1.31 $y = \ln(x^2 - 1)$
1.32 $y = (\ln x)^3$
1.33 $y = \ln x^4$
1.34 $y = \exp(-x^2)$
1.35 $C_p = 3e^{-x}$
1.36 $C_p = 4e^{-3x}$
1.37 $C_p = 20(e^{-0.2t} - e^{-2t})$
1.38 $y = e^{3x-2}$
1.39 $C_p = 6x^3 + 3e^{-x}$
1.40 $y = \ln x^{-5}$

1.8 INDEFINITE AND DEFINITE INTEGRALS INVOLVING EXPONENTIAL AND LOGARITHMIC FUNCTIONS

Many functions in pharmacokinetics have reverses. For example, the reverse of a "rate" or "slope" relationship is the equation of line or curve of "concentration or amount versus x," and the reverse of an equation of the line is the area under the concentration–time line or curve. Reversing these functions is referred to as antidifferentiation or integration and the following symbol is used to identify the operation:

$$\int f(x)dx = F(x) + C \qquad (1.7)$$

If the interval of integration is not defined, as in the above relationship, the operation is called indefinite integration and $F(x)$ is the *indefinite integral*. The *definite integral*, on the other hand, is the magnitude of an integral over a well-defined interval. Mathematically, if $F(x)$ is the integral of $f(x)$ between an upper limit of $x = b$ and lower limit of $x = a$ (ie, $a \le x \le b$), the integration is defined as

$$\int_a^b f(x)dx = F(b) - F(a) \qquad (1.8)$$

An example of a definite integral would be when we determine the magnitude of the area under the plasma concentration–time curve of a drug between time of administration ($a = 0$) and 6 hours after the injection ($b = 6$) (Figure 1.8). An example of an indefinite integral is when the area is between the time of administration ($a = 0$) and the time that the dose is totally eliminated from the body ($b = t$, where $t \cong \infty$). Both the upper and lower limits in a definite integral are real numbers. Therefore, the definite integral is a real number, whereas the indefinite integral is a function.

The basic equations of integration of exponential and logarithmic functions that are useful in future chapters are listed in Table 1.6.

APPLICATION

Consider the integration of the following equation, which corresponds to oral absorption of drug X:

$$C_p = 10(e^{-0.01t} - e^{-0.1t}).$$

TABLE 1.6 Basic Equations of Integration of Exponential and Logarithmic Functions

Function	Indefinite Integral
$f(x) = e^x$	$F(x) = \int e^x dx = e^x + C$
$f(x) = e^{ax}$	$F(x) = \int e^{ax} dx = (1/a)e^{ax} + C^a$
$f(x) = 1/x$	$F(x) = \int (dx/x) = \ln x + C^b$
$f(x) = e^{-ax}$	$F(x) = \int e^{-ax} dx = (1/-a)e^{-ax} + C$
$f(x) = 1/x$	$F(x) = \int (dx/x) = \ln|x| + C^c$

$^a a \neq 0.$
$^b x > 0.$
$^c x \neq 0.$

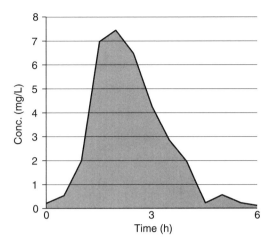

FIGURE 1.8 Area under the plasma concentration–time curve between $t = 0$ and $t = 6$ h.

Here C_p is plasma concentration in mg/L (the dependent variable y) and t is time in hours (the independent variable x). The equation itself corresponds to a skewed bell-shaped curve and the indefinite integral of the equation is

$$\text{area} = 10 \int (e^{-0.01t} - e^{-0.1t}) = 10\,((e^{-0.01t}/-0.01) + (e^{-0.1t}/0.1))$$

whereas the definite integral of the same equation over the interval $t = 0$ to $t = 2$ hours can be estimated as

$$10 \int_0^2 e^{-0.01t} - e^{-0.1t} = 10((e^{-0.02}/-0.01) + (e^{-0.2}/0.1) + (1/0.01) - (1/0.1) = 1.67 \text{ mg h/L}$$

ASSIGNMENT
Find the integral of the following equations over the interval $0 \leq x \leq \infty$. (*Note*: The integration of equations of line or curve, identified here by y or C_p will yield the equations of the area under the line or curve between 0 and ∞. The integration of equations of slope, identified by dy/dx, will provide the equation of the related lines. Assume a and b are constant and t is the independent variable x.)
1.41 $C_p = A(e^{-at} - e^{-bt})$
1.42 $C_p = Ae^{-at}$
1.43 $C_p = Ae^{-at} + Be^{-bt}$
1.44 $y = (e^{-ax} - e^{-bx})/A$
1.45 $y = 4/x$
1.46 $dy/dx = -ky$
1.47 $dy/dx = k_0$ (constant)
1.48 $y = -5/x$
1.49 $C_p = 40e^{-at} - 30e^{-bt}$
1.50 $y = 20/e^{-bx}$

Find the numerical answer to each of the following definite integrals.

1.51   Area under the curve of $C_p = 20e^{-4t} + 15e^{-0.2t}$ over the interval $0 \leq x \leq 1$

1.52   Area under the curve of $C_p = 100e^{-0.5t}$ over the interval $1 \leq x \leq 5$

1.53   Area under the curve of $C_p = 50(e^{-0.693t} - e^{-6.93t})$ over the interval $0 \leq x \leq 2$

1.54   Area under the curve of $y = (e^{2x} - e^{-0.2x})/2$ over the interval $0 \leq x \leq 3$

1.55   Area under the curve of $y = (10/e^{0.1x}) + (8/e^{0.05x})$ over the interval $0 \leq x \leq 4$

1.9 APPROXIMATING DEFINITE INTEGRALS BY THE TRAPEZOID RULE

The trapezoid rule, also called the rectangle rule, is a practical method of approximating definite integrals. In this method, instead of integrating a continuous function we divide the interval of observation into subintervals. After estimating the area of each subinterval, the total area is approximated by adding up the areas of subintervals. The approximation of the total area is closer to the real value when the subintervals are small and x values are close together.

1.9.1 Approximating the Definite Integral of an Equation by the Trapezoid Rule

The stepwise procedure is as follows:

- Identify the interval of integration and the area bounded by the interval.
- Divide the interval into a number of equal subintervals. Obviously, the approximation of the area would improve significantly if we use smaller subintervals.
- Determine the midpoints of each subinterval.
- By substituting each midpoint into the equation, estimate the corresponding y value.
- Determine the area of each subinterval by multiplying the calculated y value by the distance between the two midpoints.
- Add all calculated areas of subintervals together to determine the total area under the curve of the equation within the designated interval.

APPLICATION

Use the trapezoid rule to approximate the area under the equation

$$\int_2^{12} 20(e^{-0.2t} - e^{-2t}).$$

Assume we selected the number of subintervals as $n = 5$ and the units of the independent and dependent variables are h and mg/L, respectively.

Step 1. Find the length of each subinterval:

$$\text{length of each subinterval} = (12 - 2)/5 = 2.$$

Step 2. Find the midpoint of each interval:

$$t_{\text{midpt1}} = (2 + 4)/2 = 3$$

$$t_{midpt2} = (4 + 6)/2 = 5$$

$$t_{midpt3} = (6 + 8)/2 = 7$$

$$t_{midpt4} = (8 + 10)/2 = 9$$

$$t_{midpt5} = (10 + 12)/2 = 11$$

Step 3. Multiply the y value corresponding to each t_{midpt} by the length of subinterval to estimate the area of subinterval. Add all the areas of subintervals together to estimate the total area under the interval. The following calculation summarizes Step 3:

$$AUC_2^{12} = 20(2)[(e^{-0.6} - e^{-6}) + (e^{-1} - e^{-10}) + (e^{-1.4} - e^{-14}) + (e^{-1.8} - e^{-18}) + (e^{-2.2} - e^{-22})]$$

$$AUC_2^{12} = 57.44 \text{ mg h/L}$$

To estimate the total area from $t = 2$ h to $t = \infty$, the terminal area between $t = 12$ and $t = \infty$ should be added to the total area. One approach that is more applicable to exponential functions is to divide the last y value by the constant of the smallest exponent:

$$\text{terminal area} = 20(e^{-2.4} - e^{-24})/0.2 = 9.07 \text{ mg h/L}$$

$$AUC_2^{\infty} = 9.06 + 57.44 = 66.51 \text{ mg h/L}$$

The total area from $t = 0$ to $t = \infty$ would then be the combination of the first area from $t = 0 \rightarrow 2$ h and the area from 2 h $\rightarrow \infty$ as follows:

$$T_{midpt\ 0 \rightarrow 2} = (0 + 2)/2 = 1 \text{ h}$$

$$AUC_0^{\infty} = [20(2)(e^{-0.2(1)} - e^{-2(1)})] + 66.51 = 93.84 \text{ mg h/L}$$

The AUC approximated by the trapezoid rule is usually slightly different from the AUC estimated from the integrated equation. Compare the following answers with those for the trapezoidal rule.

$$AUC_2^{12} = 20\left[-\left(\frac{e^{-2.4}}{0.2}\right) + \left(\frac{e^{-24}}{2}\right) + \left(\frac{e^{-0.4}}{0.2}\right) - \left(\frac{e^{-4}}{2}\right)\right] = 57.778 \text{ mg h/L}$$

$$AUC_0^{\infty} = 20[(1/0.2) + (1/2)] = 90 \text{ mg h/L}$$

The difference is related to the truncation error of the trapezoid rule. For more information on the difference between the two methods you may consult textbooks/web sites of numerical analysis.

1.9.2 Approximating the Area under the Curve of Numerical Data by the Trapezoid Rule

The procedure is similar to what described earlier for estimation of the area under an equation (Section 1.9.1) with the following added considerations:

- Decide whether the approximation of area is from $a = 0$ to $b = \infty$ or from $a \geq 0$ to $b < \infty$.
- When the interval is from 0 to ∞, include the initial values of x and y and add the terminal area after the last data point.
- The general formula to determine the area between $t = 0$ and $t = \infty$ is

$$\text{AUC}_0^\infty = \sum_{i=0}^{n} [(y_i + y_{i+1})/2](x_{i+1} - x_i) + \text{AUC}_n^\infty \tag{1.9}$$

where n is the total number of observations, i identifies each measurement, $i = 0$ indicates that the interval starts from $a = 0$ and the initial values of x and y should be included, and AUC of $n \rightarrow \infty$ represents the terminal area between the last data point and infinity.

APPLICATION

The plasma concentrations of an ampicillin following oral administration of 10 mg/kg of its prodrug (equimolar to 7 mg/kg ampicillin) to a 6-month-old, 6.5-kg, 60-cm infant are listed in Table 1.7. Calculate the area under the curve from $t = 0$ to $t = 6$ h. Since $a = 0$, $b = 6$ h, and $n = 13$, the general equation for estimation of area is:

$$\text{AUC}_0^6 = \sum_{i=0}^{14} \left(\frac{C_{p_i} + C_{p_{i+1}}}{2} \right)(t_{i+1} - t_i) \tag{1.9a}$$

The related calculations are presented in Table 1.7.

TABLE 1.7 Calculations of Area under the Plasma Concentration–Time Curve of the Ampicillin in the 6-Month-old Infant Using the Trapezoidal Rule

Time (h)	Plasma Concentration (mg/L)	$t_{i+1} - t_i$	$\left(\dfrac{C_{p_i} + C_{p_{i+1}}}{2} \right)$	Area
0.00	0.00			
0.05	0.2	0.05	0.10	0.005
0.10	0.50	0.05	0.35	0.017
0.20	2.00	0.10	1.25	0.125
0.30	7.00	0.10	4.50	0.450
0.50	7.50	0.20	7.25	1.450
1.00	6.50	0.50	7.00	3.500
1.50	4.30	0.50	5.40	2.700
2.00	2.85	0.50	3.57	1.785
2.50	1.95	0.50	2.40	1.200
3.00	0.25	0.50	1.60	0.800
4.00	0.55	1.00	0.90	0.900
5.00	0.25	1.00	0.40	0.400
6.00	0.10	1.00	0.175	0.175
			$\text{AUC}_{0\,h}^{6\,h} =$	13.507 mg h/L

TABLE 1.8 Plasma Concentration versus Time Data for Assignment 1.57

Time(min)	10	20	40	60	90	120	180	240	350
C_p(mg/L)	0.24	0.60	5.00	7.80	8.20	6.50	3.80	1.90	0.44

The total area under the curve in the interval $0 \leq t \leq 6$ h is 13.507 mg h/L. Note that the unit of area under the curve when concentration with unit of mass/volume is plotted against time is expressed in mass volume/time.

ASSIGNMENT

1.56   Use the trapezoid rule to approximate the area under the curve of the first 30 minutes of Table 1.7.

1.57   Use the trapezoid rule to estimate the area under the curve of the data in Table 1.8 from $a = 0$ to $b = 350$ min.

1.58   Given the curve

$$C_p = 20_{(mg/L)}e^{-3.2(1/h)t} + 12_{(mg/L)}e^{-1.2(1/h)t} + 6_{(mg/L)}e^{-0.4(1/h)t}$$

   1. Estimate the area under the curve by the trapezoid rule from 0 to 5 hours. Select $n = 10$ subintervals.

   2. Estimate the area by integration from 0 to 5 hours.

   3. Estimate total area from 0 to ∞ by the trapezoid rule and integrated equation.

1.10 DIFFERENTIAL EQUATIONS

The equation $dy/dx = ky$ (Table 1.1, Equation 6) is an example of a differential equation. The dependent variable, y, and its first derivative, dy/dx, are both present in the equation: $(dy/dx) - ky = 0$. Therefore, as a general rule we may define differential equations as those that involve an unknown dependent variable and its first, second, or higher derivatives; for instance, $3(d^2y/dx^2) + 2(dy/dx) + y = 0$ is another example of this type of equation. Differential equations are useful mathematical tools for defining the behavior of xenobiotics in the body. Discussion of the different types of differential equations is the subject matter for courses on differential equations. In this chapter we review solutions of differential equations that have significant application in pharmacokinetics, namely, linear homogenous differential equations with constant coefficients.

Mathematical functions that relate the initial dose of a drug to its disposition in the body are common in pharmacokinetics. To derive these functions or so-called mathematical models, we start by writing the differential equations of the disposition process followed by integration with respect to initial dose. Therefore, any solution of linear differential equations of pharmacokinetics must satisfy the initial condition, that is, the dose. The initial dose by itself is a function of the route of administration. For instance, the initial condition of the systemic circulation, that is, the amount at time zero, is equal to dose after a bolus intravenous injection and equal to zero after an orally administered drug. A convenient method of integration for most differential equations is the Laplace transform (in honor of the great mathematician Pierre Simon de Laplace (1749–1827)), which provides a practical technique for integrating differential equations and finding integrated solutions that satisfy the initial conditions.

1.11 THE LAPLACE TRANSFORM METHOD OF INTEGRATION

The idea behind the Laplace transform is very simple. Every solution of any differential equation has a Laplace transform and the derivatives of the function can also be expressed in terms of Laplace transforms. This means that any complex differential equation can be converted into a linear algebraic equation and the resulting equation can then be solved by simpler methods. The final solution of the algebraic conversion is subjected to an inverse transformation that may often be facilitated by a table of Laplace transforms, yielding the desired solution of the differential equation. To learn more about the basic properties and the uniqueness theorem of the Laplace transform, consult textbooks on ordinary differential equations.

Assume our function is $y = f(t)$. The Laplace transform of this function, represented by the notation $\mathscr{L}[f(t)]$, can be obtained by multiplying the function, $f(t)$, by $e^{-st}dt$ and integrating from time 0 to ∞. Thus, the Laplace transform of the function $f(t)$ is

$$\mathscr{L}[f(t)] = \int_0^\infty e^{-st} f(t) \tag{1.10}$$

where s is the Laplace operator and the function is converted from real variable t into a function of complex parameter s.

APPLICATION

Consider the function $f(t) = 1$. The Laplace transform of $f(t) = 1$ is

$$\mathscr{L}[f(t)] = \mathscr{L}(1) = \int_0^\infty e^{-st}(1)dt = \left.\frac{e^{-st}}{-s}\right|_0^\infty = \frac{1}{s} \tag{1.11}$$

Therefore, the Laplace transform of 1 is $1/s$ and the inverse Laplace transform of $1/s$ is 1:

$$\mathscr{L}^{-1}(1/s) = 1 \tag{1.12}$$

From the above transformation it can also be concluded that the Laplace transform of any constant A is A/s and the inverse Laplace transform of A/s is A. For example, $\mathscr{L}(5) = 5/s$ and $\mathscr{L}^{-1}(5/s) = 5$.

Laplace transforms of other functions such as exponential functions of $f(t) = e^{kt}$ and $f(t) = e^{-kt}$ can be developed as follows:

$$\mathscr{L}(e^{kt}) = \int_0^\infty e^{-st}e^{kt}dt = \int_0^\infty e^{(k-s)} = \left.\frac{e^{(k-s)}}{k-s}\right|_0^\infty = \frac{1}{s-k} \tag{1.13}$$

$$\mathscr{L}(e^{-kt}) = \int_0^\infty e^{-st}e^{-kt}dt = \int_0^\infty e^{-(s+k)} = \left.\frac{e^{-(s+k)t}}{-(s+k)}\right|_0^\infty = \frac{1}{s+k} \tag{1.14}$$

Accordingly,

$$\mathscr{L}^{-1}[1/(s - k)] = e^{kt} \quad \text{and} \quad \mathscr{L}^{-1}[1/(s + k)] = e^{-kt} \tag{1.15}$$

Table 1.9 is a short list of Laplace transforms that are useful in the development of integrated equations of pharmacokinetics. A and B are constants, and k, k_1, k_2, and k_3 are rate constants in their general form and are not related to any specific rate constant. The equations are developed under the assumption that $k_1 \neq k_2 \neq k_3$, m is a power constant, and s is the Laplace parameter.

Among all theorems of Laplace transformation the following are the most useful in pharmacokinetics:

1. If $\mathscr{L}[f_1(t)] = F_1(s)$ and $\mathscr{L}[f_2(t)] = F_2(s)$, then

$$\mathscr{L}[f_1(t)] + \mathscr{L}[f_2(t)] = F_1(s) + F_2(s) \tag{1.16}$$

2. If a is a constant, then

$$\mathscr{L}[af(t)] = a\mathscr{L}[f(t)] = aF(s) \tag{1.17}$$

TABLE 1.9 A Short List of Laplace Transforms

Function	Laplace Transform
1. 1	$1/s$
2. A	A/s
3. t	$1/s^2$
4. At	A/s^2
5. t^m	$m!/(s^{m+1})$
6. e^{kt}	$1/(s - k)$
7. e^{-kt}	$1/(s + k)$
8. Ae^{kt}	$A/s - k$
9. Ae^{-kt}	$A/s + k$
10. Ate^{-kt}	$A/(s + k)^2$
11. $(A/k)(1 - e^{-kt})$	$A/[s(s + k)]$
12. $At^m e^{-kt}$	$A/(s + k)^{m+1}$
13. $(A/k_1)e^{-(k_2/k_1)t}$	$A/(k_1 s + k_2)$
14. $(A/k)t - [A(1 - e^{-kt})/k^2]$	$A/[s^2(s + k)]$
15. $(Ae^{-kt}) - (B/k)(1 - e^{-kt})$	$(As - B)/[s(s + k)]$
16. $[(B - Ak_1)e^{-k_1t} - (B - Ak_2)e^{-k_2t}]/(k_2 - k_1)$	$(As + B)/[(s + k_1)(s - k_2)]$
17. $(A/k_2 - k_1)(e^{-k_1t} - e^{-k_2t})$	$A/[(s + k_1)(s + k_2)]$
18. $(1/k_2k_1) + [(k_2e^{-k_1t} - k_1e^{-k_2t})/k_1k_2(k_1 - k_2)]$	$1/[s(s + k_1)(s + k_2)]$
or $(A/k_1 - k_2)[((1 - e^{-k_2t})/k_2) - ((1 - e^{-k_1t})/k_1)]$	$A/[s(s + k_1)(s + k_2)]$
or $A[(1/k_1k_2) + (e^{-k_1t}/k_1(k_1 - k_2)) - (e^{-k_2t}/k_2(k_1 - k_2)]$	$A/[s(s + k_1)(s + k_2)]$
19. $(A/k)t - (A(1 - e^{-kt}))$	$A/[s^2(s + k)]$
20. $(B/k_1k_2) - ((Ak_1 - B)e^{-k_1t}/k_1(k_1 - k_2)) + ((Ak_2 - B)e^{-k_2t}/k_2(k_1 - k_2))$	$(As + B)/[s(s + k_1)(s + k_2)]$
21. $[(A - k_1)e^{-k_1t}/((k_2 - k_1)(k_3 - k_1))] + [(A - k_2)e^{-k_2t}/((k_1 - k_2)(k_3 - k_2))]$ $+ [(A - k_3)e^{-k_3t}/((k_1 - k_3)(k_2 - k_3))]$	$(s + A)/(s + k_1)(s + k_2)(s + k_3)$

3. If a and b are constants, then

$$af_1(t) + bf_2(t) \text{ has Laplace transform } aF_1(s) + bF_2(s) \tag{1.18}$$

4. The Laplace transform of derivative dy/dx is the Laplace transform of y minus the value of the function at $t = 0$, that is,

$$\mathcal{L}\left[\frac{dy}{dx}\right] = s\bar{y} - y_0 \tag{1.19}$$

$\bar{y}$ is the Laplace transform of y.

1.12 DETERMINANTS AND CRAMER'S RULE

In solving the pharmacokinetic systems of linear differential equations with constant coefficients using Laplace transforms, the coefficients of the transformed functions and the constant terms of the initial conditions play an important role. Briefly, you may recall that any two-variable linear equation can be written in the form

$$ax + by = C \tag{1.20}$$

Similarly, any three-variable equation can be written in the form

$$ax + by + cz = Q \tag{1.21}$$

where a, b, and c are the constant coefficients, and Q is also a constant. In developing some of the equations of pharmacokinetics we frequently encounter systems of simultaneous linear equations of the form

$$ax + by = C$$

$$dx + ey = F \tag{1.22}$$

or

$$ax + by + cz = Q$$

$$dx + ey + fz = R$$

$$gx + hy + iz = s \tag{1.23}$$

and so on. Determinants can make the process of solving a simultaneous set of differential equations simple. The objective of this brief review is only to focus on the use of determinants in the process of solving simultaneous linear differential equations by Laplace transformation. Obviously, the applications and theorems of determinants are beyond the scope of this section.

We now define the solution of the system of equations with three variables (Equations 1.23) according to Cramer's rule. The first step is to establish the determinant of the system by using the coefficients of the variables that are unknown:

$$D = \begin{vmatrix} a & b & c \\ d & e & f \\ g & h & i \end{vmatrix} \quad (1.24)$$

The solution of this determinant is

$$D = aei + bfg + cdh - ceg - bdi - afh \quad (1.25)$$

The signs of Equation 1.25 are decided according to the rule

$$(-1)^{\text{No. of rows}+\text{No. of columns}}$$

That is,

$$\begin{vmatrix} +11 & -12 & +13 \\ -21 & +22 & -13 \\ +31 & -32 & +33 \end{vmatrix}$$

where the first number is the row number and the second is the column number. Therefore, position 32, for example, refers to the third row and second column.

According to Cramer's rule if the solution of determinant D is not zero, then the equations have a unique solution and each variable can be expressed as a fraction of two determinants. The numerator of the fraction is expressed by replacing the column of coefficients of the variable under evaluation with the constants of the system. For example, consider solving for x in the simultaneous Equations 1.23:

$$x = \frac{\begin{vmatrix} Q & b & c \\ R & e & f \\ S & h & i \end{vmatrix}}{\begin{vmatrix} a & b & c \\ d & e & f \\ g & h & i \end{vmatrix}} = \frac{Qei + bfS + Rhc - Sec - Rbi - Qfh}{aei + bfg + chd - gec - dbi - afh} \quad (1.26)$$

A similar arrangement is repeated for each of the unknowns. For instance, for y the solution is

$$y = \frac{\begin{vmatrix} a & Q & c \\ d & R & f \\ g & S & i \end{vmatrix}}{\begin{vmatrix} a & b & c \\ d & e & f \\ g & h & i \end{vmatrix}} = \frac{aRi + Qfg + dSc - cRg - Qdi - fSa}{aei + bfg + chd - gec - dbi - afh} \quad (1.27)$$

The unknowns of a system with two variables can also be determined in a similar way. For example, for simultaneous equations $ax + by = C$ and $dx + ey = F$, the following determinants can be set up:

$$x = \frac{\begin{vmatrix} C & b \\ F & e \end{vmatrix}}{\begin{vmatrix} a & b \\ d & e \end{vmatrix}} = \frac{Ce - bf}{ae - bd} \qquad y = \frac{\begin{vmatrix} a & C \\ d & F \end{vmatrix}}{\begin{vmatrix} a & b \\ d & e \end{vmatrix}} = \frac{aF - dC}{ae - bd} \qquad (1.28)$$

APPLICATION

The following is an example of the use of Laplace transforms and determinants in pharmacokinetics.

Assume a known amount of drug X is given orally to a patient at time 0 and further assume that the drug is absorbed into the body and the systemic circulation, and finally eliminated from the body. This scenario is diagrammed in Figure 1.9. A_D represents the amount of drug at the site of absorption at any time t, A is the amount in the body at time t, k_a and K are the rate constants of absorption and elimination, and A_e is the total amount eliminated from the body at time t.

By writing the related differential equations for the amount of drug at each compartment, we can develop time-dependent relationships for the amount of drug in the body, at the site of absorption, and the amount eliminated from the body. Since our independent variable is time, the differential equations define the rate of change of amount with respect to time. The rate of change in a compartment is the difference between the rates of input and output. The site of absorption is the provider compartment and has only output, and urine is the end compartment and has only input. However, the systemic circulation receives input from the gastrointestinal tract and provides input for the end compartment. The rate of input or output is the related rate constant multiplied by the amount of drug in the compartment that they originate from. The rate constants in this model have units of "time^{-1}" and the rates have units of mass/time. Thus, the rate of change in the amount of drug in different compartments can be defined as

$$dA_D/dt = -k_a A_D \qquad (1.29)$$

$$dA/dt = k_a A_D - KA \qquad (1.30)$$

$$dA_e/dt = KA \qquad (1.31)$$

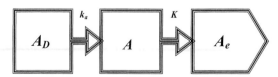

FIGURE 1.9 Schematic diagram of one-compartment model with first-order input and first-order elimination.

The Laplace transforms of Equations 1.29 to 1.31 are

$$s\overline{A}_D - A_D{}^0 = -k_a\overline{A}_D \quad \Rightarrow \quad (s + k_a)\overline{A}_D = A_D{}^0 \tag{1.32}$$

$$s\overline{A} - 0 = k_a\overline{A}_D - K\overline{A} \quad \Rightarrow \quad -k_a\overline{A}_D + (s + K)\overline{A} = 0 \tag{1.33}$$

$$s\overline{A}_e - 0 = k\overline{A} \quad \Rightarrow \quad -K\overline{A} + s\overline{A}_e = 0 \tag{1.34}$$

Here we have three simultaneous equations that can be used individually or in combination to develop the time-dependent integrated equations for each compartment.

The amount of drug at the site of absorption, A_D, at time t can be estimated from the related Laplace transform (Equation 1.32) with the initial condition of $A_D{}^0$ and the use of Table 1.9, line 9:

$$\overline{A}_D = \frac{A_D{}^0}{s + k_a} \tag{1.35}$$

Therefore,

$$A_D = A_D{}^0(e^{-k_a t}) \tag{1.36}$$

The amount of drug in the body, A, at time t, is determined from Equations 1.32 and 1.33 by using the two-by-two determinant and the Laplace table. Assuming the initial condition is zero, that is, at time zero the dose is introduced at the site of absorption and nothing has reached the systemic circulation,

$$\overline{A} = \frac{\begin{vmatrix} s + k_a & A_D{}^0 \\ -k_a & 0 \end{vmatrix}}{\begin{vmatrix} s + k_a & 0 \\ -k_a & s + K \end{vmatrix}} = \frac{(s + k_a)(0) + A_D{}^0(k_a)}{(s + k_a)(s + K) + (k_a)(0)} = \frac{A_D{}^0 \times k_a}{(s + k_a)(s + K)} \tag{1.37}$$

The inverse Laplace transform of Equation 1.37 from line 17 of Table 1.9 is

$$A = \frac{(A_D{}^0)(k_a)}{K - k_a}(e^{-Kt} - e^{-k_a t}) \tag{1.38}$$

We now determine the total amount of drug eliminated from the body, A_e, per unit of time. This can be achieved by solving Equations 1.32 to 1.34 simultaneously with the help of the three-by-three determinant:

$$\overline{A}_e = \frac{\begin{vmatrix} s + -k_a & 0 & A_D{}^0 \\ -k_a & s + K & 0 \\ 0 & -K & 0 \end{vmatrix}}{\begin{vmatrix} s + k_a & 0 & 0 \\ -k_a & s + K & 0 \\ 0 & -K & s \end{vmatrix}} = \frac{(A_D{}^0)(K)(k_a)}{s(s + k_a)(s + K)} \tag{1.39}$$

Taking the inverse Laplace transform of Equation 1.39 (Table 1.9, line 18) provides the equation of the time course of drug elimination:

$$A_e = A_D^0 K k_a \left[\frac{1}{k_a K} + \frac{K e^{-k_a t} - k_a e^{-Kt}}{k_a K (k_a - K)} \right]$$

or

$$A_e = A_D^0 \left[1 + \frac{K e^{-k_a t}}{(k_a - K)} - \frac{k_a e^{-Kt}}{(k_a - K)} \right] \tag{1.40}$$

ASSIGNMENT

1.59 Consider the model presented in Figure 1.10, which may be used in different circumstances for different applications. For this assignment assume that all free drug appears instantaneously in compartment 1. Compartment 2 is the cumulative amount of free drug eliminated via urine. Compartment 3 is the amount of metabolite, corrected for molecular weight, eliminated from the body. The excretion rate constant is k_{12}, the metabolic rate constant is k_{13}, and the elimination rate constant for metabolite(s) is k_{34}. All rate constants are assumed first-order and the overall elimination rate constant, K, is equal to k_{12} plus k_{13}. Compartment 4 is the cumulative amount of metabolite eliminated from the body. Derive the integrated equations for the following:

1. Amount of unchanged drug in the body at time t.
2. Cumulative amount of drug excreted unchanged in the urine at time t.

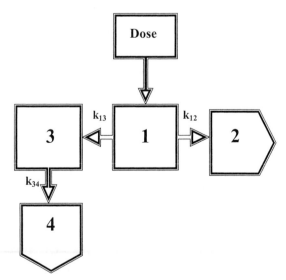

FIGURE 1.10 Schematic diagram of one-compartment model with instantaneous input and first-order excretion and metabolism.

3. Amount of metabolite in the body at time t.
4. Cumulative amount of metabolite eliminated from the body at time t.

1.13 INPUT AND DISPOSITION FUNCTIONS

A different approach in writing the Laplace transform of linear differential equations in pharmacokinetics is based on multiplying the input function of a drug into a compartment with the disposition function of the drug in that compartment. Disposition here refers to distribution and elimination. For example, consider the model of the assignment 1.59. The input function of compartment 1 is the intravenous bolus injection of drug. The input function of compartment 4 is the rate constant k_{34} multipied by Laplace transform of compartment 3. To develop the disposition functions we may consider the compartments of a model as being two types, those that have exit rates and those that are end-compartments. The compartments with exit rates are known as driving-force compartments. The end-compartments have no exit rate and are known as non driving-force compartments. The disposition function of driving-force compartments, is $1/(s + k)$, where k is the sum of the exit rate constants and s is the Laplace operator, and the disposition function of non driving-force compartments is $1/s$.

1.13.1 Input Functions

The input functions via the major routes of administration into the body are:

1. Intravenous bolus: dose (ie, $A_D{}^0$)
2. Intravenous infusion: $f(t) = k_0$ (k_0 is the zero-order rate of infusion.)
   Therefore,

$$\mathscr{L}[f(t)] = \int_0^{t_{\text{inf}}} k_0\, e^{-st}\, dt = -\frac{k_0}{s}\, e^{-st_{\text{inf}}} + \frac{k_0}{s}$$

and

$$\mathscr{L}[k_0] = \frac{k_0}{s}(1 - e^{-st_{\text{inf}}}) \qquad (1.41)$$

where t_{inf} is the time of infusion.
3. Oral absorption: $f(t) = FDk_a e^{-kat}$ (F is the fraction of dose absorbed, FD is the amount of drug absorbed and k_a is the first-order absorption rate constant.)

$$\mathscr{L}[f(t)] = FDk_a \int_0^{\infty} e^{-k_a}e^{-st} = FDk_a \int_0^{\infty} e^{-(k_a+s)} = \frac{FDk_a}{s + k_a} \qquad (1.42)$$

4. The input function from any driving-force compartment (DFC) into other compartments is (exit rate constant)$_{\text{DFC}} \times$ (Laplace transform)$_{\text{DFC}}$

TABLE 1.10 Summary of Input and Disposition Functions and Laplace Transforms of Different Compartments of Assignment 1.59

Location	Input Function	Disposition Function	Laplace Transform
Compartment 1	A_D^0	$1/(s + K)$	$\overline{A} = A_D^0/(s + K)$
Compartment 2	$k_{12}\,\overline{A}$	$1/s$	$\overline{A}_2 = k_{12}\,\overline{A}/s$
			$\overline{A}_2 = (k_{12}/s)(A_D^0/(s + K)$
Compartment 3	$k_{13}\,\overline{A}$	$1/(s + k_{34})$	$\overline{A}_3 = (k_3\,\overline{A})/(s + k_{34})$
			$\overline{A}_3 = (k_{13}A_D^0)/(s + k_{34})(s + K)$
Compartment 4	$k_{34}\,\overline{A}_3$	$1/s$	$\overline{A}_4 = (k_{34}\,\overline{A}_3)/s$
			$\overline{A}_4 = (k_{34}/s)[(k_{13}A_D^0)/(s + k_{34})(s + K)]$

Multiplication of the input and disposition functions provides the Laplace transform for a given compartment. The summary of the input and disposition functions and Laplace transforms of different compartments of Assignment 1.59 are presented in Table 1.10.

1.13.2 Disposition Function

In more complex multicompartment linear models when all peripheral compartments are interdependent with the central compartment, the disposition function of the central compartment is determined by

$$(Disp.)_s = \frac{\displaystyle\prod_{i=2}^{n}(s + E_i)}{\displaystyle\prod_{i=1}^{n}(s + E_i) - \sum_{j=2}^{n}\left[k_{1j}k_{j1}\prod_{\substack{m=2\\m\neq j}}^{n}(s + E_m)\right]} \tag{1.43}$$

where $(Disp)_s$ = the disposition function of the central compartment as a function of Laplace operator, s; n = number of driving-force compartments; E_i = overall exit rate constant from ith compartment; k_{1j} = first-order rate constant from the central compartment to jth compartment (a receiver peripheral compartment); k_{j1} = first-order rate constant from jth compartment to central compartment; Π = continued product of $s + E_i$ starting from ith compartment that is not prohibited; $\sum$ = summation of the two rate constants multiplied by the continued product of $s + E_m$ when m is not prohibited.

APPLICATION

Consider how Equation 1.43 can be applied to a more complex model such as Figure 1.11. All four compartments are considered driving-force compartments; they are interdependent with the central compartment (compartment 1) and they exit to the outside environment, not necessarily the same environment. The overall exit rate constants are as follows:

Compartment 1 $E_1 = k_{10} + k_{12} + k_{13} + k_{14}$
Compartment 2 $E_2 = k_{20} + k_{21}$
Compartment 3 $E_3 = k_{30} + k_{31}$
Compartment 4 $E_4 = k_{40} + k_{41}$

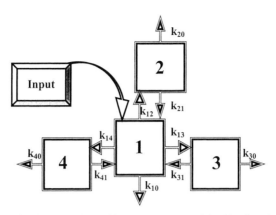

FIGURE 1.11 Schematic diagram of a multicompartment model with all peripheral compartments connected to the central compartment.

The disposition function of compartment 1 according to Equation 1.43 is

$$(\text{Disp.})_{s,1} = \frac{(s + E_2)(s + E_3)(s + E_4)}{\begin{aligned}&(s + E_1)(s + E_2)(s + E_3)(s + E_4) - k_{12}k_{21}(s + E_3)(s + E_4)\\&- k_{13}k_{31}(s + E_2)(s + E_4) - k_{14}k_{41}(s + E_2)(s + E_3)\end{aligned}} \tag{1.44}$$

Following substitution of the miniature rate constants for E_1, E_2, E_3, and E_4 in the denominator of Equation 1.44, mathematical manipulation, and giving expressions of α, β, γ, and δ as the hybrid rate constants of the new combination of miniature rate constants, the equation changes to the following disposition function:

$$(\text{Disp.})_{s1} = \frac{(s + E_2)(s + E_3)(s + E_4)}{(s + \alpha)(s + \beta)(s + \gamma)(s + \delta)} \tag{1.45}$$

Multiplication of the disposition function (Equation 1.45) with any of the input functions yields the Laplace transform of the central compartment. For example, the Laplace transform of Compartment 1 assuming intravenous bolus as the input is

$$\mathscr{L}(A_1) = \text{input} \times (\text{Disp.})_{s1} = \frac{\text{dose}(s + E_2)(s + E_3)(s + E_4)}{(s + \alpha)(s + \beta)(s + \gamma)(s + \delta)} \tag{1.46}$$

To determine the inverse Laplace transform of Equation 1.46 we may use a more extensive table of Laplace transforms or use the method of partial fractions as described in Section 1.13.3.

1.13.3 Determination of Inverse Laplace Transform by Method of Partial Fractions

When the denominator of the Laplace transform of a compartment contains more s terms than the numerator and has no repeated term, its inverse Laplace transform can be estimated by substituting the hybrid rate constants for each s term in the numerator and denominator followed by multiplication by the related exponential function. For example, the inverse Laplace transform of the central compartment (Equation 1.46), using the partial fractions method, is

$$A_1 = \frac{\text{dose}(E_2 - \alpha)(E_3 - \alpha)(E_4 - \alpha)}{(\beta - \alpha)(\gamma - \alpha)(\delta - \alpha)} e^{-\alpha t} + \frac{\text{dose}(E_2 - \beta)(E_3 - \beta)(E_4 - \beta)}{(\alpha - \beta)(\gamma - \beta)(\delta - \beta)} e^{-\beta t}$$

$$+ \frac{\text{dose}(E_2 - \gamma)(E_3 - \gamma)(E_4 - \gamma)}{(\alpha - \gamma)(\beta - \gamma)(\delta - \gamma)} e^{-\gamma t} + \frac{\text{dose}(E_2 - \delta)(E_3 - \delta)(E_4 - \delta)}{(\alpha - \delta)(\beta - \delta)(\gamma - \delta)} e^{-\delta t} \quad (1.47)$$

where A_1 is the amount in the central compartment at time t. The four exponential terms of the equation are created when s in the Laplace transform of the compartment is set respectively equal to $-\alpha$, $-\beta$, $-\gamma$ and $-\delta$ followed by multiplication of each term by their corresponding exponential terms.

1.13.4 Input Disposition Function of Peripheral Compartments

Once the Laplace transform of the central compartment is established, by using the method of substitution the Laplace transforms of the peripheral compartments can be determined. For instance, consider Compartment 2 of Figure 1.11. The related equations are

$$\frac{dA_2}{dt} = k_{12}A_1 - k_{21}A_2 - k_{20}A_2$$

$$\frac{dA_2}{dt} = k_{12}A_1 - E_2A_2 \qquad \text{(where } E_2 = k_{21} + k_{20}\text{)}$$

$$\mathscr{L}\left[\frac{dA_2}{dt}\right] = s\overline{A}_2 - 0 = k_{12}\overline{A}_1 - E_2\overline{A}_2$$

$$\overline{A}_2 = \frac{k_{12}\overline{A}_1}{(s + E_2)} = \frac{k_{12}[\text{dose}(s + E_2)(s + E_3)(s + E_4)]}{(s + E_2)(s + \alpha)(s + \beta)(s + \gamma)(s + \delta)} = \frac{k_{12}[\text{dose}(s + E_3)(s + E_4)]}{(s + \alpha)(s + \beta)(s + \gamma)(s + \delta)}$$

Therefore, by using the method of partial fraction the integrated equation can be obtained as follows:

$$A_2 = \frac{k_{12}[\text{dose}(E_3 - \alpha)(E_4 - \alpha)]}{(\beta - \alpha)(\gamma - \alpha)(\delta - \alpha)} e^{-\alpha t} + \frac{k_{12}[\text{dose}(E_3 - \beta)(E_4 - \beta)]}{(\alpha - \beta)(\gamma - \beta)(\delta - \beta)} e^{-\beta t}$$

$$+ \frac{k_{12}[\text{dose}(E_3 - \gamma)(E_4 - \gamma)]}{(\alpha - \gamma)(\beta - \gamma)(\delta - \gamma)} e^{-\gamma t} + \frac{k_{12}[\text{dose}(E_3 - \delta)(E_4 - \delta)]}{(\alpha - \delta)(\beta - \delta)(\gamma - \delta)} e^{-\delta t}$$

In the above relationships, the input function into the second compartment is k_{12} multiplied by the Laplace transform of the first compartment.

1.14 FIRST-DERIVATIVE TEST OF MAXIMUM

Graphs of plasma concentrations of drugs that are absorbed through absorption sites that are separated from the systemic circulation by a barrier are usually bell-shaped. The early part of the curve has a positive slope and the terminal portion has a negative slope. The change from positive to negative slope occurs at the maximum point of the graphs. Therefore, when the first derivative is positive the curve rises, and when it is negative the curve falls. When the first derivative is equal to zero, the curve changes the direction from rising to falling and the slope at that instant of time is equal to zero (Figure 1.12). This concept is used in pharmacokinetics to determine the maximum plasma concentration and the related time. Consider the following application of this mathematical concept.

APPLICATION

The following equation is the pharmacokinetic model of an orally administered dose of drug X:

$$C_p = 20 \text{ mg}/L(e^{-0.05(h^{-1})t} - e^{-0.2(h^{-1})t})$$

The graph of this equation is bell-shaped and concave downward. Taking its first derivative, setting it equal to zero, and solving for t will determine the instant of time when the slope is equal to zero and C_p is maximum.

$$\frac{dC_p}{dt} = -e^{-0.05t} + 4e^{-0.2t} = 0$$

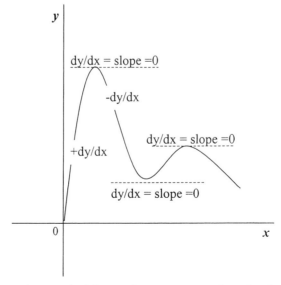

FIGURE 1.12 The maximum and minimum of a curve, representing a function, occur at the x values where the first derivative of the function is equal to zero. The maximum point is between positive and negative slopes, and the minimum point is between negative and positive slopes. A function may have more than one maximum and minimum.

When $dC_p/dt = 0$, t corresponds to T_{max}

$$4e^{-0.2T_{max}} = e^{-0.05T_{max}}$$

$$\ln 4 - 0.15T_{max} = 0$$

$$T_{max} = 9.242 \text{ h}$$

Therefore, the first derivative at $t < 9.242$ h is positive, represents the rising of the curve, and that at $t > 9.242$ is negative, which indicates the downward portion of the curve. For example, the slopes of the curve at $t = 5$ h and $t = 12$ h are

$$\frac{dC_p}{dt} = -e^{-0.05(5)} + 4e^{-0.2(5)} = 0.693$$

$$\frac{dC_p}{dt} = -e^{0.05(12)} + 4e^{-0.2(12)} = -0.187$$

1.15 GEOMETRIC SERIES

Another useful mathematical concept in pharmacokinetics is the geometric series. This concept is used in connection with multiple dosing kinetics. A geometric series is a series for which the ratio of each two consecutive terms is a constant function of the summation. For example, assume that we are walking for a good cause toward a finish line that is 10 miles away. We start off by going walking two thirds of the distance. We rest and then we continue for two thirds of the remaining one third of the 10 miles. We continue, each time walking two thirds of the remaining distance. Therefore, at each time the remaining distance is one third of the previous remaining distance; after n interludes the remaining distance is $(1/3)^n$. On $n + 1$ times the distance walked is $(2/3)(1/3)^n$ and the distance remaining is $(1/3)^{n+1}$. Thus, after $n + 1$ times we have

$$10[(2/3) + (2/3(1/3)) + (2/3(1/3)^2) + (2/3(1/3)^3) + \cdots + (2/3(1/3)^n) + (2/3(1/3)^{n+1})] = 10$$

This can be written as $10[(2/3)(S_n (1/3) + (1/3)^{n+1})] = 10$, where S_n stands for the series. By canceling 10 from both sides, the equation changes to $[(2/3)(S_n (1/3) + (1/3)^{n+1})] = 1$, which can further be reduced to

$$(1 - 1/3)S_n(1/3) = 1 - (1/3)^{n-1}$$

Therefore, $S_n(1/3) = (1 - (1/3)^{n+1})/(1 - 1/3)$, and if we replace $1/3$ by x, the equation changes to the following algebraic equation:

$$S_n(x) = \frac{1 - (x)^{n+1}}{1 - (x)} \tag{1.48}$$

APPLICATION

Assume drug X is given to a patient on a multiple dosing regimen. The dose is injected intravenously in a fixed dosing interval (τ) equal to the half-life of the drug, and the target steady-state accumulation, similar to the 10-mile distance in the preceding example, is known. The following equation represents the time course of a single dose in the body:

$$C_p = 10(mg/h)e^{-0.1155t}$$

The following are the related multiple dosing functions based on the general equation of geometric series:

$$S_n(e^{-0.1155t}) = \frac{1 - e^{-n(0.1155)\tau}}{1 - e^{-0.1155\tau}}$$

Therefore,

$$C_{p_{max}} = 10\left(\frac{1 - e^{-n(0.1155)\tau}}{1 - e^{-0.1155\tau}}\right)$$

$$C_{p_{min}} = 10\left(\frac{1 - e^{-n(0.1155)\tau}}{1 - e^{-0.1155\tau}}\right)e^{-0.1155\tau}$$

As n approaches ∞ the above equations change to

$$S_n(e^{-0.1155t})_{n\to\infty} = \frac{1}{1 - e^{-0.1155\tau}}$$

$$(C_{p_{max}})_{ss} = \frac{10}{1 - e^{-0.1155\tau}}$$

$$C_{p_{max}} = \frac{10e^{-0.1155\tau}}{1 - e^{-0.1155\tau}}$$

The use of these functions is discussed in detail in Chapter 10.

1.16 KINETICS AND RATE EQUATIONS

We may define the behavior of a system, chemical or biologic, by either principles of dynamics or principles of kinetics. The dynamic evaluation is the study of "initial" and "end" states of the system. Therefore, time as an independent variable and the rate of the process or processes that lead to the end state are not included in the evaluation. In other words, dynamic evaluation, despite its name, is static. The data obtained in this type of study determine the dynamics of the system or process, similar to the principles of thermodynamics or pharmacodynamics or toxicodynamics. Kinetics, on the other hand, is the study of time-dependent processes and the time dependency of the change(s) from initial to end state in terms of related rates and mechanisms. In pharmacokinetics we often encounter mass fluxes of drugs from outside of the body into the systemic circulation, drug exchanges among different organs or tissues, biotransformation of drugs, or elimination of drugs from the body. The goal, contrary to pharmacodynamics, is to determine the rates of these processes. Therefore, the rate processes in pharmacokinetics are referred to orderly changes that take place at a definable rate proceeding from an initial condition to a different end state. For example, a drug is given to a patient at an initial time and we are interested in learning how long and at what rate it would take for different biological processes to handle the drug and ultimately eliminate it from the body. Hence, the initial and end states are known and the interest is in quantitative evaluation of the rates at which biologic processes occur. The same expressions and mathematical forms that are used in chemical kinetics are applied to biologic systems and used in pharmacokinetics. In Sections 1.16.1 and 1.16.2 we review the reaction orders and the mathematical forms that are developed for simple irreversible and isothermal reactions that are applied in pharmacokinetics (Figures 1.13 and 1.14).

1.16.1 First-order Process

In a first-order process the rate is proportional to the first power of the concentration or amount of substance under evaluation. To develop rate laws we may start with the simple expression that "rate is proportional to the amount or concentration of the substance," or

$$\text{rate} \propto [A]$$

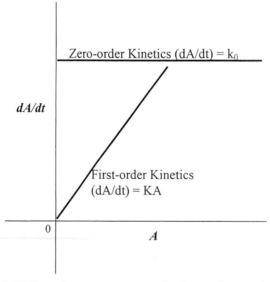

FIGURE 1.13 Plots of rate versus amount for first- and zero-order kinetics.

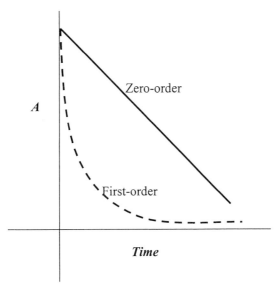

FIGURE 1.14 Plots of amount or concentration versus time for first- and zero-order kinetics.

An equals sign and proportionality constant, K, can replace the proportionality sign and the rate can be expressed as a differential equation of dA/dt:

$$\frac{dA}{dt} = \pm KA \tag{1.49}$$

The plus sign symbolizes a positive outcome for the process, such as "formation" or "accumulation," and the minus sign represents a negative outcome, such as "decomposition" or "disappearance." The differential, dA/dt, is a theoretical relationship and it is not meant to be measured experimentally. However, the integrated rate equations encompass the times of sampling and measurement and are practical for evaluation of the kinetics of a process. The integrated equations of first–order kinetics, with either positive or negative rate, can be derived and presented as follows:

$$\int_0^\infty \frac{dA}{A} = \pm K \int_0^\infty dt$$

Therefore,

$$\ln A = \pm Kt + \text{constant}$$

$$\text{at} \quad t = 0, \text{constant} = \ln A_{t=0} = \ln A_0$$

Therefore,

$$\ln A = \ln A_0 - Kt \quad \text{or} \quad \ln(A/A_0) = \pm Kt \tag{1.50}$$

As $\ln A = 2.303 \log A$

$$\log A = \log A_0 \pm (K/2.303)t \quad \text{or} \quad \log(A/A_0) = \pm (K/2.303)t \tag{1.51}$$

Also, from $e^{\ln A} = A$ it follows that $e^{\ln A} = e^{\ln A_0} e^{\pm Kt}$ will be equal to

$$A = A_0 e^{-Kt} \tag{1.52}$$

Equation 1.49 establishes the units of the rate, dA/dt, as "mass/time" and the units of the rate constant, K, as "time^{-1}". Furthermore, Equations 1.50 and 1.51 imply that for first-order process, plots of $\ln A$ or $\log A$ versus time will be linear with a slope equal to $\pm K$ (for Equation 1.50) or $\pm K/2.303$ (for Equation 1.51) and a y intercept equal to $\ln A_0$ or $\log A_0$, respectively. The equations also indicate that for first-order kinetics, plots of $\ln(A/A_0)$ or $\log(A/A_0)$ versus time will pass through the origin with a slope $\pm K$ or $\pm K/2.303$. Equation 1.52 indicates that a plot of A versus t on semilog paper is a straight line with a y intercept of A_0 and a slope of $\pm K/2.303$ (Figure 1.15).

An important aspect of first-order kinetics is definition of the equations $\ln(A/A_0) = \pm Kt$ or $\log(A/A_0) = \pm Kt/2.303$. They mean that the time required for a first-order process to proceed to a certain level, for example, 50% complete or 90% complete, is independent of the amount or concentration of a drug. This property is used to estimate the half-life of a drug. The half-life, $T_{1/2}$, is the time in which a process is half-complete, or it is the time required for one-half of the initial amount or concentration of a drug to be used in a process. The latter definition is used to develop the following equation for $T_{1/2}$:

$$\text{At } t = T_{1/2}, \quad A = A_0/2$$

$$\ln \frac{A_0}{2} = \ln A_0 \pm \frac{KT_{1/2}}{2.303}$$

$$\log A_0 - \log \frac{A_0}{2} = \log \frac{A_0/2}{A_0} = \log 2 = 0.301$$

$$KT_{1/2} = 0.693$$

Therefore,

$$T_{1/2} = 0.693/K \quad \text{or} \quad K = 0.693/T_{1/2} \tag{1.53}$$

1.16.2 Zero-order Process

Processes in which the rate is independent of concentration or amount of drug are considered zero-order kinetic processes. The rate, therefore, is determined by factors other than drug itself. An example of this type of kinetics is when a high concentration of a drug saturates the enzyme system responsible for the metabolism of the drug and the metabolism proceeds at a constant rate, which is the maximum rate of metabolism. Under

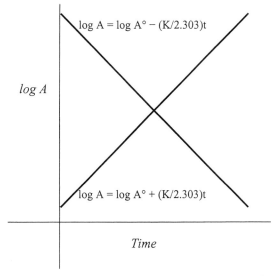

The plot shows:
$\log A = \log A^\circ - (K/2.303)t$
$\log A = \log A^\circ + (K/2.303)t$
with y-axis labeled *log A* and x-axis labeled *Time*.

FIGURE 1.15 Linear plots of log amount or concentration versus time for first-order kinetics.

this condition the enzyme system determines the rate. Another example is when an infusion pump infuses solution of a drug intravenously and the pump determines the constant rate of input. The rate equation of a zero-order process is expressed as

$$\frac{dA}{dt} = \pm k_0 \tag{1.54}$$

where k_0 is the zero-order rate or rate constant, which has the units of mass/time. Integration of the above equation yields

$$A = A_0 \pm k_0 t \tag{1.55}$$

where A is the amount at time t and A_0 is the initial amount. The plot of A versus t on a linear graph is a straight line with y intercept of A_0 and slope of k_0.

The half-life of a zero-order process, contrary to first-order kinetics, is not a constant. It is a variable that is directly proportional to 50% of the initial amount or concentration of the drug and is inversely proportional to the zero-order rate:

$$A_0 - \frac{A_0}{2} = k_0 T_{1/2}$$

$$T_{1/2} = \frac{A_0}{2k_0} \tag{1.56}$$

Second- and higher-order kinetics and their applications are beyond the scope of this textbook.

BIBLIOGRAPHY

1. Benet LZ. General treatment of linear mammillary models with elimination from any compartment as used in pharmacokinetics. *J Pharm Sci* 61(4):536, 1972;61:536.

2. Benet LZ, Turi JS. Use of a general partial fraction theorem for obtaining inverse Laplace transforms in pharmaceutical analysis. *J Pharm Sci* 1971;60:1593.

3. Brauer F, Nohel JA. *Ordinary Differential Equations.* Menlo Park, CA: Benjamin, 1973:392.

4. Gardiner WC. *Rates and Mechanisms of Chemical Reactions.* New York: Benjamin, 1969:20.

5. Gibaldi M, Perrier D. *Pharmacokinetics.* 2nd ed. New York: Marcel Dekker, 1982:419.

6. Hamming RW. *Introduction to Applied Numerical Analysis.* New York: McGraw–Hill, 1971:173.

7. Johnson FH, Eyring H, Stover GJ. *The Theory of Rate Processes in Biology and Medicine.* New York: Wiley, 1974:373.

8. Rescigno A, Serge G. *Drug and Tracer Kinetics.* New York: Blaisdell, 1966:1.

9. Thomas GB. *Calculus and Analytic Geometry, Part 1: Functions of One Variable and Analytic Geometry.* Alternate ed. Reading, MA: Addison–Wesley, 1972:1.

10. Rudin W. *Principles of Mathematical Analysis.* 2nd ed. New York: McGraw–Hill, 1969:187, 201, 53.

11. Vaughn DP, Trainor A. Derivation of general equations for linear mammaillary models when the drug is administered by different routes. *J Pharmacokinet Biopharm* 1975;3:230.

CHAPTER 2

GENERAL INTRODUCTION TO PHYSIOLOGIC MODELING AND COMPARTMENTAL ANALYSIS

And indeed all things that are known have number.
For without this nothing whatever could possibly be thought of or known.
PYTHAGORAS (STOBAEUS SELECTIONS 1.21.7C)

OBJECTIVES

- To introduce the concept of pharmacokinetics.
- To review different approaches in pharmacokinetic modeling and analysis.
- To introduce the principles of compartmental and physiologic modeling.
- To understand the utility of the various approaches in pharmacokinetic analysis.

2.1 INTRODUCTION

The study of the kinetics of absorption, distribution, metabolism, and excretion of drugs and their corresponding pharmacologic response is referred to as *pharmacokinetics*. Therefore, the scope of this knowledge is the quantitative analysis of how living systems handle xenobiotics rather than how drugs act on living systems. The study of drug action belongs primarily to the field of pharmacology. The knowledge of pharmacokinetics is based on concentration curves of drugs or their metabolite(s) in the body and other relevant kinetic data. Based on the observed data a relationship is then hypothesized that is usually stated in mathematical form between the variables of measurements. The relationship is then tested to see how closely it agrees with observed data. The mathematical relationship that is developed based on relevant kinetic data is called a *pharmacokinetic model*. Therefore, pharmacokinetic models are mathematical relationships that are used to explain and predict the overall behavior of a drug in the body. There are three popular approaches to the study of the pharmacokinetics of a compound in living systems:

■ Physiologic pharmacokinetics uses the anatomic arrangements of organs and different regions in living systems with their subtle processes and process control.

■ Classic compartmental analysis is based on dividing living systems into plausible compartments with no anatomic significance that may include lumped regions of the body.

■ Noncompartmental analysis is the option that somewhat avoids the assumptions associated with the other two approaches and employs the statistical concept of moments. This approach is discussed in Chapter Seventeen.

2.2 PHYSIOLOGIC MODELS

The basic idea behind physiologic modeling is to incorporate quantitative parameters of anatomic regions in the mathematical description of disposition of a compound. These parameters include blood flow, tissue volumes, binding, transport, and elimination from an organ. As there are parallelisms in the anatomy of mammalian systems, such as having all organs between arterial and venous blood or most organs having comparable fractions of the body weight, the physiologic models are usually developed in experimental animals and, then, by changing the physiologic parameters, they can be extrapolated to humans. Therefore, the important features of this approach in pharmacokinetic modeling are:

■ To provide a detailed and quantitative portrayal of drug disposition in a variety of species.

■ To extrapolate the results from animals such as mice, rats, dogs, and primates upward to humans. This extrapolation is called *scaling up* and may also be applicable, in certain cases, in the opposite direction, that is, scaling down to lower species.

■ To predict drug levels in different organs.

■ To facilitate simulation of drug disposition in disease states.

■ To assess cancer risk in humans following exposure to carcinogens.

■ etc.

To develop a physiologic model, a diagram similar to Figure 2.1 is considered with relevant organs to describe the disposition of a compound. The number of organs or regions included in the model is determined by the physicochemical characteristics of a compound such as lipid solubility, binding, or ionization and preferential uptake by an organ. For example, for a highly lipid-soluble drug fat tissues are important and included in the model, and for a water-soluble drug with no uptake by the fat tissues this region would be excluded. Therefore, the in vitro determination of physical pharmacy parameters such as partition coefficient is important in the selection of the appropriate model. A diagram of the model is presented in Figure 2.1.

Another important characteristic of physiologic modeling is the presentation of each organ or region in terms of its subcompartments; for example, the disposition of a drug in a region can be defined not only in the blood of capillaries but also in interstitial fluid and intracellular volume. Obviously, having too many subcompartments may make the analysis cumbersome.

When the uptake of drug from blood of capillaries into interstitial and intracellular subcompartments is rapid and the three regions are essentially in equilibrium, as in the uptake of highly lipid-soluble compounds, the limiting factor of uptake is blood flow. Thus,

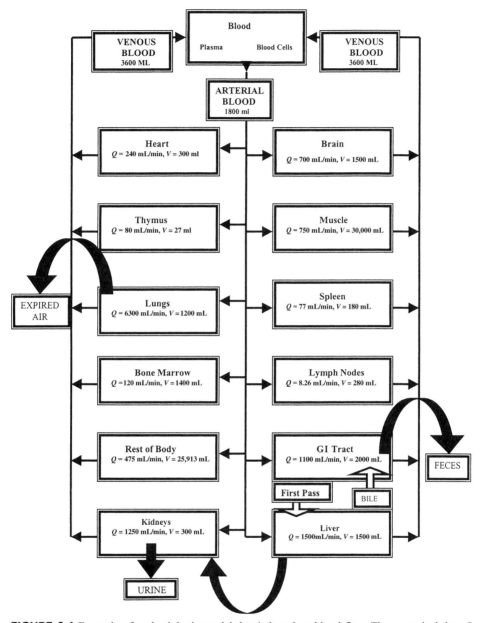

FIGURE 2.1 Example of a physiologic model that is based on blood flow. The numerical data Q (blood flow) and V (organ volume) are from References 1–7 and 10–12. Solid arrows represent blood flow.

the faster a drug gets into an organ, the faster the organ takes it up. Under this condition the uptake of the drug is considered a *blood flow-limited process* because the organ or the region is capable of not only taking up the drug rapidly but also holding large quantities of the drug. Flow-limited models are usually presented as in Figure 2.1. On the other hand, if the transfer of a drug between extracellular (ie, blood and interstitial fluid) and intracellular fluids is limited by the permeation of the drug through the cell membrane, the process is considered a *membrane-limited* or *permeability-limited process.*

Once the relevant body regions have been identified in a physiologic model, the mass balances for blood and the organs can be written by considering the rates of input and the rates of output. For example for a flow-limited model, as in Figure 2.1, the mass balance of parent drug in the blood is

rate of change of amount of drug in blood = rate of input from organs into blood
$$- \text{ rate of output into organs} + \text{dose as a function of time}$$

The related differential equation is

$$V_B \frac{dC_{Blood}}{dt} = \left[Q_{brain} \frac{C_{brain}}{R_{brain}} + Q_{heart} \frac{C_{heart}}{R_{heart}} + Q_{liver} \frac{C_{liver}}{R_{liver}} + Q_{kidney} \frac{C_{kidneys}}{R_{kidneys}} + Q_{fat} \frac{C_{fat}}{R_{fat}} + \cdots \right]$$

$$- [Q_{brain} + Q_{heart} + Q_{liver} + Q_{kidneys} + Q_{fat} + \cdots]C_{blood} + \text{dose}(t) \qquad (2.1)$$

where C is concentration, Q is blood flow, V is volume, and R is tissue/blood distribution ratio. Multiplication of Q (volume/time) by C (mass/volume) yields the units of rate in terms of mass/time. R has no units and multiplication of V (volume) by dC/dt (mass/volume time) also yields the units of mass/time. Equation 2.1 requires that the dose be included as a function of time.

The mass balance of parent compound in organs of elimination such as the liver or kidneys is

rate of change of amount of drug in the organ
$$= \text{rate of input} - \text{rate of output} - \text{rate of elimination}$$

The related differential equations are

Liver: $$V_{liver} \frac{dC_{liver}}{dt} = Q_{liver} \left[C_{blood} - \frac{C_{liver}}{R_{liver}} \right] - Cl_m \frac{C_{liver}}{R_{liver}} \qquad (2.2)$$

Kidney: $$V_{kidney} \frac{dC_{kidney}}{dt} = Q_{kidney} \left[C_{blood} - \frac{C_{kidney}}{R_{kidney}} \right] - Cl_r \frac{C_{kidney}}{R_{kidney}} \qquad (2.3)$$

Lung: $$V_{lung} \frac{dC_{lung}}{dt} = Q_{lung} \left[C_{blood} - \frac{C_{lung}}{R_{lung}} \right] - Cl_l \frac{C_{lung}}{R_{lung}} \qquad (2.4)$$

where Cl_m, Cl_r, and Cl_l are metabolic, renal, and lung clearances with units of volume/time

The differential equations for other organ or regions follow the general equation of

rate of change of amount of drug in the organ = rate of input − rate of output

That is,
$$V_{organ} \frac{dC_{organ}}{dt} = Q_{organ} \left[C_{blood} - \frac{C_{organ}}{R_{organ}} \right] \qquad (2.5)$$

For membrane-limited model the differential equation of each organ is then expressed in terms of two rate equations: rate of change of drug concentration in extracellular fluid and rate of change of drug concentration in the tissue portion of the organ, that is, intracellular fluid. This means that each organ in Figure 2.1 is subdivided into two compartments of extracellular and intracellular fluids, as shown in Figure 2.2.

Therefore, the related differential equations of an organ in a membrane-limited model are written as follows:

1. For the blood compartment or extracellular fluid of an organ or region,

rate of change of drug concentration in blood or extracellular compartment of an organ
= rate of input − rate of output + membrane transport

$$V_{blood} \frac{dC_{blood}}{dt} = Q_{blood}[C_{input} - C_{output}] + P(C_{tissue} - C_{blood}) \qquad (2.6)$$

where P is the membrane permeability and $C_{tissue} - C_{blood}$ is the concentration gradient across the membrane.

2. For the tissue portion or intracellular fluid of the organ or region,

rate of change of drug in the tissue or intracellular compartment
= rate of uptake ± rate of secretion or elimination

$$V_{tissue} \frac{dC_{tissue}}{dt} = P(C_{blood} - C_{tissue}) + Cl_{secretion}(C_{tissue}) - Cl_{elimination}(C_{tissue}) \qquad (2.7)$$

where P is the membrane permeability and Cl is the clearance term.

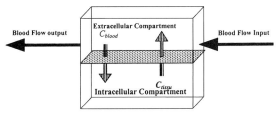

FIGURE 2.2 Schematic representation of an organ in membrane-limited models. C_{blood} is the concentration of drug in the blood and extracellular fluid and C_{tissue} is the concentration in the intracellular part of the tissue or organ. Dark arrows represent blood flow in and out of the organ and lined arrows signify the mass transfer between the two intracellular and extracellular compartments.

The analysis of experimental data according to physiologic modeling is based mostly on simulation of the time course of drug in different anatomic regions. The simulation is achieved by substituting in the equations of a selected model the physiologic constants and parameters of the organs (blood flow, weight, etc), the input function of the experimental conditions, and the physicochemical parameters of the compound. The simulation provides the predicted concentrations of the drug. The observed data (ie, the experimental values) are then judged based on their closeness to the predicted values. From the predicted and observed concentration–time profiles other pharmacokinetic parameters such as clearances, area under plasma concentration–time curve, and half-life can be estimated. Physiologic models provide the versatility of identifying and treating potentially saturable processes such as capacity-limited metabolism and active secretion for an organ of elimination such as the liver or kidneys. Under these conditions the clearance of the organ is no longer a constant.

A practical aspect of the model is its use in scaling up the data from small vertebrates to larger species in animal kingdom. For instance if a model is selected based on the behavior of a compound in experimental animals such as mice and rats, it can be scaled up to humans by replacing the physiologic, anatomic, and biochemical parameters of the animal with those of humans. Thus, a new curve can be simulated for humans based on the behavior of the drug in experimental animals. Obviously, in scaling up to humans, certain parameters such as the partition coefficient of the drug or membrane permeability are assumed to be the same among different species.

2.3 CLASSIC COMPARTMENTAL ANALYSIS

This approach is fundamentally different from physiologic modeling and it is more practical in clinical situations. To establish the intent of this approach let us consider the following background. Assume you administered a drug to a patient through one of the routes of administration but with the intention of achieving a systemic effect. To achieve the systemic effect you have made the tacit assumption that the drug will appear in the blood and distribute by the systemic circulation to different regions in the body including the receptor sites. Along with the overall distribution of the drug in the body certain physiologic processes take place that influence the concentration of drug in blood or plasma and at the receptor site. Among these processes protein binding, storage in adipose tissues, metabolism by the liver, excretion by the kidney, interaction with receptor sites, elimination by other organs, and sometimes enterohepatic recirculation are the most important factors (Figure 2.3). The interaction of drug with macromolecules such as plasma proteins and enzymes and various tissues is reversible and follow the law of mass action. Thus the free dug in the blood or plasma can eventually reach a quasi-equilibrium with the drug bound to macromolecules and tissues. If the equilibrium between blood or plasma and tissues is achieved very rapidly, as is the case for highly perfused tissues such as liver, heart, and kidneys, these tissues will be considered a part of the systemic circulation.

In compartmental analysis, we look at the mathematical description of the time course of drug concentration in the systemic circulation. In other words we look at the decline in concentration of drug in the body by using a biologic sample as our indicator. The major biologic samples that may be collected noninvasively in humans and that can provide

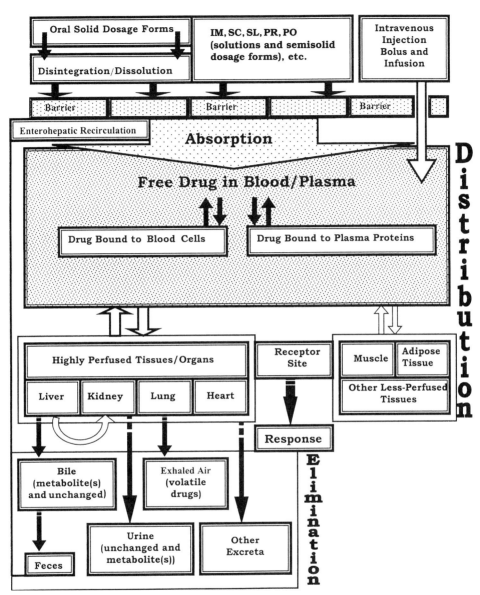

FIGURE 2.3 General diagram of physiologic processes of absorption, distribution, and elimination (metabolism and excretion) that highlights the basic premise of the compartmental analysis in pharmacokinetics.

useful information about the effects of all processes involved in ADME of drug are blood and urine. Other biologic samples may also provide useful information. For example, in the case of highly volatile drugs, exhaled air is an important sample, and, depending on the type of drug and significance of information, saliva or milk may also be used. Bile is an important biologic sample; however, its collection in humans is not practical, and feces usually do not provide useful information about the biliary elimination of drugs due to the difficulties associated with the extraction of drug from fecal particles and interference of by-products of microbial degradation of the drug in the large intestine. The collection of bile in experimental animals, known as bile cannulation, is a routine procedure for determination of biliary elimination and the *in vivo* metabolism profile of drugs.

Theoretically, the receptors would be the ultimate biologic sites at which to measure the amount of drug bound to receptor, and obviously it would be the ultimate way of optimizing the dose or dosing regimen for a drug. The problem with this theory is that measurement of drug associated with receptor sites for majority of drugs is not possible and most often the receptor site is not clearly well understood. Therefore, we have to rely on biologic samples that are accessible and the drug concentrations of which are in equilibrium with the drug associated with the receptor. The only biologic sample that fits these criteria is blood. In blood we have the options of measuring total concentration of drug in blood or plasma (ie, bound and unbound (free) drug), and measuring only the concentration of free drug. It is important to remember that the amount of drug bound to plasma proteins, blood cells, or peripheral tissues is not free for interaction with the receptor site. Hence, no pharmacologic response should be expected from drug bound to proteins of plasma or residing in tissues. Therefore, measuring the concentration of free dug in plasma would be more realistic in predicting the changes in free concentration at the receptor site. The free concentration or amount of drug at its receptor site, according to the following equilibrium equation that represents the reversible interaction between a drug and receptor consistent with the law of mass action, is proportional to the concentration or amount of the drug bound to the receptor site. The concentration or amount of drug bound to receptor is responsible for the response and therapeutic outcome:

$$\text{free drug + receptor} \rightleftharpoons \text{drug–receptor} \longrightarrow \text{response}$$

Based on the above reasoning, the following are the assumptions of compartmental analysis:

- Only free drug interacts with its receptor site to provide the pharmacologic response.
- The concentration of free drug in circulatory system is proportional to the concentration of free drug at the receptor site and therefore proportional to the amount of drug associated with the receptor.

It is worth noting that for some drugs that are highly bound to plasma proteins, such as diphenylhydantoin (phenytoin), where the concentration of free dug is too low to be measured accurately, the total concentration of drug, that is, bound and unbound, is measured in routine clinical therapeutic drug monitoring.

The next step is to develop the mathematical description of compartmental models based on the above assumptions, taking into account the unique physicochemical characteristics of each drug and disposition of drug in the body with regions of different features and functions. As the systemic circulation is connected to peripheral tissues and organs, it is assumed that changes in the concentration of free drug in plasma, or in some instances the total concentration of drug in plasma, reflect changes in the concentration of drug in the peripheral compartments. Thus, the concentration–time curve of drug in

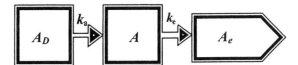

FIGURE 2.4 One-compartment model with first-order input and first-order output.

plasma can provide important information about the ways the body handles the drug. The basic approach in this quantification is to summarize the data of the concentration–time curves of free drug and/or its metabolite(s) by mathematical equations or models. These mathematical relationships are based on conceiving the body as discrete compartments. This means that the body may be divided into one or more compartments without making any anatomic assumptions about the specific content of these compartments. Diagrams of some of the examples are presented in Figures 2.4 to 2.8.

The compartments of these models have no relation to any physiologic system or anatomic regions. Contrary to the physiologic models, the inputs and outputs into these compartments are not identified as blood flow or diffusion fluxes, but are defined in general forms of zero- or first-order kinetics. The compartments may be assumed as various organs or tissues that altogether handle a drug like a homogeneous compartment, and thus the sampling from the compartment, if it is feasible, is from a well-mixed amount of drug in the volume of that compartment. The highly perfused tissues, because of their high blood flow rate and fast equilibrium with blood concentration, are usually considered a part of the central compartment. Thus, the central compartment in many of the compartmental models is composed of the systemic circulation and highly perfused tissues. The central compartment is also the major sampling compartment. To include other regions of the body that reach equilibrium with drug concentration in systemic circulation at a much

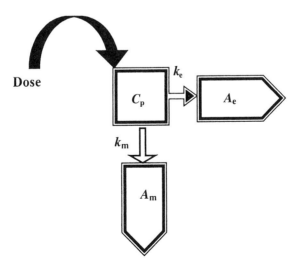

FIGURE 2.5 One-compartment model with instantaneous input and first-order metabolism and excretion.

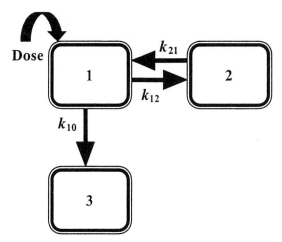

FIGURE 2.6 Two-compartment model with instantaneous input and first-order elimination.

slower rate, or when the drug is taken up preferentially by a particular organ or region, more complex models with two, three, or four compartments must be used. However, the important operating rule is to include the minimum number of compartments consistent with the behavior of the drug, the physiologic reality, and the ease of calculating the relevant parameters. Determination of the optimum number of compartments for a drug is usually handled by curve fitting the plasma concentration of the drug versus time. Simultaneous curve fitting of the drug levels in plasma and urine, or in plasma and bile, or in plasma, urine, and bile is also highly recommended. The curve-fitting task is usually handled with specialized pharmacokinetic software. Most curve-fitting computer programs use special statistical tests to determine the optimum number of compartments in this type of modeling. The curve-fitting procedure is a highly developed and sophisticated mathematical and statistical procedure and its description is beyond the scope of this textbook. It is important to remember that extensive information on pharmacokinetic models of therapeutic and nontherapeutic agents have been published in health science-related journals that can provide meaningful information in practice and research. Determination of the number of compartments is important only when the pharmacokinetics of a new agent, or the effect of disease states or drug–drug interaction on the pharmacokinetics of available compounds, is under investigation.

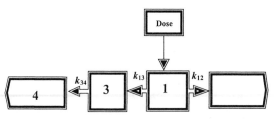

FIGURE 2.7 One-compartment model with respect to parent compound (compartment 1) and one-compartment model with respect to metabolite(s) (compartment 3).

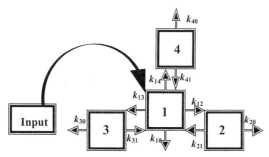

FIGURE 2.8 Multicompartment mammillary model with a central compartment (compartment 1), three peripheral compartments (compartments 2–4), and distribution rate constants of k_{12}, k_{21}, k_{13}, k_{31}, k_{14}, k_{42}. Elimination from the compartments is identified as k_{10}, k_{20}, k_{30}, and k_{40}.

In compartmental analysis it is important to distinguish between linear and nonlinear pharmacokinetics. As was mentioned earlier under physiologic modeling, nonlinear pharmacokinetics exists when a drug is absorbed or eliminated by mechanisms that are potentially saturable. Nonlinear processes are usually governed by the Michaelis–Menten equation which is discussed in detail in the section related to drug metabolism (Chapter 5). In nonlinear pharmacokinetics, also known as dose-dependent pharmacokinetics, the half-life and clearance, which are usually independent of the drug concentration in plasma or blood and are considered constant, become variable and their values depend on the dose and plasma concentration. The dose dependency of pharmacokinetics is a source of variability of therapeutic outcomes of drugs and it is difficult to predict the behavior of a drug in different individuals. Linear pharmacokinetics, known as dose-independent pharmacokinetics, exists when all biologic processes (ie, ADME) are governed by first-order kinetics, and the half-life and clearance are considered constant in this type of kinetics.

The topic of dose-independent pharmacokinetic analysis is discussed in detail in Chapters 7 to 18.

2.4 NONCOMPARTMENTAL ANALYSIS

In recent years a different type of pharmacokinetic analysis has become popular that is based purely on the observed data and statistical moment theory. As no particular model is assumed in this type of analysis, the topic is not included in this chapter. The principle of noncompartmental analysis is discussed in detail in Chapter 17.

BIBLIOGRAPHY

1. Bischoff KB. Current applications of physiological pharmacokinetics. *Fed Proc* 1980;39:2456.
2. Bishchoff KB. Physiological pharmacokinetics. *Bull Math Biol* 1986;48:309.
3. Bischoff KB, Dedrick RL, Zaharko DS, Longstreth JA. Methotrexate pharmacokinetics. *J Pharm Sci* 1971;60:1128.
4. Chow H-H. A physiologically based pharmacokinetic model of zidovudine (AZT) in the mouse: Model development and scale-up to human. *J Pharm Sci* 1997;86:1223.

5. Dedrick RL, Bischoff KB, and Zaharko DS. Interspecies correlation of plasma concentration history of methotrexate (NS-740). *Cancer Chemother Rep* 1970;54:95.

6. Gallo JM, Lam FC, Perrier DG. Area method for the estimation of partition coefficient for physiological pharmacokinetic model. *J Pharmacokinet Biopharm* 1987;15:271.

7. Harrison LI, and Gibaldi M. Physiologically based pharmacokinetic model for digoxin disposition in dogs and its preliminary application to humans. *J Pharm Sci* 1977;66:1679.

8. Jacquez JA. Compartmental Analysis in Biology and Medicine: Kinetics of Distribution of Tracer-labeled Materials. New York: *Elsevier,* 1972:1.

9. Metzler CM. Estimation of pharmacokinetic parameters: Statistical considerations. *Pharmacol Ther* 1981;13:543.

10. Nakashima E, Yokogawa K, Ichimura F, Kurata K, Kido H, Yamaguchi N, Yamana T. A physiologically based pharmacokinetic model for biperiden in animals and its extrapolation to human. *Chem Pharm Bull* 1987;35:718.

11. Ritchel WA, Banerjee PS. Physiologic pharmacokinetic models: Application, limitations and outlook. *Methods Exp Clin Pharmacol* 1986;8:603.

12. Rowland M. Physiologic pharmacokinetic models and interanimal species scaling. *Pharmacol Ther* 1985;29:49.

13. Wagner JG. Fundamentals of Clinical Pharmacokinetics. Hamilton, IL: *Drug Intelligence,* 1975:4.

CHAPTER 3

ROUTES OF ADMINISTRATION AND DRUG ABSORPTION

No thing happens at random but all things as a result of a reason and by necessity.
AETIUS (STOBAEUS SELECTIONS 1.25.4)

OBJECTIVES

- To review the general principles of absorption from the GI tract and other routes of administration.

- To determine the conditions under which absorption of drugs follows first-order kinetics.

- To discuss the major physiologic factors associated with the absorption of drugs that may influence the plasma concentration–time profile and pharmacologic response.

- To review mechanisms of absorption in relation to the routes of administration.

3.1 INTRODUCTION

Absorption, distribution, metabolism, and excretion (ADME) are the important biological processes in evaluation of the pharmacokinetics of drugs. These processes that are influenced by the physicochemical nature of drugs and the route of administration determine the onset of action, duration of action, and intensity of the pharmacologic response. Routes of administration such as the parenteral route avoid the absorption process and provide an immediate onset of action. For drugs that diffuse through a barrier, a delay in the onset action may occur, the magnitude of which depends on the complexity of the barrier and the physicochemical characteristics of the drug and the dosage form.

The ensuing sections in this chapter are brief reviews of the routes of administration and the absorption process. The purpose is to differentiate between the routes where drugs are placed in the vascular system for immediate distribution and the routes where drug must be absorbed through a barrier before reaching the systemic circulation.

3.2 ROUTES OF ADMINISTRATION

We may classify the routes of administration into four categories.

FIRST CATEGORY
These drugs must pass through a barrier to reach the systemic circulation. The purpose of using these routes is to achieve a systemic rather than a local effect.

A. Oral routes
  1. Oral administration
  2. Sublingual
  3. Buccal

B. Inhalation

C. Injection into the body but not into the vascular system
  1. Subcutaneous
  2. Intramuscular
  3. Intradermal

D. Administration through a natural orifice
  1. Nasal
  2. Rectal
  3. Vaginal

SECOND CATEGORY
These drugs are injected directly into the systemic circulation (ie, the absorption process is bypassed and the drug is distributed immediately).

A. Injection into the vascular system
  1. Intravenous
  2. Intraarterial*

---

*Specialized route of administration that is not used routinely.

THIRD CATEGORY
The topical routes are in this category. These drugs are placed on the skin with the intention of achieving a systemic effect. Absorption through the skin, because of the presence of the outermost horny layer of skin (stratum corneum), is more complex than the routes of administration in the first category. In addition to the physicochemical characteristics of the drug and the dosage form, environmental factors such as humidity, temperature, and physiologic condition of the skin play important roles in the absorption process. The absorption of drugs, even highly lipophilic drugs, is not immediate and the concentration of drug in plasma gradually rises after a threshold of low concentration.

A. Topical routes
  1. Transdermal
  2. Cutaneous

FOURTH CATEGORY

Drugs administered by these specialized routes of administration achieve local and targeted therapy. Although the goal is a local and targeted effect, a portion of drug may reach the systemic circulation.

A. Injections
1. Intralesional
2. Epidural (also referred to as peridural and extradural)
3. Intrathecal
4. Intracisternal
5. Intracardiac
6. Intraventricular
7. Intraocular
8. Intraarticular
9. Intraperitoneal
10. Intraarticular

B. Administration through a natural orifice
1. Intraauricular
2. Intrauterine
3. Intraurethral
4. Ophthalmic

In the following sections we review only those routes of administration where drugs have to cross a barrier to reach the systemic circulation for general distribution. The routes of administration that bypass the absorption process and the routes used to achieve a local effect are not discussed in this chapter.

3.2.1 Oral Absorption

Absorption from the GI tract into the systemic circulation entails the permeation of drug from the lumen to the gut wall and subsequent diffusion through the capillary wall into the blood. Discussion of the anatomy and physiology of the GI tract is beyond the scope of this text and you are encouraged to consult the appropriate chapters in anatomy and physiology textbooks.

3.2.1.1 Factors Influencing GI Absorption: Among the various factors that influence the absorption of drugs by this route the following, because of the influence they exert on the pharmacokinetics of an orally administered drug, are considered important.

I. Various regional pH of GI tract and pK_a of the drug

II. Gastric emptying process

III. Intestinal motility or small intestinal transit time (SITT)

IV. First-pass extraction
   A. Hepatic
   B. Gastrointestinal microflora
   C. Intestinal metabolic enzymes such as cytochrome P450 3A4 (CYP3A4).
   D. P-glycoprotein (Pgp)

V. Food

VI. Disease states

VII. Other factors

3.2.1.2 Effect of Various pH of GI Tract on Absorption of Drugs: Orally administered drugs pass through two different environments: the gastric environment and the small intestinal environment. Aside from their anatomic differences, gradual changes in their pH influence the absorption of weakly acidic and basic drugs. Gastric pH is highly acidic during the fasting state and is comparable to the pH of 0.15 M HCl containing pepsin. During a meal, however, because of the buffering capacity of the nourishment, gastric pH becomes more alkaline. Therefore, gastric pH varies during the day. The alkaline environment of the small intestine remains essentially consistent and similar during life. The pH of this environment increases from 5.5–6.0 in the duodenum to about 9–11 in the ileum.

Many drugs are either weakly acidic or basic compounds, and according to the pH partition theory only the un-ionized forms of the molecules are capable of partitioning through a membrane. Therefore, the low pH of the stomach increases the concentration of un-ionized weakly acidic drugs and the high pH of the intestine forms the un-ionized weakly basic drugs. Thus, weakly basic drugs in the stomach and weakly acidic drugs in the intestine are in the ionized form. The Henderson–Hasselbalch equation can be used to relate the pK_a of a drug and pH of the GI tract to the ratio of the ionized to un-ionized species.

$$([\text{un-ionized}]/[\text{ionized}])_{\text{acidic}} = 10^{(pK_a - pH)} \qquad (3.1)$$

$$([\text{un-ionized}]/[\text{ionized}])_{\text{basic}} = 10^{(pH - pK_a)} \qquad (3.2)$$

For example, consider drug A with a pK_a of 3 and drug B with a pK_a of 8 that are placed at pH 2 and 7.
   At pH $\cong$ 2

$$([\text{un-ionized}]/[\text{ionized}])_{\text{drug A}} = 10^{(3-2)} = 10$$

$$([\text{un-ionized}]/[\text{ionized}])_{\text{drug B}} = 10^{(2-8)} = 10^{-6}$$

Therefore, at pH 2, for every 10 un-ionized molecules of drug A with pK_a 3, only one molecule would be ionized. The ratio changes significantly for drug B with pK_a 8, where for every one un-ionized molecule 10^6 molecules would be ionized. At pH 7 the ratios for drug A and B are 10^{-4} and 10^{-1}, respectively. Thus, at higher pH the weakly basic drugs are more un-ionized and acidic drugs are more ionized, and the opposite is true at low pH.

It should be noted that although weakly acidic drugs are mainly in the un-ionized form in the stomach they are absorbed mostly from intestine. The reasons are the limited surface area, impermeability of the stomach wall to small hydrophilic molecules, and short residence of drugs in the stomach. Thus, it is only reasonable to assume that most of the weakly acidic drugs are also absorbed from the small intestine. The onset of action, however, is more immediate for acidic drugs.

3.2.1.3 Gastric Emptying: The gastric emptying process essentially is regulated by neural and hormonal control. The process is a carefully regulated task that is coordinated between contractile movement in the stomach and small intestine. Briefly, the upper part (proximal) of the stomach receives the ingested food following mastication (chewing) and deglutition (swallowing). A sustained contraction is initiated and the contents of the upper part are pressed toward the lower part (distal) of the stomach. The proximal stomach is responsible for transfer of gastric contents known as chyme from the stomach to the upper part of the small intestine (duodenum). The lower part of the stomach triturates the contents, prevents the duodenal reflux, and allows only liquids and small particles to pass into the duodenum. Peristaltic contractions of both the proximal and distal stomach are under the neural control of vagus nerves and release of acetylcholine. Acetylcholine interacts with the appropriate receptor of the stomach muscle to stimulate the contraction and relaxes during swallowing. Furthermore, several hormones participate in the stimulation or inhibition of the contraction. For example, cholecystokinin inhibits the contraction of the proximal stomach, whereas it stimulates the contraction of the distal stomach; secretin and somatostatin both inhibit the contractions of the proximal and distal stomach.

The gastric emptying rate is the rate at which the stomach empties its contents into the duodenum. The delay in gastric emptying rate has been shown to be responsible for the delay in onset of action of certain drugs and dosage forms. According to the pH partition theory the weakly basic drugs are expected to be in ionized form in the stomach and therefore the slower rate of gastric emptying would delay the onset of action of basic drugs. The following factors influence the gastric emptying rate:

1. Drugs that block gastric muscle receptors for acetylcholine delay the emptying rate (eg, propantheline).
2. The high acidity of gastric chyme also delays the emtying rate.
3. The chemical composition of chyme within the stomach determines the gastric emptying rate. In humans, liquids are emptied with a half-life of approximately 12 minutes and digestible solids at a half-life of about 2 hours depending on the chemical composition of the chyme. Carbohydrates are emptied faster than proteins, and proteins faster than fats.
4. If the amount of carbohydrates, proteins, or fats is converted to caloric content, the rate of caloric transfer to the duodenum remains approximately the same. Therefore, the gastric emptying rate is controlled by the caloric content of the stomach such that the number of calories transferred to the small intestine remains constant for different nutrients over time, emptying being slower if the meal is rich in calories.
5. The gastric emptying rate can be modulated by meal size. For example, changing the solid meal size from 300 to 1692 g increases the half-life from 77 to 277 minutes; however, the size of the meal produces a pressure that stimulates the gastric emptying.

6. Simulation of the small intestinal receptors (ie, duodenojejunal receptors sensitive to osmotic pressure) by hypertonic or hypotonic solutions slows the gastric emptying rate.
7. The temperature of the solid or fluid intake may affect the gastric emptying rate. Temperatures above or below the physiologic 37°C would proportionately reduce the gastric emptying rate.
8. Other factors such as anger and agitation may increase the rate, whereas depression, trauma, and injury have been suggested to reduce the gastric emptying rate. Position of the body, such as standing or lying on the right side, may facilitate the transfer of contents to the small intestine by increasing pressure in the proximal part of the stomach.

3.2.1.4 Intestinal Motility (Small Intestinal Transit Time): The major site of absorption in the GI tract is the small intestine. The stomach and colon have a small absorptive area and the colon has a lumen full of bacteria. The small intestine is approximately 300 to 400 cm long and is an alkaline environment. It begins with the pyloric sphincter, continues with the duodenum, jejunum, and proximal and distal portions of ileum, and ends with the ileocecal valve into the large intestine. In the duodenum, the pH is approximately 6 and increases gradually throughout the intestine. The small intestine is highly rich in digestive enzymes such as lipase, protease, amylase, esterase, and nucleases. In addition, bile, which is rich in micelles of bile salts, is added to the contents of the small intestine. Small intestinal motility is mostly segmental contraction consisting of mixing contraction and propulsive contraction.

Intestinal motility has two different patterns of digestive and interdigestive activities. The interdigestive activity cycle starts with about 30 to 40 minutes of no activity in both stomach and intestine, followed by increasing contractions that are circular and migrate along the small intestine (peristaltic). This pattern of contraction removes everything that is left in the small intestine. Finally, the contractions diminish frequency and intensity and the cycle repeats. One entire cycle may take between 90 and 120 minutes in healthy and normal subjects. The ingestion of food suspends the interdigestive cycle and establishes the intestinal motility pattern for the digestive cycle. The digestive cycle comprises mainly mixing contractions with a few propulsive contractions. Small intestinal transit time (SITT) during the digestive cycle is rather difficult to determine, and considering the variability among individuals and types of food, it may not be as accurate as would be expected. One report, however, has indicated that the SITT for 95% ($SITT_{95}$) of healthy individuals is about 80 minutes, with a standard deviation of 70 minutes. Esophageal-duodenal-jejunal-ileal transit time in normal subjects fed mashed potatoes labeled with sulfur has been reported to be 378 ± 90 minutes.

Most of the factors that affect gastric emptying time, such as the presence of fats and the volume of food, also influence intestinal motility. For example, a large meal rich in fats requires longer and stronger intestinal contractions.

3.2.1.5 First-Pass Hepatic Extraction: After absorption through the epithelium drugs and nutrients enter into the submucosal capillaries that take them to the intestinal vein. The intestinal vein, after joining with the veins from the spleen and pancreas, transport the drug and nutrients through the hepatoportal vein system to the liver. In the liver, reticuloendothelial cells absorb the nutrients and small particles and droplets, and hepatocytes metabolize free drugs and nutrients. Enzymatic activity is the most important determinant of the extent of first-pass extraction by the liver. The amount of drug that is eliminated by first-pass metabolism can be estimated in terms of fraction or percentage removal, known as *extraction ratio* (ER), which is the ratio of the rate of metabolism of drug by the liver to the rate of input of drug into the liver (Figure 3.1):

$$\text{rate of input} - \text{rate of output} = \text{rate of extraction}$$

$$\text{rate of extraction/rate of input} = \text{extraction ratio}$$

or

$$(Q_{\text{liver}} \times C_{\text{liver}})_{\text{input}} - (Q_{\text{liver}} \times C_{\text{liver}})_{\text{output}} = Q_{\text{liver}}(C_{\text{liver}_{\text{input}}} - C_{\text{liver}_{\text{output}}}) \tag{3.3}$$

$$\frac{Q_{\text{liver}}(C_{\text{liver}_{\text{input}}} - C_{\text{liver}_{\text{output}}})}{(Q_{\text{liver}} \times C_{\text{liver}})_{\text{input}}} = \frac{C_{\text{liver}_{\text{input}}} - C_{\text{liver}_{\text{output}}}}{C_{\text{liver}_{\text{input}}}} = \text{ER} \tag{3.4}$$

where Q is the blood flow, C is concentration of drug, and ER is the extraction ratio.

The amount that will be available for systemic effect can therefore be estimated in terms of the fraction that escapes first-pass metabolism in the liver:

$$F_{\text{available}} = 1 - \text{ER} \tag{3.5}$$

The above equations are based on first-order metabolism and it is assumed that the extraction ratio is constant for a given compound. In the case of nonlinear metabolism, because of the limited capacity of enzyme(s) for metabolism, the extraction ratio will be a dose-dependent variable that decreases with increasing dose. Therefore, the fraction available for systemic effect (ie, bioavailability) increases significantly with increasing dose.

3.2.1.6 Gastrointestinal Metabolism by Microflora: Gastrointestinal microflora are prokaryotic and eukaryotic microorganisms of different kinds that become inhabitants of the GI environment soon after birth. They colonize not only the large intestine but also the distal portion of the ileum. All mammals, including humans, are symbiotic with microbial cells. Examples of indigenous GI microflora in humans are *Bifidobacterium, Bac-*

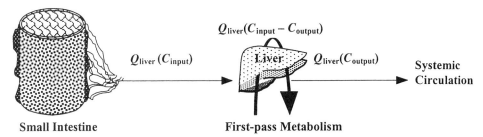

FIGURE 3.1 Schematic presentation of absorption of drug into the capillaries of small intestine leading to the hepatoportal vein and the liver, where first-pass metabolism occurs. The amount that escapes first-pass metabolism enters into the systemic circulation.

teroides fragilis, and *Bacteroides thetaiotaomicrone*. In many instances they are vital for the life of the host. To survive in the GI environment, they carry out biochemical reactions that are mostly hydrolysis, and because the GI tract is practically an oxygen-free environment, no oxidation or reduction is expected. They are also capable of breaking down conjugated metabolites such as glucuronides, sulfates, glutathiones, and other forms of conjugates. Other effects of microflora on the GI tract are reduction of intestinal transit time and hydrolysis of macromolecules and dietary polymers in the large intestine.

The small intestine is free of bacteria until the distal portion of the ileum, where microflora begin to increase in number and variety. If the active ingredient of a dosage form is not completely absorbed before reaching the distal portion of the ileum, microflora would metabolize it and the metabolic products would be absorbed. Considering the diversity of the microflora, their metabolic by-products may vary from individual to individual and therefore may reduce the availability, efficacy, and safety of the therapeutic agents.

3.2.1.7 Gastrointestinal Metabolism by CYP450 Isozymes (CYP3A4): Among the important enzymes responsible for metabolism of xenobiotics in the body, cytochrome P450 (CYP450) isozymes are the most important and investigated group of enzymes. The role of CYP450 isozymes and the diversity of their subfamilies and functions are discussed in Chapter 5. A subfamily of CYP450 known as CYP3A is involved in the metabolism of more than 50% of all xenobiotics. A member of the CYP3A subfamily, CYP3A4, is the major CYP450 in the human liver. It constitutes on average about 30% of liver CYP450 and it may increase to 60% in an induced liver. In the epithelial barrier of the small intestine the amount of CYP3A4 constitutes about 70% of total CYP450 present in the small intestine. Therefore, it plays a major role in intestinal first-pass metabolism of drugs that are considered substrates for CYP3A4. The systemic availability of these drugs is influenced significantly by the presence of this enzyme not only in the intestine but also in the liver. Obviously the presence of inhibitors or inducers of the enzyme system would increase or decrease the availability of the drugs, respectively.

3.2.1.8 Effect of P-glycoprotein: P-glycoprotein (Pgp) belongs to a large protein family of membrane active transporters that exist in different regions of the body and are known as the ATP-binding cassette (ABC) transporter superfamily. In the GI tract, this protein is present in the luminal membrane of intestinal epithelial cells where it acts as an efflux transporter. It is a versatile membrane transporter that acts on a wide range of endogenous and exogenous compounds. It is designated P-glycoprotein in recognition of its role in drug "permeability" across the cell membrane. Its impact on the physiologic state in the presence of its substrates and modulators is still challenging scientists around the world. Pgp is a part of the body's defense mechanism that extrudes a variety of structurally different xenobiotics from cells. Therefore, by pumping the xenobiotics out of the cells this protein reduces the systemic availability of drugs given orally. Pgp is the focal point in the challenging area of multidrug resistance in cancer chemotherapy. It has been shown through many in vitro and in vivo studies that this transmembrane protein influences efflux of a number of structurally unrelated drugs, including widely used antineoplastic agents such as anthracyclines, calcium channel blocker such as verapamil, and chemopreventive agents such as tamoxifen. The overexpression of this glycoprotein in tumor cells causes an increase in outward pumping of chemotherapeutic agents. It has been suggested that because of the proximity of Pgp to CYP3A4 and the similarity of their interactions with various compounds in the intestine, their functions at the intestinal barrier not only are of equal value but also complement each other (Figure 3.2).

3.2.1.9 Effect of Food on GI Absorption: In general the effect of foods on absorption of drugs is based on their influence on the rate and extent of absorption. In certain situations the rate of absorption may change, be delayed or accelerated, in the presence of food, but the extent of absorption remains unchanged. There are, however, cases in which the extent of absorption is reduced, but the rate remains unchanged. Obviously, any change in the rate of absorption is likely to affect the onset of pharmacologic response, whereas changing the extent of absorption may influence the duration of action.

The therapeutic agents whose extent of absorption is decreased by the presence of food include compounds that are unstable in gastric fluid and, because of the presence of fat or low pH, remain longer in the stomach. Drugs may interact irreversibly with food components and not be absorbed, or they may interact reversibly and be absorbed later in their passage through the small intestine. Absorption of drugs that are poorly soluble in GI fluids may be increased in the presence of food because of the secretion of bile salts. The secretion of bile salts is the direct result of food intake, which releases the contents of the gallbladder into the small intestine. The classic examples of this type of drug are griseofulvin and cyclosporin; their extent of absorption is dependent on the presence of bile

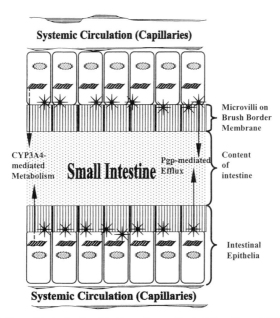

FIGURE 3.2 Depiction of intestinal epithelia and coordinated function of CYP3A4 and P-glycoprotein (Pgp) in reducing the absorption of parent drug.

salts. Another example is the increase in extent of absorption of midazolam, triazolam, nifedipine, and cyclosporine when ingested with grapefruit juice.

3.2.1.10 Effect of Disease States: Discussion of the effect of pathophysiologic factors of disease states on the process of absorption is beyond the scope of this chapter. It is, however, important to indicate that certain disease states such as ulcerative colitis and Crohn's disease (inflammatory bowel diseases) may reduce the extent of absorption of drugs significantly. Furthermore, it has been reported that gastric emptying can be delayed for patients with diabetes mellitus. Therefore, depending on the type of disease, different changes in the process of absorption of drugs are expected.

3.2.1.11 Other Factors Influencing Oral Absorption of Drugs: A number of nonphysiologic factors may influence the absorption of drugs:

- Drugs may exist as a racemic mixture of R and S enantiomers. Different enantiomers have different rates and extents of absorption and may have different pharmacologic responses.
- Formulation of different dosage forms of a drug may result in different rates and extents of absorption. For example, a controlled-release oral dosage form has a different profile of absorption than the conventional solid dosage forms prepared by direct compression.
- Physicochemical properties of drugs such as hydrophobicity and hydrophilicity affect absorption. Drugs with a higher partition coefficient are usually absorbed faster and more completely. For example, the hydrophobic β blockers propranolol and metoprolol have faster rates of absorption and greater extents of absorption than the hydrophilic counterpart β blockers atenolol and nadolol. The type of salt or crystal of a drug may have different solubility and hence change the absorption behavior of a drug.
- The timing of administration of drugs relative to food intake is also an important factor that may influence the absorption of drugs. For example, taking penicillin G or erythromycin 1 hour before a meal or 2 hours after a meal improves the rate and extent of absorption of these drugs. In this particular case the reason is a reduction in gastric emptying time and length of exposure to the acidic environment of the stomach. The rate and extent of absorption of some compounds, such as halofantrine, are improved by taking the drug with fatty foods.
- Finally, disintegration and dissolution of solid dosage forms may also become rate limiting in the absorption of drugs.

3.2.2 Basic Mechanisms of GI Absorption

The basic mechanisms involved in the transport of drugs across the GI tract absorptive epithelia into the systemic circulation are as follows:

    I. Passive diffusion
      1. Transcellular diffusion
      2. Paracellular diffusion

II. Carrier-mediated transcellular diffusion (also known as facilitated diffusion)

III. Transcellular diffusion subject to P-glycoprotein efflux

IV. Active transport

V. Pinocytosis

Two other mechanisms may possibly be involved in the absorption of drugs from the GI tract:

VI. Solvent drag

VII. Ion-pair absorption

3.2.2.1 Passive Diffusion: Transcellular and Paracellular: Passive diffusion plays a major role in a large number of physiologic processes. Most therapeutic agents are transported across the GI tract membrane by passive diffusion. The driving force in this type of diffusion is the concentration gradient between the GI environment and the systemic circulation. This means that the concentration of drug is greater at the site of absorption. Considering the large volume of systemic circulation and small volume of GI tract fluid, the concentration of drug at the site of absorption is greater than the concentration of free drug in systemic circulation (Figure 3.3).

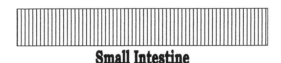

Small Intestine

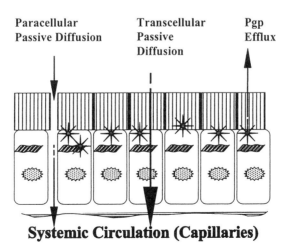

FIGURE 3.3 Representation of paracellular and transcellular passive diffusion and exsorption role of P-glycoprotein (Pgp) through the intestinal epithelium.

If we define the rate of absorption as dA/dt, where dA represents theoretical mass of drug that absorbs across the membrane per time dt, and dC/dx as the concentration gradient term, then according to Fick's First Law of Diffusion the rate of absorption can be stated as

$$\frac{dA}{dt} = -(D_{coeff})(\text{area})\,\frac{dC}{dx} \tag{3.6}$$

where D_{coeff} is the diffusion coefficient, (area) is the surface area available for diffusion, and dC is the change in concentration across the thickness of the barrier, dx.

Equation 3.6 is usually represented as

$$\frac{dA/dt}{(\text{area})} = J = -D_{coeff}\,\frac{dC}{dx} \tag{3.7}$$

Equation 3.7 is known as Fick's First Law and J is the flux. Equation 3.6 can also be presented in the following form that includes concentrations of drug at the site of absorption and systemic circulation:

$$\frac{dA}{dt} = \left(\frac{(D_{coeff})(\text{area})}{x}\right)\Delta C \tag{3.8}$$

where x is the thickness of the barrier and ΔC is the difference in concentrations between the GI tract and systemic circulation, that is, $\Delta C = C_{GI} - C_{blood}$.

When $C_{GI} > C_{blood}$

$$\frac{dA}{dt} = \left(\frac{(D_{coeff})(\text{area})}{x}\right)C_{gut} \tag{3.9}$$

$(D_{coeff} \times \text{area})/x$ is defined as the permeability constant, P. Therefore, Equation 3.9 can also be presented as

$$\frac{dA}{dt} = P(C_{gut}) \tag{3.10}$$

which is linear first-order kinetics.

3.2.2.2 Carrier-mediated Transcellular Diffusion (Also Known as Facilitated Diffusion): When absorption resembles passive diffusion but is mediated by a carrier, it is called carrier-mediated or facilitated diffusion (Figure 3.4). Large hydrophilic molecules that do not dissolve in the lipid moiety of the barrier and are larger than the barrier's pores may use this type of transport. The general concept is that the membrane contains macromolecules that act as carrier and facilitate the non-energy-requiring passage of the drug through the membrane. Therefore, the rate of this passage depends on the following factors:

a. Concentration gradient of the drug.
b. Quantity of the macromolecule (ie, carrier) present for the absorption.

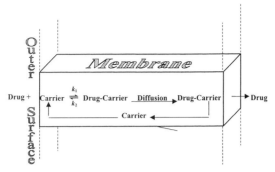

FIGURE 3.4 Diagram of carrier-mediated transport through membrane.

c. Rate of reversible interaction of drug with the carrier (ie, both interaction and splitting).
d. Diffusion coefficient of the drug–carrier complex through the membrane

Obviously any of the above factors can become a rate-limiting step in the absorption process.

Although facilitated transport is a non-energy-requiring process that does not proceed against a concentration gradient, there is a marked contrast with passive diffusion: because the process is dependent on the amount of carrier present in the barrier a saturation phenomenon may occur. Therefore, the kinetics of absorption may become nonlinear at high concentrations of drugs. It is important to note that only a few exogenous compounds use facilitated transport. Among them are endocrine steroids (receptor-facilitated cellular absorption) and Vitamin B_{12} (glycoprotein-facilitated intestinal transport).

3.2.2.3 Transcellular Diffusion Subject to P-glycoprotein Efflux: As was discussed in Section 3.2.1.8, Pgp with a molecular weight of 170-kDa is an ATP-dependent, efflux membrane transporter that interacts with a large number of xenobiotics. This protein is distributed in a number of tissues, particularly in the epithelial cells of the GI tract, liver, kidney, and pancreas and in the capillary endothelia of brain and testes. Its major physiologic role is to prevent cell death by pumping the drug out of the cell against a concentration gradient. This protein is known to be responsible for multidrug resistance (MDR) because of its role in reducing intracellular concentrations of drugs and preventing drugs from reaching their targets. The role of Pgp in limiting drug absorption from the GI tract is of special importance. The pumping of drug out of the intestinal epithelium against a concentration gradient results in reduced drug absorption and bioavailability.

3.2.2.4 Active Transport: In active transport, similar to facilitated transport, carriers are used to transfer selected molecules. The carriers are proteins, and, contrary to facilitated transport, they require energy for the absorption. Active transport occurs mostly against a concentration gradient and only at certain sites such as the intestines, liver, and kidneys. Because the process requires energy and the concentration of protein carriers is limited, active transport is apt to produce saturation. Furthermore, the protein carriers are subject to competitive inhibition by compounds of similar structure. Pathways of active transport in the intestine exist for the purpose of transferring certain nutrients such as uracil, choline,

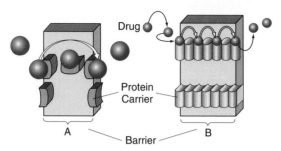

FIGURE 3.5 Hypothetical mechanisms of active transport: (A) direct hypothesis, (B) shuttling hypothesis.

folate derivatives, and bile salts. Drug molecules that are structurally similar to these nutrients use the same pathways for absorption. For example, the anticancer drug 5-fluorouracil (5FU) uses the uracil pathway, and methotrexate, another anticancer drug, uses the folate derivative pathway.

The exact mechanism of active transport has not been fully elucidated. Obviously the carriers are quite specific for a given compound. There are, however, certain postulations that have been accepted as plausible scenarios. For example, a protein carrier may pick up a drug molecule, go through the energy-requiring conformational change, and rotate 180° and release the drug at the opposite side (Figure 3.5A). Another scenario is that protein carrier could be a very large molecule with binding sites and functional groups across its surface, and therefore it is capable of shuttling the drug molecule between the binding sites to the opposite side (Figure 3.5B)

3.2.2.5 Pinocytosis: In this type of absorption drugs with large molecules such as proteins or lipophilic carriers such as liposomes or droplets of microemulsion may cross the membrane by physically forcing themselves through the membrane or by the membrane's sucking in the drug molecule or drug–carrier complex. The process is initiated when the membrane engulfs the molecule or particle and then the membrane breaks off and forms a membrane-coated particle. The coated particle or molecule is then transported across the barrier to the opposite side where the drug or particle is released (Figure 3.6).

We know very little about physiologic significance of pinocytosis. It is not considered a major mechanism of drug absorption although it could be responsible for the uptake of small quantities of macromolecules.

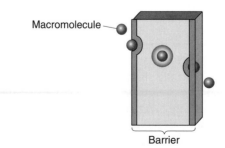

FIGURE 3.6 Pinocytotic transport of particles or large molecules through the membrane.

3.2.2.6 Solvent Drag: The speculation in this type of mechanism is that the absorption of drug is a function of the physicochemical characteristics of its solvent. Therefore, the permeation of solvent will transport the dissolved molecules of drug along through the membrane.

3.2.2.7 Ion-pair Absorption: According to pH partition theory, ionized forms of drugs cannot readily diffuse through a biologic barrier; however, many ionized drugs, such as quaternary ammonium compounds and sulfonic acids, are absorbed after oral administration. The mechanism(s) of absorption of ionized molecules is not quite clear. One explanation is the hypothesis of ion-pair absorption. According to this hypothesis, oppositely charged molecules may interact and form a neutral complex. The neutral complex then crosses the biologic barrier by passive diffusion. As the formation of a neutral complex is a simple chemical equilibrium, an excess of one ion can increase the formation of the complex. Thus, the formation and absorption of the complex depend on the concentration of one or both ions and this dependency contributes to the erratic absorption of drug. This means that formation of the complex is the rate-limiting step in the absorption process. The breakdown of the complex is also based on chemical equilibrium. Once the neutral complex is inside the membrane a new equilibrium is established and all three species—positive, negative, and neutral—are present in the membrane at the same time. As the charged molecules leave the barrier more of the neutral complex breaks down into charged molecules (Figure 3.7). This hypothesis has not been fully supported in vivo by the experimental data.

3.2.3 Absorption from Other Significant Routes of Administration

3.2.3.1 Sublingual and Buccal Absorption: Sublingual/buccal absorption takes place in the highly vascular region of the mouth between the cheeks or under the tongue. The absorption occurs in the presence of saliva with a pH approximately between 6 and 7. Ab-

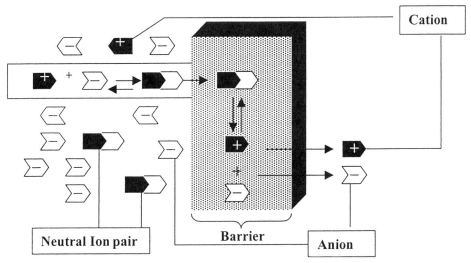

FIGURE 3.7 Diagram of hypothesis of formation, equilibrium, and breakdown of neural ion-pair complex.

sorption of drugs occurs through the mucosa into the systemic circulation only by passive diffusion and is limited by the molecular weight of the drug. There has been no report on the presence of active absorption, facilitated transport, or pinocytosis at this site. This is a useful route of administration for drugs that are unstable in the low pH of the stomach, destroyed by enzymes of the GI tract, or subjected to first-pass effect; however, the flow of saliva itself, 0.5 ml/min, may wash away the drug from the site of absorption into the stomach. Therefore, the volume of the dosage form may also play an important role in sublingual/buccal absorption and its bioavailability. It has been advocated that absorption from the GI tract gradually diminishes with age, but sublingual/buccal absorption maintains its consistency.

3.2.3.2 Inhalation: Drugs taken by this route of administration are mostly in the form of aerosols or gases. Absorption of substances by inhalation is from the membrane or mucosa of the nose, pharynx, trachea, bronchi, bronchioles, alveolar sacs, and alveoli. Therefore a large surface area is usually available for absorption of drugs. This route of administration is used for local as well as systemic effect. Absorption of lipid-soluble and volatile gases such as ether and chloroform is very rapid, and the onset of systemic anesthetic action is rather instantaneous. Water-soluble gases do not penetrate farther than nasopharyngeal region. Aerosols, on the other hand, are dispersed solid particles or droplets. Absorption of drugs from aerosols is dependent on the deposition of these particles or droplets. The size of particles and the pattern of airflow limit their migration through the pulmonary system. Larger particles (5–30 μm) are retained in the nasopharyngeal region by inertial impaction. Small particles (1–5 μm) are retained in the trachea and bronchial and bronchiolar regions by sedimentation. Smaller particles (1 μm) penetrate deep into the pulmonary tree, reach the alveolar sacs, and dissolve in the available fluid. Therefore, absorption of small particles that are trapped in the fluid occurs mainly by passive diffusion. Particles may also directly penetrate the epithelial membrane and be absorbed by pinocytosis.

Drugs that are administered by inhalation to produce a systemic effect avoid the low pH of the stomach and first-pass elimination in the liver; however, the absorption and bioavailability of drugs administered by this route, because of the random removal of particles by exhalation, may be inconsistent. It is worth noting that the maximum air capacity of the lungs is about 5700 cm^3 and the total air that moves in and out of the lungs in active normal breathing is approximately 4500 cm^3; therefore, the lungs retain 1200 cm^3 of air. The number of breaths per minute is approximately 12 to 20. At rest the volume of air is reduced to 500 cm^3. Air velocity is very high in the nasopharyngeal region and decreases as air reaches the alveolar region. Hence, if the particles do not become impacted they are removed by exhalation from the site of absorption. There is always a greater tendency for smaller particles to be exhaled. Needless to say, a cough or sneeze, with an air velocity of 75 to 100 miles per hour, can remove a significant number of particles from the site of absorption, particularly if it occurs immediately after administration of the drug.

3.2.3.3 Subcutaneous Absorption: The subcutaneous route of administration is usually used for injection of small volumes of vaccines or drugs such as insulin and local anesthetics. This route is also used to implant prolonged-release dosage forms such as polymeric rods and pellets. When drugs are introduced into the subcutaneous region they travel by passive diffusion to reach the primary absorption membrane, the capillary wall. If the compound is lipophilic, it can diffuse directly through the capillary membrane by transcellular passive diffusion. Water-soluble drugs diffuse through cleft pores and vesicular channels of the membrane by paracellular passive diffusion. There has been no report to indicate that other mechanisms of absorption such as pinocytosis and active or facilitated transport take place at this site. The rate-limiting steps in the absorption of drugs after subcutaneous administration, for the purpose of achieving a systemic effect, are the release of drug from the dosage forms and the blood flow to the region. Therefore, factors that cause vasoconstriction of capillaries, such as cooling and administration of vasoconstrictors, reduce the absorption of drugs from this site significantly.

3.2.3.4 Intramuscular Absorption: Absorption from muscle is similar to absorption from the subcutaneous region. Lipophilic compounds are absorbed very rapidly by transcellular passive diffusion, whereas lipid-insoluble molecules are absorbed by paracellular passive diffusion through cleft pores and vesicular channels. The rate of absorption is dependent on the following factors:

- In general drugs are absorbed faster from deltoid than gluteal muscle.
- Absorption of drugs from gluteal muscle of individuals with lower fat/muscle ratio is faster than that of individuals with a higher ratio.
- Local uptake of lipid-soluble compounds is greater in individuals with a higher fat/muscle ratio than in individuals with a lower ratio.
- Absorption of drugs into the systemic circulation from muscle is dependent on blood flow. Muscle blood flow at rest is about 3 to 4 mL/min per 100 g of muscle. This increases to a maximum of 80 to 90 mL/min per 100 g of muscle. Therefore, absorption of drugs from the muscle of active individuals is faster than that of patients who are confined to bed.
- Drugs injected into the muscle or subcutaneous region, in contrast to the GI tract, have no time limit for residence and both regions are used for controlled-release dosage forms.
- If drugs are injected in the form of solution, emulsion, or suspension the maximum volume cannot exceed 10 mL.

In general, the intramuscular route administration may be used for drugs that are not stable in the GI tract or are incompletely absorbed; however, incomplete absorption may also occur in the muscular environment because of precipitation or decomposition of drugs. Furthermore, conditions such as hypotension and circulatory diseases may also reduce the rate and extent of absorption.

3.2.3.5 Intraperitoneal Absorption: A thin membrane called the peritoneum covers the abdominal cavity and its organs. With its large surface area and blood-rich capillaries this membrane is the site of absorption or exsorption of drugs for intraperitoneal administration. Drug absorbed into the blood of the peritoneal capillary network reaches the portal circulation, which must pass through the liver before distribution in the body. Therefore, the drug may undergo hepatic first-pass elimination. In humans intraperitoneal exchange of drugs is used in continuous ambulatory peritoneal dialysis. Drugs added to dialysate (dialysis solution) are absorbed into the systemic circulation by passive diffusion or can be removed from the systemic circulation into a dialysate that contains no drug.

3.2.3.6 Intradermal Absorption: The site of injection is below the stratum corneum. This route is not used to achieve a systemic effect. Intradermal injection is often used for allergy testing of therapeutic agents or for a few vaccines that are intended for local reaction.

3.2.3.7 Intranasal Absorption: The nasal route has received a great deal of attention as a convenient mode of administration for achieving systemic effect. The nasal passage is covered by highly specialized and unique epithelia such as olfactory epithelium, brush cells, goblet cells, ciliated cells, and basal cells. An important characteristic of this site of absorption is the capability of the epithelia to metabolize xenobiotics. A number of isozymes of cytochrome P450 such as CYP1A1, CYP2B1, and CYP4B1 have been identified in the nose of several different species. Therefore, nasal metabolism may reduce the bioavailability of drugs. The surface area for absorption begins in the nostril and ends in the pharynx. Absorption of drugs from this site is also by passive diffusion. Lipid-soluble gases are absorbed or metabolized by epithelia. Insoluble particles are usually removed and swallowed following their deposition. Water-soluble gases or particles are dissolved in mucus, pass through the epithelium, and enter into the capillaries. Other factors that may affect the absorption of drugs from this site are blood flow to the region; viscosity of the mucus and its flow rate, pH and size of dose, and environmental factors such as humidity and temperature.

3.2.3.8 Rectal Absorption: The rectum, with a length of 15 to 20 cm and surface area of 200 to 400 cm^2, is located in the terminal portion of the pelvic colon. This site of absorption has a pH between 7.4 and 8.0 with limited buffer capacity and temperature of 37°C. It is a highly vascular region. The superior rectal artery is the main artery and its venous network comprises the upper rectal vein, middle rectal vein, and lower rectal vein system. The upper rectal vein is linked to the hepatoportal vein system; the middle and lower veins enter into the inferior vena cava. Therefore, drugs that are absorbed from the upper part of the rectum enter the upper rectal vein and are subject to first-pass metabolism in the liver before distribution. Drugs that are absorbed in the middle and lower rectal veins avoid the liver and distribute in the body following absorption into the systemic circulation. The mechanisms of absorption at this site are transcellular and paracellular passive diffusion. There is no active site for absorption and there is no proof of carrier-mediated transport. Some advantages of using this route of administration are as follows:

- It is a stable environment for the absorption of drugs. The pH, viscosity, and temperature are constant, rectal motility is very low, and the residence time of drugs is rather long and limited by defecation. Overall, the condition is most suitable for administration of controlled-release dosage forms.
- The lymphatic circulation of the rectal region is significant and therefore drugs that are targeted toward the lymph can be administered rectally.
- The rectum has no enzymes and thus no metabolism takes place at this site; however, the metabolic activity of gut flora continues to pose a problem.
- It is an alternative route for drugs that have low bioavailability following oral administration.
- It is a convenient route for patients, such as infants, who cannot take solid dosage forms orally.

This route has several shortcomings:

■ First-pass elimination of drug absorbed from the upper part of rectum.
■ Unsuitability with irritant drugs.
■ Inconsistent bioavailability.

3.2.3.9 Intravaginal Absorption: Absorption occurs from the highly vascular region of the vagina. The pH of this environment in the adult population is usually acidic between 4 and 5. The lower pH has been attributed to the fermentation of normally secreted glycogen to lactic acid by bacteria that usually colonize this site. Most vaginal dosage forms are intended for local effect; however, this site can be used effectively to achieve systemic effect, for example, with progesterone-containing dosage forms. Absorption from this site is by transcellular and paracellular passive diffusion. No active absorption or carrier-mediated transport has been reported for this site.

3.2.3.10 Transdermal Absorption: The mechanism of percutaneous absorption of xenobiotics, though based on diffusion, is not similar to the aforementioned routes of absorption because of the complexity of the barrier. The physiologic role of skin is to protect the body, reduce loss of water and heat, and prevent the absorption of foreign substances including xenobiotics; however, polar and nonpolar drugs, if administered in an appropriate manner, can be absorbed to some extent through the skin and enter the systemic circulation. The skin is composed of three major regions:

■ The epidermis consists of the stratum corneum, stratum granulosum, spinosum, and germinativum
■ Appendages include sweat and sebaceous glands and hair follicles.
■ The dermis is composed of connective tissues, fat, capillaries, and glands.

The epidermis with its outer layer called the stratum corneum, or horny layer, is the rate-limiting layer in the absorption process. The stratum corneum is composed of densely packed keratin and is the layer that prevents absorption. The openings in the skin provided by the appendages constitute approximately 1% of the total surface area of the skin. Transfer of drugs through these openings is fast but does not constitute a significant amount as compared with absorption from the remaining 99% surface area. Therefore two major mechanisms, transepidermal penetration and transappendageal absorption, govern the absorption of drugs through the skin. The dermis is the layer above the subcutaneous region. When drugs reach the dermis they can diffuse freely toward the capillaries, the subcutaneous region, and finally the systemic circulation. The rate and extent of transdermal absorption are dependent on the following factors:

A. Skin-related factors
   1. Integrity of skin and whether it is normal or diseased
   2. Frequency of administration
   3. Location of administration
   4. Area of administration
   5. Skin biotransformation due to the presence of enzymes

   a. CYP450 isozymes
      i. CYP1A1
      ii. CYP2A1
      iii. CYP1B1
      iv. CYP2B1
   b. Enzymes of phase II metabolism
      i. UDP-glucuronosyl transferase
      ii. π and α isozymes of glutathione transferase
   c. Catabolic enzymes
      i. Proteases
      ii. Lipases
      iii. Glycosidases
      iv. Phosphatases

B. Drug-related factors
   1. Partition coefficient of drug
   2. Particle and molecular size
   3. Viscosity of dosage forms
   4. Diffusion coefficient of drug in the dosage form.
   5. Diffusion coefficient of drug in the skin

C. Environmental factors
   1. Temperature
   2. Humidity
   3 Air current

D. Addition of penetration enhancers in dosage form such as
   1. Alcohol or other organic solvents
   2. Surfactants (eg, sodium lauryl sulfate)
   3. Prohibited compounds such as dimethylsulfoxide (DMSO), dimethylformamide (DMF), dimethyl acetamide (DMA)

ASSIGNMENT (EXTRA CREDIT)
EC-3.1 Read the following review article and answer the questions of this assignment:
Yu DK. The contribution of P-glycoprotein to pharmacokinetic drug–drug interaction. *J Clin Pharmacol* 1999;39:1203–11.

QUESTIONS
   I. Discuss the roles of CYP3A and Pgp in the following combination therapies:

   ■ Tamoxifen and digoxin
   ■ Lidocaine and dexamethasone
   ■ Ketoconazole and tamoxifen
   ■ Verapamil and hydrocortisone

   II. Explain the use and significance of the Caco-2 cell monolayer in the evaluation of Pgp.
   III. Name the biologic barriers of the body that contain significant amounts of Pgp.

IV. Considering the role of Pgp and CYP3A, what would be necessary for the development of new drugs?

V. What precautions are required with respect to taking the following medications with grapefruit juice:

- Verapamil
- Amiodarone
- Paclitaxel

EC-3.2 Answer the following questions after reading the article by Marathe et al:

Marathe PH, Sadefer EP, Kollia E, Greene DS, Barhaiya RH, Lipper RA, Page RC, Doll WJ, Ryo UY, Digenis GA. *In vivo* evaluation of the absorption and gastrointestinal transit of avitriptan in fed and fasted subjects using gamma scintigraphy. *J Pharmacokinet Biopharm* 1998;26:1–20.

QUESTIONS

- Describe the experimental protocol.
- Discuss the effect of intrasubject variations in gastric emptying on the extent of absorption of avitriptan.
- How would you explain the cause of the double-peak phenomenon for avitriptan?
- Is the cause of the double-peak phenomenon observed for drugs such as cimetidine and ranitidine the same as that for avitriptan?
- Summarize your evaluation of data on subject 6. Are the data on subject 6 significantly different from others?

EC-3.3 Based on the data presented in the paper by O'Reilly et al (No. 16 in the Bibliography) prepare a 10-minute presentation and/or a written report underscoring the following points:

- Gastric emptying behavior of particulate dosage forms before, during, and after a meal.
- Differences between gastric emptying of encapsulated particles and predispersed particles (sprinkled onto the food).
- Relationship between gastric emptying and duration of action of particulate dosage forms.

BIBLIOGRAPHY

1. Amlacher R, Härtl A, Neubert R, Stockel U, Wenzel K. Influence of ion-pair formation on the pharmacokinetic properties of drugs: pharmacokinetic interactions of bretylium and hexasalicylic acid in rabbit. *J Pharm Pharmacol* 1991;43:794.
2. Burks TF, Galligan JJ, Porreca F, Barker WD. Regulation of gastric emptying. *Fed Proc* 1985; 44:2897.
3. Christian PE, More JG, Sorenson JA, Coleman RE, Welch DM. Effect of meal size and correction technique on gastric emptying time: studies with two tracers and opposed detectors. *J Nucl Med* 1980;21:883.
4. Ehle FR, Robertson JB, Van Soest PJ. Influence of dietary fibers on fermentation in human large intestine. *J Nutr* 1982;112:156.

5. Finegold SM, Sutter VL, Mathisen GE. Normal indigenous intestinal flora. In: Hentges DJ, editor. Human Intestinal Microflora in Health and Disease. New York, Academic Press, 1983:3.

6. Gibaldi M. Limitation of classical theories of drug absorption. In: Prescott LE, Nimmo WS, editors. Drug Absorption. Lancaster: MTP Press Limited Falcon House, 1981:1.

7. Guyton AC, Hall JE. Textbook of Medical Physiology. 9th ed. Philadelphia: WB Saunders, 1996:793.

8. Hall SD, Thummel KE, Watkins PB, Lown KS, Benet LZ, Paine MF, Mayo RR, Turgeon DK, Baily DG, Fontana RJ, Wrighton SA. Molecular and physical mechanism of first-pass extraction. *Drug Metab Disp* 1999;27:161.

9. Härtl A, Amlacher R, Neubert R, Hause C. Influence of ion-pair formation of bretylium and hexylsalicylic acid on their blood levels in dogs. *Pharmazie* 1990;45:295.

10. Hayton WL. Rate-limiting barriers to intestinal drug absorption: a review. *J Pharmacokinet Biopharm* 1980;8:321.

11. Kim RB, Fromm MF, Wandel C, Leake B, Wood AJJ, Roden DM. The drug transporter P-glycoprotein limits oral absorption and brain entry of HIV-1 protease inhibitors. *J Clin Invest* 1998;101:289.

12. Lown KS, Baily DG, Fontana RJ, Janardan SK, Adair CH, Fortlage LA, Brown MB, Guo W, Watkins PB. Grapefruit juice increases felodipine oral availability in humans by decreasing intestinal CYP3A4 protein expression. *J Clin Invest* 1997;99:2545.

13. Lown KS, Mayo RR, Leichtman AB, Hsiao H-L, Turgeon DK, Schmiedlin-Ren P, Brown MB, Guo W, Rossi SJ, Benet LZ, Watkins PB. Role of intestinal P-glycoprotein (mdr1) in interpatient variation in the oral bioavailability of cyclosporin A. *Clin Pharmacol Ther* 1997;62:248.

14. Nimmo WS. Gastric emptying and drug absorption. In: Prescott LE, Nimmo WS, editors. Drug Absorption. Lancaster: MTP Press Limited Falcon House, 1981:11.

15. Oberle RL, Amidon GL. The influence of variable gastric emptying and intestinal transit rates on the plasma level curve of cimetidine: an explanation for double peak phenomenon. *J Pharmacokinet Biopharm* 1987;15:529.

16. O'Reilly S, Wison CG, Hardy JG. The influence of food on the gastric emptying of multiparticulate dosage forms. *Int J Pharm* 1987;34:213.

17. Pond SM, Tozer TN. First-pass elimination: basic concepts and clinical consequences. *Clin Pharmacokin* 1984;9:1.

18. Rabinson PH, Moran T, McHugh PR. Inhibition of gastric emptying and feeding by fenfluramine. *Am J Physiol* 1986;250:R764.

19. Savage DC. Gastrointestinal microflora in mammalian nutrition. *Annu Rev Nutr* 1986;6:155.

20. Ueda K, Yoshida A, Amachi T. Recent progress in P-glycoprotein research. *Anticancer Drug Des* 1999;14:115.

21. van der Ohe M, Camillari M. Measurements of small bowel and colonic transit: indications and methods. *Mayo Clin Proc* 1992;67:1169.

22. Welling PG. Effect of food on drug absorption. *Annu Rev Nutr* 1996;16:383.

CHAPTER 4

DISTRIBUTION OF DRUGS IN THE BODY

Things taken together are whole and not whole,
being brought together and brought apart, in tune and out of tune;
out of all things there comes a unity, and out of a unity all things.
ARISTOTLE (ON THE WORLD 5.396B20)

OBJECTIVES

■ To review the general principles of drug distribution.

■ To discuss the major physiologic factors involved in drug distribution.

■ To review the extent of protein binding and the related graphic analysis.

■ To discuss physiologic barriers in drug distribution

4.1 INTRODUCTION

After gaining access to the systemic circulation through one of the routes of administration, drugs distribute in different tissues and organs of the body. Depending on their physicochemical characteristics a series of physical and physiologic processes occur simultaneously that shape the distinctive pattern of their distribution in the body. An example of physical processes is the simple dilution of drug in intracellular and extracellular fluids, and examples of physiologic processes are protein binding, tissue uptake, and permeation of drug through different barriers in the body. Thus, in general the distribution of drugs can be influenced by factors such as:

■ Blood flow.
■ Extent of binding to plasma proteins.
■ Physicochemical characteristics of drugs.
■ Degree and extent to which drugs penetrate through physiologic barriers.
■ Extent of elimination which continuously removes the drug from the body and competes with the distribution phenomena (Chapter 5).

Let us review these factors in more detail.

4.2 BLOOD FLOW

Blood flow is the volume of blood that reaches a site in the body per unit of time; the units are volume/time and the magnitude differs from region to region. Total blood flow is 5000 mL/min, which corresponds to cardiac output at rest. Cardiac output is the volume of blood pumped by the heart per minute. In addition to cardiac output, an important factor in blood flow is the volume of blood in various parts of systemic circulation. The heart usually holds 7% of the total blood; the pulmonary system, 9%; arteries, about 13%; arterioles and capillaries, 7%; and veins, venules, and venous system, the remaining 64%. The capillaries with their permeable walls allow the exchange of drugs, nutrients, and so on with the interstitial fluid of organs/tissues and merge with the venules, which gradually converge into larger veins. During this transcapillary exchange drug is transported across the capillary wall into the tissue. This transport may result from the difference in pressures, such as osmotic pressure and hydrostatic pressure, between the inside and outside of the capillary, or may result mainly from a concentration difference between the drug across the capillary wall. Distribution of a drug to a region of the body depends on the blood flow to that region and how fast the drug is transferred from the site of administration to the region. Table 4.1 summarizes the differences in volumes and blood flows of different organs/tissues of the human body for a 30- to 39-year-old man of 70-kg body weight and 1.73-m^2 body surface area.

The blood flow essentially determines how fast a drug can be delivered to a body region and reflects the relative rate at which an organ/tissue may be expected to come into equilibrium with blood. The amount of drug that can be stored or distributed in a tissue, however, depends on the size of the tissue and the physicochemical characteristics of the drug, such as partition coefficient between organ and blood.

Depending on the physicochemical characteristic of drugs, transcapillary exchange and

TABLE 4.1 Blood Flow to Different Organs/Tissues at Rest for a 30- to 39-Year-old Man of 70-kg Body Weight and 1.73-m^2 Body Surface Area

Organ/Tissue	Volume (L)	Blood Flow (mL/min)	Blood Flow (mL/min)/ 100 mL Tissue	Volume of Blood in Equilibrium with Tissue (mL)
Adrenals	0.02	100	500	62
Kidneys	0.30	1240	410	765
Thyroid	0.02	80	400	49
Gray matter	0.75	600	80	371
Heart	0.30	240	80	148
Liver + portal system	3.90	1760	45	976
Red marrow	1.40	120	9	74
Muscle	30	600	2	370
Fat	10	200	2	123
Fatty marrow	2.20	60	2.70	37
Bone cortex	6.40	0	0	0
Total		5000		

storage in tissue are either a blood flow-limited phenomenon known as perfusion-limited distribution or a transfer-limited phenomenon known as permeability-limited distribution.

4.2.1 Transcapillary Exchange of Drugs: Perfusion-limited and Permeability-limited Distribution

To differentiate between the two types of distribution, let us assume that the capillary resembles a hollow cylinder of length L and radius r in which blood flows with a velocity of v in the positive direction x. The concentration of drug in the tissue around the capillary is C_{tissue} and the concentration in the blood is C_{blood}. The drug diffuses across the capillary membrane because of the concentration gradient between blood and tissue. If we consider a segment of the direction between x and $x + \Delta x$, the difference in mass flux of the drug between the beginning and the end of the Δx segment would be equal to the mass flux across the capillary wall. This equality can be written in the following form where the cross-sectional area of the capillary is πr^2 (r is the radius of the cross-sectional circle), the surface area of diffusion is $2r\pi\Delta x$, and the permeability constant for drug in the capillary membrane is P:

$$v[C_{blood}(x + dx) - C_{blood}(x)]\, \pi r^2 = P[C_{tissue} - C_{blood}(x)]2r\pi\Delta x \tag{4.1}$$

As the limit of $\Delta x \rightarrow 0$, Equation 4.1 changes to the form

$$\pi r^2 v(dC_{blood}/dx) = -2r\pi P[C_{blood} - C_{tissue}] \tag{4.2}$$

The cross-sectional area times the velocity, $\pi r^2 v$, is equal to blood flow, Q. The surface area of the whole length of capillary under observation, S, is equal to $2r\pi L$. Therefore, Equation 4.2 can be written as

$$\frac{dC}{dx} = -\frac{PS}{QL}(C_{blood} - C_{tissue}) \tag{4.3}$$

C_{blood} at time zero is equal to the concentration in arterial blood, $C_{arterial}$. Integration of Equation 4.3 yields the equation

$$C_{blood}(x) - C_{tissue} = (C_{arterial} - C_{tissue})e^{-PSx/QL} \tag{4.4}$$

Setting $x = L$ and $C_{blood}(L) = C_{venous}$, Equation 4.4 changes

$$C_{venous} = C_{tissue} + (C_{arterial} - C_{tissue})e^{-PS/Q} \tag{4.5}$$

Also, the mass flux across the capillary wall into the tissue, J_{tissue}, in terms of net mass current leaving the capillary per length L, would be

$$J_{tissue} = 2r\pi P\int_0^L [C_{blood}(x) - C_{tissue}]dx = QC_{arterial} - QC_{venous} \tag{4.6}$$

Substituting Equation 4.5 into Equation 4.6 yields

$$J_{\text{tissue}} = (C_{\text{arterial}} - C_{\text{tissue}})Q(1 - e^{-PS/Q}) \qquad (4.7)$$

Capillary clearance is then defined as

$$\text{clearance} = \frac{J_{\text{tissue}}}{C_{\text{Arterial}} - C_{\text{tissue}}} = Q(1 - e^{-PS/Q}) \qquad (4.8)$$

Capillary clearance may be defined as the volume of blood from which drug is diffused into the tissue per units of time. The extraction ratio of the distribution is then defined as

$$\text{extraction ratio} = E = 1 - e^{-PS/Q} \qquad (4.9)$$

Equation 4.9 may also be defined as

$$E = \frac{C_{\text{arterial}} - C_{\text{venous}}}{C_{\text{arterial}} - C_{\text{tissue}}} \qquad (4.10)$$

indicating that the extraction ratio is an equilibration fraction between the drug concentration in the tissue and arterial capillaries and the venous side of the capillaries. Comparison of Equations 4.5 and 4.10 demonstrates further that capillary clearance is equal to blood flow multiplied by the extraction ratio.

$Q > PS$, or $C_{\text{arterial}} \approx C_{\text{venous}}$, would indicate that the drug is not highly lipophilic, the extraction ratio is less than one, and the distribution of the drug is limited by how fast it diffuses through the capillary membrane. This is called diffusion-limited distribution or permeability-limited distribution, and the mass transfer into the tissue is defined by

$$J_{\text{tissue}} = PS(C_{\text{arterial}} - C_{\text{tissue}}) \qquad (4.11)$$

The driving force for the transfer of drug into tissue is the concentration gradient.

$Q < PS$, or $C_{\text{venous}} \approx C_{\text{tissue}}$ (ie, the concentration of drug in the tissue is in equilibrium with the concentration on the venous side of the capillaries) indicates that the drug is highly lipophilic. The extraction ratio is equal or close to one, and because the uptake of drug by the tissue is thermodynamically much more favorable than its presence in the blood, distribution is limited by how fast the drug can be delivered to the tissue. When the drug reaches the tissue, uptake is immediate. This type of distribution is called perfusion-limited distribution or blood flow-limited distribution, and the mass transfer into the tissue can be defined as

$$J_{\text{tissue}} = Q(C_{\text{arterial}} - C_{\text{tissue}}) \qquad (4.12)$$

Blood flow is the principal factor in distribution, and the concentration gradient plays very little or no role in mass transfer of drug.

4.3 BINDING OF DRUGS TO PROTEINS

The binding of drugs to plasma proteins influences their distribution in the body significantly. The binding creates a drug–protein complex with a molecular size equal to the sum of molecular weights of the drug and protein. Therefore, the small molecules of drug associated with proteins can no longer permeate easily through the barriers and thus its distribution is different from that of unbound drug. Also, because its functional groups have interacted with the functional groups of protein it can no longer interact with the functional groups of membrane or intracellular receptors. Therefore, binding to protein not only affects the distribution of drug in the body, but also influences therapeutic outcome. This is the main reason for using the concentration of unbound drug in plasma for pharmacokinetic analysis and design or adjustment of dosing regimen for optimum therapeutic outcome.

The protein binding of drugs when administered concomitantly may be different from that of drugs administered individually. Thus, the distribution of drugs given individually may be different from their distribution when given in combination. This change in protein binding is considered a possible outcome of drug–drug interactions and is the result of displacement of one drug from plasma proteins by another drug. Similar displacement can also occur at the cellular level, with other proteins and enzymes of tissues. The displacement causes an increase in the free fraction of drug in plasma and a proportionate elevation in the drug concentration at receptor sites. It is important to remedy this problem by adjusting the dosage regimen of drugs when they are coadministered. The change in protein binding of drugs is a major concern, especially for drugs with a narrow therapeutic range.

4.3.1 Proteins of Plasma That Are Involved in Drug–Protein Interactions

The major protein of plasma is albumin. It is a large protein with a molecular weight of 69,000 Da and a catabolic half-life of approximately 17 to 18 days. This protein is produced exclusively by the hepatocytes of the liver. It is the major plasma and tissue protein responsible for binding most drugs. This protein, despite its large molecular size, and in addition to being circulated in the vascular system, can also diffuse into the extravascular compartment. Albumin possesses both negatively and positively charged binding sites. Interactions of drugs with this protein occur by hydrogen binding, hydrophobic binding, and van der Waals forces. A wide variety of factors such as pregnancy, surgery, age, sex, and interethnic and racial differences affect interactions of drugs with this protein. The kidneys do not filter albumin, and therefore, drugs that are bound to albumin also remain unfiltered. Thus, the degree of binding has significant influence not only on the distribution of a drug, but also on its renal elimination. Furthermore, the degree of binding influences the metabolism of a drug. Only free drug can be taken up by the hepatocytes in the liver. Therefore, the greater the percentage of bound drug, the lower the hepatic uptake and rate of metabolism of a drug. As was mentioned earlier, the degree of a drug's binding to plasma albumin can also be significantly affected by concomitant administration of drugs that displace the drug from its binding site on albumin, resulting in an increase in the plasma concentration of free drug.

Other proteins of plasma are fibrinogen, globulins such as γ globulin and β_1 globulin (ie, transferrin), ceruloplasmin and α and β lipoproteins. Fibrinogen and its polymerized form, fibrin, are involved in formation of blood clots. Globulins are mainly γ globulins, which are antibodies and interact with specific antigens. Transferrin is involved in the transport of iron, ceruloplasmin is involved in the transfer of copper, and α and β lipoproteins are carriers of lipid-soluble compounds.

4.3.2 Estimation of Parameters of Protein Binding

The binding of drugs to plasma proteins is usually determined in vitro at physiologic pH and temperature. The techniques of determination include equilibrium dialysis, dynamic dialysis, ultrafiltration, gel filtration chromatography, ultracentrifugation, microdialysis, and a few recently developed fast methodologies for high-throughput experiments. The objective of all these techniques is to estimate the concentration of free drug that is in equilibrium with the drug–protein complex. The selected methodology and conditions of experiment should be such that the stability of the complex and equilibrium is preserved and the concentration of free drug is not overestimated by breakdown of the complex during measurement. After all, most drug–protein complexes are held together by weak chemical interactions such as electrostatic interactions, van der Waal's forces, and hydrogen binding, which tend to separate at nonphysiologic pH, temperature, and osmotic pressure.

In the conventional method of dialysis, plasma or protein solution with a pH of 7.2 to 7.4 is spiked with different concentrations of drug. The mixture in then dialyzed at 37°C through a dialysis membrane with molecular cutoffs $\approx$ 12,000 to 14,000 Da against an equivalent volume of phosphate buffer ($\approx$ 67 mM, pH 7.2–7.4), made isotonic with NaCl. The dialysis membrane is used in the form of a bag that holds protein and drug and the bag is placed in the buffer solution. A modified version of the bag is a prefabricated two compartments unit that is separated by dialysis membrane. The equilibrium of free drug across the membrane is usually achieved in about two to three hours. The concentration of free drug is measured in the buffer side i.e., outside of the bag or compartment separated by membrane, which is assumed to be equal to the concentration of free drug inside the bag or compartment. The concentration of free drug inside the bag or compartment is assumed to be in equilibrium with the drug bound to protein. The protein can be either the albumin solution or blank plasma sample containing albumin. The binding parameters of the drug, such as free faction or association constant can then be determine by the following application of the Law of Mass Action.

$$\text{drug + protein} \;\underset{k_2}{\overset{k_1}{\rightleftharpoons}}\; \text{drug–protein}$$

$$K_a = \frac{C_{DP}}{C_D \times C_{Pr}} = \frac{k_1}{-k_2} \tag{4.13}$$

where K_a is the association constant, C_D is the concentration of free drug in moles, C_{Pr} is the concentration of protein with free binding sites, C_{DP} is the concentration of drug–

protein complex, and k_1 and k_2 are the rate constants of forward and reverse reactions, respectively. The reciprocal of the association constant is known as the dissociation constant:

$$K_D = \frac{C_D \times C_{Pr}}{C_{DP}} = \frac{k_2}{k_1} = \frac{1}{K_a} \tag{4.14}$$

The magnitude of the association constant, K_a, represents the extent of drug–protein binding. Drugs that bind extensively to plasma proteins usually have a very large association constant.

On the basis of Equation 4.14 we can determine the following relationships for the concentration of a drug–protein complex:

$$C_{DP} = K_a C_D C_{Pr} \tag{4.15}$$

When the concentration of total protein (C_{PT}) at the start of an in vitro experiment is known and the concentration of drug–protein complex (C_{DP}) is estimated experimentally, the concentration of free protein (C_{Pr}) that is in equilibrium with the drug–protein complex can then be determined as

$$C_{Pr} = C_{PT} - C_{DP} \tag{4.16}$$

Substituting Equation 4.16 for C_{Pr} in equation 4.15 yields

$$C_{DP} = K_a C_D (C_{PT} - C_{DP}) \tag{4.17}$$

$$C_{DP}(1 + K_a C_D) = K_a C_D C_{PT} \tag{4.18}$$

which can be manipulated to

$$\frac{C_{DP}}{C_{PT}} = \frac{K_a C_D}{1 + K_a C_D} \tag{4.19}$$

Setting C_{DP}/C_{PT} (number of moles of drug bound per mole of protein at equilibrium) equal to r (ie, $r = C_{DP}/C_{PT}$), changes the equation to

$$r = \frac{K_a C_D}{1 + K_a C_D} \tag{4.20}$$

When there are n identical binding sites per mole of protein, the equation is multiplied by n:

$$r = \frac{n K_a C_D}{1 + K_a C_D} \tag{4.21}$$

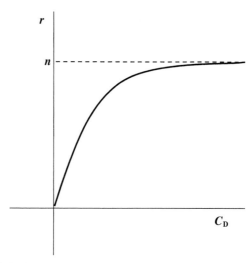

FIGURE 4.1 Langmuir isotherm (Equation 4.20), with y axis as the number of moles of drug bound per moles of protein and x axis as the concentration of free drug.

Equation 4.21 is known as the Langmuir equation, and a plot of r versus C_D yields a hyperbolic isotherm (Figure 4.1). To change Equation 4.21 to a simple straight-line equation we may use one of the following approaches:

1. By taking the reciprocal of Equation 4.21,

$$\frac{1}{r} = \frac{1}{nK_aC_D} + \frac{1}{n} \tag{4.22}$$

Equation 4.22, known as a double reciprocal, indicates that a plot of $1/r$ versus $1/C_D$ is linear with slope $= 1/nK_a$ and y intercept $= 1/n$ (Figure 4.2).

2. By rearrangement of Equation 4.21 a different linear equation can be obtained:

$$\frac{r}{C_D} = nK_a - rK_a \quad \text{or} \quad \frac{r}{C_D} = K_a(n - r) \tag{4.23}$$

A plot of r/C_D versus r, known as a Scatchard plot, is also a straight line with slope $= -K_a$ and y intercept $= nK_a$ (Figure 4.3).

3. Equation 4.21 can also be rearranged to provide a straight-line relationship in terms of the concentrations of free and bound drug:

$$\frac{C_{DP}}{C_{PT}} = \frac{nK_aC_D}{1 + K_aC_D} \tag{4.24}$$

$$\therefore C_{DP} + C_{DP}K_aC_D = nC_{PT}K_aC_D$$

$$\frac{C_{DP}}{C_D} = nK_aC_{PT} - K_aC_{DP} \tag{4.25}$$

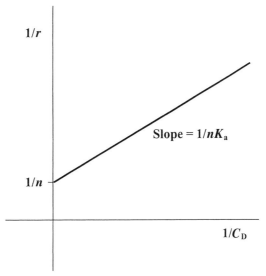

FIGURE 4.2 Plot of Equation 4.21 describing the relationship between the reciprocal of r (moles of drug bound per mole of protein) and reciprocal of C_D (free concentration of drug). The y intercept is the reciprocal of the number of binding sites per mole of protein, and "slope/y intercept" is the equilibrium association constant. This plot is also known as a Klotz double-reciprocal plot.

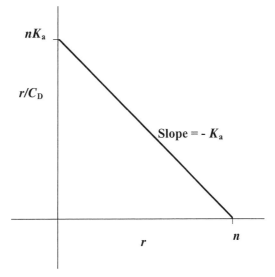

FIGURE 4.3 Scatchard plot describing the relationship between r/C_D and r (Equation 4.23), with a slope equal to the association constant, K_a; x intercept equal to the number of binding sites, n; and y intercept equal to nK_a.

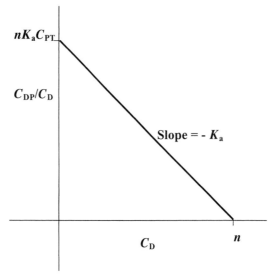

FIGURE 4.4 Linear plot of C_{DP}/C_D (ratio of bound to free drug) versus C_{DP} (concentration of bound drug), with slope $= -K_a$ and y intercept $= nK_aC_{PT}$.

Thus, a plot of C_{DP}/C_D versus C_{DP} is linear with slope $= -K_a$ and y intercept $= nK_aC_{PT}$. This equation is used when the concentration of protein is unknown and the estimate of K_a is based on the measurable concentration of drug in the buffer compartment. The determination of drug bound to protein is based on estimation from the free fraction (Figure 4.4).

The Scatchard plot (Equation 4.23, Figure 4.3) yields a straight line when there is only one type of binding site. However, there is more than one type of binding site on a molecule of protein, the related Langmuir equation is

$$r = \frac{n_1 K_{a1} C_D}{1 + K_{a1} C_D} + \frac{n_2 K_{a2} C_D}{1 + K_{a2} C_D} + \cdots + \frac{n_n K_{an} C_D}{1 + K_n C_D} \tag{4.26}$$

where n_1 and K_{a1} are the parameters of one type of identical binding sites, n_2 and K_{a2} are the parameters of the second type of identical binding sites, and so on. For example, the –COO$^-$ of an aspartic acid or glutamic acid residue can be one type of binding site, and the –S$^-$ of a cysteine residue or –NH$^{2\pm}$ of a histidine residue, the second type of binding site. When the drug molecule has affinity for two types of binding sites, the Scatchard plot of r/D versus r is not a straight line and the plot resembles the curve presented in Figure 4.5. Extrapolation of the initial and terminal linear segments of the curve, however, yields two straight lines that correspond to:

$$r/D = n_1 K_{a1} + r K_{a1}$$

$$r/D = n_2 K_{a2} + r K_{a2}$$

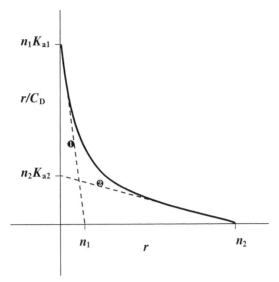

FIGURE 4.5 Scatchard plot of binding to a protein with two different classes of binding sites. The curve represents the first two terms of Equation 4.26 that can be analyzed as two straight lines that are the extensions of linear segments of the initial and terminal portions of the curve. Line 1 represents the high-affinity, low-capacity binding site, and line 2 represents the low-affinity, high-capacity binding site.

As the affinity and capacity of the two binding sites are different, the line with greater y intercept and smaller x intercept is identified as the high-affinity, low-capacity sites, whereas the line with smaller y intercept and greater x intercept represents the low-affinity, high-capacity binding sites.

4.4 EFFECT OF PHYSICOCHEMICAL PROPERTIES OF DRUGS ON DISTRIBUTION

As was discussed earlier, lipophilic drugs permeate through capillaries much faster than polar compounds. This permeation is more significant in highly perfused organs, particularly the liver and kidneys. The accumulation of lipophilic compounds in adipose tissue is also significant. The ability of a lipophilic compound to permeate through the capillary wall or partition into an organ/tissue is expressed in terms of its partition coefficients in a defined organic solvent–water system. The octanol–water system has been accepted as a reliable in vitro reference because the partition coefficients of drugs estimated by this system correlate with their biologic activity. Storage of large amounts of highly lipophilic drugs in adipose tissue creates a redistribution pattern in which the plasma concentrations of drugs decline and the drug retained in the fatty tissue is released into the systemic circulation for redistribution, elimination, and also reuptake by the fatty tissues. Thus, the redistribution may create a lingering pharmacologic response, such as long-term drowsiness in the use of certain barbiturates and anesthetics.

The degree of ionization also plays an important role in distribution of xenobiotics. Most drugs are salts of weak bases or acids and according to pH partition theory only the un-ionized forms of drugs can penetrate through the capillary wall and cellular membrane. Therefore, the pK_a of drugs and pH of the surrounding are also important in the permeation of drug in tissue and calculation of the partition coefficient.

4.5 PHYSIOLOGIC BARRIERS

Several physiologic barriers affect the distribution of drugs in the body. The function of these barriers is essentially to protect different regions of the body from foreign substances.

4.5.1 Placental Transfer

The placenta has many functions. For example, it receives nutrients and oxygen from maternal arteries for distribution through fetal capillaries and disposes fetal waste products and carbon dioxide into maternal veins. It also regulates the complex hormonal levels during pregnancy. The barrier between the fetal systemic circulation and maternal blood changes during pregnancy. This barrier, made up of various cell layers, is thicker at the early phase of pregnancy and gradually becomes thinner near term. The change in the barrier makes diffusion of nutrients and xenobiotics more selective at the beginning and near term. A number of nutrients such as glucose are transported by facilitated transport, and nutrients such as purines and pyrimidines are transported against concentration gradient. Xenobiotics, in general, distribute through the placenta by passive diffusion. Molecules that resemble purines and pyrimidines may permeate and distribute by active transport. An important characteristic of the placenta is its first-pass effect because of the presence of metabolic enzyme system. Therefore, a lower fetal plasma concentration would be expected for drugs that are substrates for the placenta metabolic enzyme system.

4.5.2 Blood–Brain Barrier

The distribution of drugs into the brain is limited by the blood–brain barrier. The tight junctions of endothelial cells of cerebral capillaries create this barrier. Transfer of drugs by pinocytosis through this tight barrier is very rare, and the transport of water-soluble drugs or nutrients requires specific carrier or receptor. The permeation of lipophilic compounds occurs by passive diffusion, and therefore their passage is dependent on their partition coefficients. The higher the partition coefficient, the easier the passage through the barrier. This permeation, however, is not absolute, even for lipophilic compounds. It has been established that brain endothelial cells contain significant amounts of P-glycoprotein (Pgp), which acts as an active drug efflux pump. This transporter protein, which has affinity for a wide range of totally unrelated molecules, plays an important role in reducing and preventing the passage of drugs into the brain. Therefore, Pgp, in association with the tightly joined capillary endothelial cells, severely restricts the distribution of therapeutic agents intended for the treatment of brain diseases.

4.5.3 Blood–Testis Barrier

This physiologic barrier restricts exchange of drugs between the blood and testis tissue and interstitial fluids. Mainly the capillary endothelium and the Sertoli cells create this barrier. The Sertoli cells, which have an important role in spermatogenesis, are tightly joined together and form an additional layer to the endothelium of capillaries. Furthermore, the testis, because of the presence of metabolizing enzyme systems such as cytochrome P450 isozymes, is capable of metabolizing molecules that succeed in crossing the barrier. Therefore, the barrier itself and gonadal metabolism limit the distribution of drugs into this organ. Furthermore, Pgp is localized significantly in testicular endothelium and contributes to the exclusion of a wide range of xenobiotics.

4.5.4 Blood–Aqueous Humor Barrier

The blood–aqueous humor barrier may not have a major impact on the overall distribution of drugs but, similar to other barriers, limits the distribution of drugs to some extent. When drugs are administered systemically (eg, intravenously, orally) a fraction of the dose may diffuse into the anterior chamber of the eye; however, some compounds do not appear there at all. This restriction applies mostly for small hydrophilic compounds and large-molecular-weight proteins and polymers. Similar to the blood–brain barrier, the presence of tight junctions of capillary endothelium and Pgp glycoprotein impede the free exchange of drugs between blood and aqueous humor.

4.5.5 Blood–Lymph Barrier

The balance of body water is maintained by the lymphatic system. This system drains the extra volume of interstitial fluids with all their waste products and protein, known as lymph, into the blood circulation. The lymphatic system, similar to the blood system, is formed by lymphatic capillaries that join together and form lymphatic vessels. The vessels usually follow the same route as the blood vessels. They go through successive sets of lymph nodes to filter the lymph and finally join blood vessels at the junction of the jugular and left subclavian veins. Because of its extensive network, the lymphatic system plays an important role in the distribution of lipophilic compounds administered orally. Small polar molecules are usually excluded from the distribution by the blood–lymph barrier, mostly because of the anatomy of lymphatic capillaries; however, some large-molecular-weight proteins have been demonstrated to cross this barrier.

APPLICATION

4.1 The total albumin concentration used in an experiment is 2×10^{-4} M. The concentrations of drug selected for the experiment (C_D) are listed in Table 4.2, as are estimates of the concentrations of drug–protein complex (C_{DP}). By using double-reciprocal and Scatchard plots (Table 4.2) calculate the association constant and number of binding sites.

Double-reciprocal plot:

Assuming ideal data and using the slope relationship yields,

$$\text{slope} = (0.2083 - 0.8334)/(62.54 - 1010.10) = 6.597 \times 10^{-4} \text{ M}$$

TABLE 4.2 Data Related to Application 4.1

C_D (M)	9.9×10^{-4}	2.67×10^{-3}	6.00×10^{-3}	1.6×10^{-2}
C_{DP}	2.4×10^{-4}	4.8×10^{-4}	7.2×10^{-4}	9.6×10^{-4}
Double-reciprocal Calculations				
r	1.2	2.4	3.6	4.8
$1/r$	0.8334	0.4167	0.2778	0.2083
$1/C_D$	1010.10	374.53	166.67	62.54
Scatchard Plot Calculations				
r/C_D (M^{-1})	1212.12	898.88	600.00	300.19

As $1/r = (1/nK_aC_D) + (1/n)$,

$$\text{y intercept} = 1/n = 0.8334 - (6.597 \times 10^{-4} \times 1010.10) = 0.167$$

Therefore,

$$K_a = (1/(6.597 \times 10^{-4}))(0.167) - 253.145 \text{ L/mol}$$

$$n = 1/0.167 = 6$$

Using regression analysis yields

$$y = 0.1681 + (6.58 \times 10^{-4})\, x$$

Therefore,

$$n = 1/0.1681 = 5.9488$$

$$K_a = 0.1681 \times (1/(6.59 \times 10^{-4})) = 255.08 \text{ L/mol}$$

Scatchard Plot:
   Using the slope relationship:

$$\text{slope} = (300.19 - 1212.12)/(4.8 - 1.2) = -253.31 = -K_a$$

$$K_a = 253.31 \text{ M}^{-1}$$

$$\text{y intercept} = nK_a = 1212.12 + 1.2(253.31) = 1516.092 \text{ mol/L}$$

$$n = 1516.092/253.31 = 5.985$$

Using regression analysis:

$$y = 1511.47 - 252.89x$$

$$K_a = 252.89 \text{ M}^{-1}$$

$$n = 1511.47/252.89 = 5.976$$

TABLE 4.3 Data Related to Application 4.2

C_D (μmol/L)	4.590	9.792	26.316	77.724
C_{DP} (μmol/L)	13.928	27.234	46.206	70.533
r	0.612	1.102	2.065	3.060
r/C_D (L/μmol)	0.1334	0.1125	0.0784	0.0394
C_{DP}/C_D	3.034	2.781	1.755	0.907

4.2 The binding of a drug to plasma proteins was evaluated using dynamic dialysis. The data are reported in Table 4.3. By using the Scatchard plot calculate n and K_a:

$$\text{slope} = (0.0394 - 0.1334)/(3.060 - 0.612) = -0.0384 \text{ L/}\mu\text{mol} = -K_a$$

$$K_a = 0.0384 \text{ L/}\mu\text{mol}$$

$$n = ((r/C_D) + rK_a)/K_a$$

$$n = (0.1334 + (0.612 \times 0.0384))/0.0384 = 4.08$$

By using Equation 4.25 calculate K_a (the related calculations are presented in Table 4.3):

$$\text{slope} = (0.907 - 3.034)/(70.533 - 13.928) = -0.0375 \text{ L/}\mu\text{mol} = -K_a$$

$$K_a = 0.0375 \text{ L/}\mu\text{mol}$$

4.3 The binding of a drug to albumin was investigated by the method of equilibrium dialysis. Albumin (1.2×10^{-3} M) mixed with drug (0.5×10^{-3} M) was allowed to equilibrate for 3 hours. The measurement of the drug in the buffer compartment indicated a concentration of 0.2×10^{-3} M.

Determine the number of moles of drug bound per total protein: $C_D = 0.2 \times 10^{-3}$ M in the buffer compartment that is in equilibrium with C_D of the compartment containing albumin. $C_D + C_{DP}$ in the albumin compartment $= (0.5 - 0.2) \times 10^{-3} = 0.3 \times 10^{-3}$ M. Therefore,

$$C_{DP} = (0.3 \times 10^{-3} \text{ M}) - (0.2 \times 10^{-3}) = 0.1 \times 10^{-3} \text{ M}$$

$$r = (0.1 \times 10^{-3} \text{ M})/(1.2 \times 10^{-3} \text{ M}) = 0.0833$$

Calculate the free and bound fractions:

$$\text{free fraction (ff)} = (0.2 \times 10^{-3})/(0.3 \times 10^{-3}) = 0.67$$

$$\text{bound fraction (bf)} = 0.1 \times 10^{-3} \text{ M}/(0.3 \times 10^{-3}) = 0.33$$

ASSIGNMENT

4.1 Given the data in Table 4.4 calculate the number of binding sites and association constant.

TABLE 4.4 Data Related to Assignment 4.1

r	0.736	1.472	2.112	2.496
C_D (mol/L)	3.2×10^{-5}	9.28×10^{-5}	1.792×10^{-4}	3.2×10^{-4}

4.2 The albumin binding of drug X was evaluated by using equilibrium dialysis. The total albumin used in the experiment was 1×10^{-4} M. The concentration of drug added to the protein was 2×10^{-3} M. If the concentration of free drug in the buffer compartment after achieving equilibrium is 6×10^{-4} M, what are the bound fraction, free fraction, and moles of drug bound per mole of protein?

4.3 The plasma protein binding of a drug was studied by microdialysis under physiologic conditions and the data in Table 4.5 were reported.
  1. By using the Scatchard plot, determine n and K_a.
  2. Repeat the calculations by using Equation 4.25.

4.4 $y = 0.2 + 0.002x$ is the regression equation of double-reciprocal analysis of binding of a drug to albumin. Determine K_a and the number of binding sites. Assume the units of concentration are micromoles per liter.

4.5 $y = 500 - 250x$ is the Scatchard equation of binding drug Z to plasma proteins. Determine the association constant and number of binding sites. The concentration was reported as millimoles per liter.

ASSIGNMENT (EXTRA CREDIT)
EC-4.1 Review the following article and answer the questions.
Påhlam I, Gozzi P. Serum protein binding of tolterodine and its major metabolites in human and several animal species. *Biopharm Drug Disp* 1999;20:91.

QUESTIONS

1. Discuss in detail the method of equilibrium dialysis used in the study.
2. To which protein of plasma does tolterodine bind predominantly?
3. What are your conclusions about the data presented in Table 4.6 which is taken from Table 1 of the article.

TABLE 4.5 Data Related to Assignment 4.3

C_D (μmol/L)	4.8	10.24	27.52	81.23
C_{DP} (μmol/L)	14.56	28.48	48.32	73.76
r	0.640	1.152	2.16	3.20
r/C_D	0.133	0.112	0.078	0.039

TABLE 4.6 Data Related to Assignment EC-4.1

Matrix	f_u (%)
AAG 0.75 g/L	10 ± 0.7
HSA 45 g/L + AAG 0.75 g/L	2.7 ± 0.1

AAG: α_1-acid glycoprotein; HSA: Human serum albumin.

4. Discuss the differences in serum protein binding of tolterodine between humans and other species (mouse, rat, rabbit, cat, dog).

BIBLIOGRAPHY

1. Aarons LJ, Rowland M. Kinetics of drug displacement interactions. *J Pharmacokinet Biopharm* 1981;9:181.
2. Mattos C, Ringe D. Locating and characterizing binding sites on proteins. *Nat Biotechnol* 1996;14:595.
3. Shary WL, Aarons LJ, Rowland M. Representation and interpretation of drug displacement interactions. *Biochem Pharmacol* 1978;27:139.
4. Krüger-Thiemer E, Diller W, Bünger P. Pharmacokinetic models regarding protein binding of drugs. *Antimicrob Agents Chemother* 1966;1965:183.
5. Wagner JG. Simple model to explain effects of plasma protein binding and tissue binding on calculated volumes of distribution, apparent elimination rate constants and clearances. *Eur J Clin Pharmacol* 1976;10:425.
6. McNamara PJ, Levy G, Gibaldi M. Effect of plasma protein and tissue binding on the time course of drug concentration in plasma. *J Pharmacokinet Biopharm* 1979;7:195.
7. Verbeeck RK, Cardinal JA, Wallace SM. Effect of age and sex on the plasma binding of acidic and basic drugs. *Eur J Clin Pharmacol* 1984;27:91.
8. Yacobi A, Stoll RG, DiSante AR, Levy G. Intersubject variation of warfarin binding to protein in serum of normal subjects. *Res Commun Chem Pathol Pharmacol* 1976;14:743.
9. Greenblatt DJ, Sellers EM, Koch-Weser J. Importance of protein binding for the interpretation of serum or plasma drug concentration. *J Clin Pharmacol* 1982;22:259.
10. Koch-Weser J, Sellers EM. Binding of drugs to serum albumin *N Engl J Med* 1976;294:311.
11. Rowland M. Plasma protein binding and therapeutic monitoring. *Ther Drug Monit* 1980;2:29.
12. Edwards DJ, Lalka D, Cerra F, Slaughter RL. Alpha acid glycoprotein concentration and protein binding in trauma. *Clin Pharmacol Ther* 1982;31:62.

CHAPTER 5

ELIMINATION OF DRUGS FROM THE BODY

*We must distinguish the causes and accounts of coming to be and perishing
that are common to everything that comes to be and perishes naturally.
We must also ask what growth and alteration are and whether alteration
and coming to be should be taken to have the same nature.*
ARISTOTLE (BOOK I—ON GENERATION AND CORRUPTION)

OBJECTIVES

- To review the general principles of drug elimination and clearance.
- To discuss the major physiologic factors involved in drug elimination.
- To review the biliary and urinary elimination of drugs.
- To discuss biotransformation of xenobiotics, Phase I and Phase II metabolism, and the Michaelis–Menten equation.
- To review different graphic approaches for estimation of Michaelis–Menten parameters.

5.1 INTRODUCTION

The body eliminates xenobiotics predominantly by excretion and metabolism. Excretion represents the elimination of unchanged drug through the major route of excretion, namely, the kidneys. Excretion may also occur through other routes such as bile/feces, sweat, milk, saliva, and exhaled air. Metabolism or biotransformation, on the other hand, is the process of conversion of drugs to pharmacologically inactive metabolites. Metabolites are formed by biochemical processes classified as Phase I and Phase II reactions, which are discussed in the related section in this chapter. The major site of metabolism is the liver, although other sites such as the skin and GI tract can become the major site of metabolism for certain drugs or dosage forms. The ultimate outcome of metabolism is conversion of drugs into more water-soluble compounds for biliary and urinary elimination.

5.2 RATE OF ELIMINATION

The general equation for describing the rate of elimination of a drug by an organ of elimination can be defined as

rate of elimination = rate of input into the organ − rate of output from the organ

The rate of input is the rate of drug delivery to the organs of elimination in the arterial inflow, and the rate of output is its exit in the venous outflow. Therefore, the rate of elimination with units of mass/time is the product of blood flow and arteriovenous concentration differences. The above general equation can be used to define a specific elimination process. For example, for renal excretion,

rate of excretion = (blood flow × arterial drug concentration)

$$- \text{(blood flow} \times \text{venous drug concentration)}$$

The preceding relationship can be written as

$$\frac{dA_e}{dt} = QC_{\text{arterial}-\text{kidney}} - QC_{\text{venous}-\text{kidney}} = Q(C_{\text{arterial}-\text{kidney}} - C_{\text{venous}-\text{kidney}}) \quad (5.1)$$

For hepatic metabolism,

rate of metabolism = (blood flow × arterial drug concentration)

$$- \text{(blood flow} \times \text{venous drug concentration)}$$

$$\frac{dA_m}{dt} = QC_{\text{arterial}-\text{liver}} - QC_{\text{venous}-\text{liver}} = Q(C_{\text{arterial}-\text{liver}} - C_{\text{venous}-\text{liver}}) \quad (5.2)$$

5.3 EXTRACTION RATIO

If we divide the rate of elimination by the rate of input, a number with no units (a fraction) is obtained that is known as extraction ratio (E). This ratio represents the ability of an organ to extract a drug from the input during transit through the organ. In other words, the extraction ratio is the fraction of input that does not leave the organ via the output.

extraction ratio = rate of elimination/rate of input

It can also be written as

$$E = \frac{Q(C_{\text{Arterial}} - C_{\text{venous}})}{QC_{\text{Arterial}}} = \frac{C_{\text{Arterial}} - C_{\text{Venous}}}{C_{\text{Arterial}}} \quad (5.3)$$

As blood flow is constant and equal, it can be cancelled from numerator and denominator. Equation 5.3 indicates that when the concentration of output (ie, C_{venous}) approaches the input (ie, C_{arterial}), the extraction ratio approaches zero, which is indicative of a lack of extraction/elimination by the organ. As the concentration of output approaches zero, however, no drug or very little drug escapes the elimination process. Thus, the extraction ratio is a value between zero and one. The extraction ratio of a drug remains constant as long as the elimination of drug follows first-order kinetics.

The fraction of drug that escapes extraction and leaves the organ via the output is the fraction that is available for distribution to the rest of the body and is expressed as

$$F = 1 - E \tag{5.4}$$

5.4 CLEARANCE

Normalizing the rate of elimination of an organ with respect to the concentration of arterial input (ie, dividing the rate of elimination by concentration of input) provides a constant known as the *clearance* of the organ.

clearance = rate of elimination/concentration of input

Writing the above relationship in form of an equation yields

$$\text{clearance} = \frac{Q(C_{\text{Arterial}} - C_{\text{Venous}})}{C_{\text{Arterial}}} = QE \tag{5.5}$$

On the basis of Equation 5.5, clearance is only a constant of proportionality that describes the relationship between the rate of elimination of a drug and its concentration:

rate of elimination = clearance × concentration

or

concentration = rate of elimination/clearance

The rate has units of mass/time and concentration has units of mass/volume. Therefore, clearance is expressed in units of volume/time:

(mass/time)/(mass/volume) = volume/time

Because, according to Equation 5.5, clearance is also the product of blood flow (with units of volume/time) and extraction ratio (with no units), it is often expressed as a virtual volume of blood from which the drug is completely removed per unit of time. As long as the elimination of a drug follows first-order kinetics, the clearance of the drug remains constant; however, when elimination is capacity-limited, it changes with time and concentration and becomes a variable.

Total body clearance of a drug (Cl_T) is the sum of all clearances occurring simultaneously by different organs in the body:

$$Cl_t = Cl_r + Cl_m + \cdots \tag{5.6}$$

where Cl_r is renal clearance, Cl_m is hepatic clearance, and so on. Total body clearance is usually estimated with the following model independent equation that presumes first-order elimination:

$$Cl_T = \frac{F \times \text{Dose}}{\text{AUC}} \tag{5.7}$$

where F is the fraction of dose available in the systemic circulation. Its value is equal to one for intravenous bolus injection; for other routes such as oral, rectal, and intramuscular injection, it may become less than one. AUC is the area under the plasma concentration–time curve estimated by trapezoidal or log trapezoidal rules. The model dependent equations of clearance are discussed in Chapters 6 and 11.

The estimation of clearance is usually based on the concentration of free drug in plasma. As the extraction ratio in Equation 5.5 cannot exceed one, it may be concluded that clearance cannot exceed the blood flow of the eliminating organ. For many drugs, however, the magnitude of clearance exceeds blood flow. One explanation is that the uptake of drug by blood cells is significant and the organ of elimination extracts the drug not only from the plasma but also from blood cells. Under this condition it is more desirable to express blood clearance rather than plasma clearance. Analytical determination of the concentration of drug in whole blood is not an easy task. There are limitations that hinder an accurate assessment of the concentration in blood. One approach in overcoming this problem is to adjust the plasma levels with a correction factor (CF) that is based on the blood hematocrit (H) and drug concentrations in plasma (C_p) and blood cells (C_{BC}):

$$CF = (1 - H) + \frac{C_{BC}}{C_p} \tag{5.8}$$

A different in vitro approach is to incubate equal and known concentrations of drug with blood and phosphate buffer, pH 7 to 7.2, separately and simultaneously. After incubation, the concentrations of drug in the plasma portion of the blood and in the buffer are determined. Based on the assumption that the concentration of drug in the buffer sample is equal to the concentration in whole blood, the ratio of buffer concentration to plasma concentration is used as the correction factor to convert plasma clearance to blood clearance:

blood clearance = plasma clearance × (buffer concentration/plasma concentration)   (5.9)

In contrast to total body clearance, intrinsic clearance is the intracellular clearance of a drug without the influence of blood flow. For example, when biotransformation occurs by one or more enzymatic reactions within the hepatocytes, intrinsic clearance is then a measure of all intracellular metabolic clearances according to the Michaelis–Menten equation.

5.5 RENAL EXCRETION

The clearance of any organ of elimination is a measure of the overall efficiency of the organ. The combined physiologic processes of the organ contribute to the magnitude of its clearance. For example, renal excretion, being a major route of elimination of xenobiotics and their water-soluble metabolites, comprises physiologic events such as filtration in the glomerulus and active and passive reabsorption and secretion in the proximal and distal tubules (Figure 5.1). The capillary wall of the glomerulus with its large pores is 25 times more permeable than regular capillary walls; in association with cardiac contraction, this facilitates the transcapillary passage of water, nutrients, ions, and both ionized and un-ionized drug molecules. The glomerular filtration rate (GFR) is about 125 mL/min, or 7.5 L/h, or 180 L/d. The composition of the filtrate is similar to that of plasma but without the large-molecular-weight proteins. The filtrate travels from Bowman's capsule toward the collecting duct and eventually the bladder; during this journey the body reabsorbs water, nutrients, and ions and secretes other solutes. Ultimately from the 180 L/d original filtrate, only about 1 L/d reaches the bladder and leaves the body as urine.

The proximal tubule has epithelial cells with a brush border that contain energy-dependent transport mechanism including P-glycoprotein. Therefore, active reabsorption and secretion of drugs occur in the tubules, and secretion of some may influence the secretion of others that compete for the same transport sites. Lipid-soluble molecules are reabsorbed by passive diffusion. The reabsorption of weak acids or bases is dependent on the pH of the filtrate and the pK_a of the drug. At low filtrate pH weak acids are un-ionized and reabsorbed, whereas at higher pH they remain ionized in the filtrate and are excreted as such in the urine.

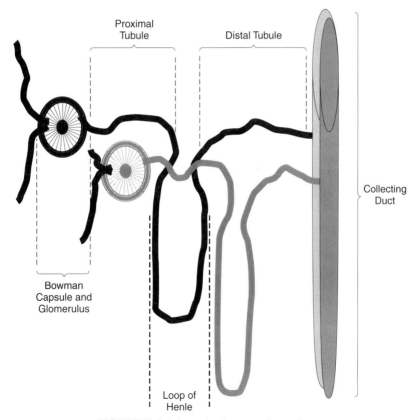

FIGURE 5.1 Schematic diagram of a nephron.

As long as the processes of filtration, reabsorption, and secretion of a drug occur by passive diffusion and follow first-order kinetics, renal clearance is a constant of proportionality that relates the rate of excretion to the plasma concentration of free drug:

$$Cl_{renal} = \frac{dA_e}{C_p} \tag{5.10}$$

The rate of excretion is the combined rates of filtration, reabsorption, and secretion:

$$\frac{dA_e}{dt} = \frac{d(A)_{filtration}}{dt} + \frac{d(A)_{secretion}}{dt} - \frac{d(A)_{reabsorption}}{dt} \tag{5.11}$$

Collecting urine samples and measuring the unchanged drug or its metabolites can determine only the renal clearance. The details of the calculation of renal clearance from urine data are discussed in Chapter 9.

5.6 METABOLISM OF XENOBIOTICS

Drug metabolism is another principal mechanism for elimination of drugs from the body. It takes place in a number of tissues, but the major site of metabolism is the liver. The ultimate purpose of the process of metabolism is biotransformation of drugs into water-soluble compounds. This biotransformation occurs with the help of a number of proteins, or enzyme systems, in the body. The outcome of biotansformation is the formation of chemically modified molecules of drug known as metabolites. The metabolites either can be water-soluble and leave the body or can be highly reactive and require further metabolism to become water-soluble. The reactive metabolites may also interact with cellular components such as membranes and macromolecules and cause repairable or nonrepairable lesions. Water-soluble metabolites leave the body by urinary and/or biliary elimination. The metabolic pathways catalyzed by the enzyme systems occur in two distinct phases known as Phase I and Phase II metabolism.

5.6.1 Phase I Metabolism

Phase I reactions include transformation of the molecular structure of drugs by creation of a new functional group(s) and/or modification of an existing functional group(s). The products of Phase I metabolism can be toxic or nontoxic substances. Any enzymatic reaction that forms nonreactive and nontoxic metabolites is also known as a detoxification pathway.

EXAMPLES OF PHASE I OXIDATIVE REACTIONS
- Oxidation of carbon–carbon double bonds
- Oxidation of alcohols
- Oxidation of aromatic carbons
- Oxidation of nitrogen-containing functional groups
- Oxidative deamination

- Oxidative N-, O-, and S-dealkylation
- Other oxidative reactions

One group of enzymes responsible for Phase I oxidative reactions is the cytochrome P450 (CYP450) enzymes. CYP450 is a large group of microsomal enzymes with the potential to catalyze dehydrogenation, hydroxylation, epoxidation, oxygenation, and dealkylation. To represent the diversity of the CYP450 enzymes a new nomenclature has been created to identify different families and subfamilies. This nomenclature is based on the amino acid sequence of the protein and their assignment to different gene families (1, 2, 3, 4, etc). When 40 to 55% of the amino acids of different CYP450 enzymes are identical they are placed in one family. Each family may have one or more subfamily. When more than 55% of the amino acids are identical, they become members of the same subfamily. The nomenclature combines a number corresponding to a specific gene family with a letter identifying the subfamily and finally a number cataloging the member of the subfamily. The four families are:

- Family 1: CYP1A
- Family 2: CYP2A, CYP2B, CYP2C, CYP2D, CYP2E
- Family 3: CYP3A
- Family 4: CYP4A

From this classification it is apparent that CYP1, CYP3, and CYP4 gene families have one subfamily and CYP2 gene family has five subfamilies. Some important members of the subfamilies are:

- Members of subfamily CYP1A: CYP1A1 and CYP1A2
- Members of subfamily CYP2A: CYP2A1, CYP2A5, CYP2A6,
- Members of subfamily CYP2B: CYP2B1, CYP2B2, CYP2B6,
- Members of subfamily CYP2C: CYP2C8, CYP2C9, CYP2C18, CYP2C19,
- Members of subfamily CYP2D: CYP2D6 and CYP2E1.
- Members of subfamily CYP3A: CYP3A4, CYP3A5 and CYP3A7.
- Members of subfamily CYP4A: CYP4A9 and CYP4A11.

The following are examples of drugs metabolized by members of the subfamilies:

Acetaminophen	CYP1A2, CYP2E1, CYP3A4
Theophylline	CYP1A2, CYP2E1, CYP3A4
Phenytoin	CYP2C9
Tamoxifen	CYP3A4
Tolbutamide	CYP2C9
Diazepam	CYP2C19 and CYP3A4
Nicotine	CYP2A6
Cyclophosphamide	CYP2B6
Propranolol	CYP2C19 and CYP2D6
Taxol	CYP2C8 and CYP3A4

OTHER EXAMPLES OF ENZYMES OF PHASE I OXIDATION
- Flavin monooxygenases (microsomal enzyme)
- Alcohol dehydrogenase (cytosolic enzyme)

- Monoamine oxidase (mitochondrial enzyme)
- Diamine oxidase (cytosolic enzyme)
- Aldehyde dehydrogenase (cytosolic enzyme)
- Xanthine oxidase (cytosolic enzyme)

EXAMPLES OF REDUCTIVE REACTIONS
- Reduction of nitrogen-containing functional groups such as azo- and nitro-
- Reduction of alcohol group
- Reduction of carbon–carbon double bond
- Reduction of carbonyl group
- Reduction of disulfide bond
- Reduction of sulfoxide
- Reduction of quinone
- Reductive dehydrogenation

EXAMPLES OF ENZYMES RESPONSIBLE FOR REDUCTIVE REACTIONS
- NADPH-quinone oxidoreductase (cytosolic enzyme)
- NADPH-carbonyl reductases
- Glutathione reductase
- Glutathione S-transferase
- CYP450

EXAMPLES OF HYDROLYSIS REACTIONS OF PHASE I METABOLISM
- Hydrolysis of esters and ethers
- Hydrolytic cleavage of C–N single bond
- Hydration and dehydration of multiple bonds
- Hydrolytic cleavage of nonaromatic heterocycles

EXAMPLES OF ENZYMES RESPONSIBLE FOR HYDROLYSIS
- Epoxide hydrolase (microsomal and cytosolic enzyme)
- Carboxylesterase (microsomal and cytosolic enzyme)
- Peptidase (blood and lysosomes)

5.6.2 Phase II Metabolism: Conjugation

The metabolites of phase II metabolism, also known as detoxification pathways, are called conjugates. Conjugates are formed by the interaction of the functional group(s) of a parent drug or its phase I metabolites with a moiety such as glucuronide or sulfate with the help of enzyme systems known as transferases. Conjugates are water-soluble hydrophilic compounds that are easily eliminated from the body through the urine or bile.

EXAMPLES OF PHASE II REACTIONS
- Methylation
- Acylation
- Sulfate conjugation

■ Glucuronide conjugation
■ Glutathione conjugation
■ Cysteine conjugation
■ Mecapturic acid conjugation

EXAMPLES OF ENZYMES RESPONSIBLE FOR PHASE II METABOLISM
■ UDP-glucuronosyltransferases (microsomal enzyme)
■ Aryl sulfotransferase (cytosolic enzyme)
■ Alcohol sulfotransferase (cytosolic enzyme)
■ Estrogen sulfotranferase (cytosolic enzyme)
■ Bile salt sulfotransferase (cytosolic enzyme)
■ Phenol *O*-methyltransferase (cytosolic enzyme)
■ Catechol *O*-methyltransferase (cytosolic enzyme)
■ *N*-acetyltranferases (cytosolic enzyme)
■ Glutathione *S*-transferase (microsomal and cytosolic enzyme)

The metabolites of Phase I metabolism are known as primary metabolites and the conjugates are referred to as secondary metabolites. The parent drug or primary metabolites of one drug may inhibit or induce Phase I and/or Phase II metabolism of another drug. The inhibition or induction of metabolism is another important reason for drug–drug interaction, which may influence the safety and efficacy of drugs. The effect of drug–drug interaction on enzyme systems is similar to the effect of one drug on the protein binding of another drug (Chapter 4), except that effect of drug on the metabolism of another drug may change the predictable metabolic profile of a drug and increase the concentration of parent compound and/or one or more toxic metabolites.

5.6.3 Kinetics of Drug Metabolism (Michaelis–Menten Kinetics)

The interaction of drugs with enzymes takes place according to the scheme

$$\text{enzyme [E]} + \text{drug [D]} \underset{K_2}{\overset{K_1}{\rightleftharpoons}} \text{enzyme–drug [E·D]} \xrightarrow{K_3} \text{metabolite [M]} + \text{enzyme [E]}$$

To develop an equation for this interaction we assume that the reaction takes place under equilibrium or a steady state. The following equations are based on the assumption of equilibrium:

$$K_{eq} = \frac{[E·D]}{[E][D]} = \frac{k_1}{k_2} \tag{5.12}$$

Therefore,

$$[E·D] = K_{eq} [E][D] \tag{5.13}$$

where K_{eq} is the equilibrium rate constant, [E] is the concentration of free enzyme, [D] is the concentration of free drug, and [E·D] is the concentration of the enzyme–drug complex.

The concentration of free enzyme at any time, [E], is defined as the concentration of total enzyme at the start [E_t] minus the concentration of enzyme associated with the enzyme–drug complex, [E·D].

$$[E] = [E_t] - [E·D] \tag{5.14}$$

Substituting Equation 5.14 in 5.13 yields

$$[ED] = K_{eq}\,[D]\,([E_t] - [E·D]) \tag{5.15}$$

Therefore,

$$[E·D]\left(\frac{1}{K_{eq}} + [D]\right) = [D][E_t] \tag{5.16}$$

or

$$[E·D] = \frac{[E_t][D]}{1/K_{eq} + [D]} \tag{5.17}$$

As the rate of formation of metabolite is $k_3[E·D]$, the rate of metabolism, v, is defined as

$$v = \frac{k_3[E_t][D]}{1/K_{eq} + [D]} \tag{5.18}$$

In Equation 5.18, $k_3[E_t]$ represents the maximum rate of metabolism, V_{max}, and $1/K_{eq}$ is the Michaelis constant, K_M, under the assumption of equilibrium. Therefore,

$$v = \frac{V_{max}C_D}{K_M + C_D} \tag{5.19}$$

where C_D is the concentration of free drug, [D].

Under the steady-state condition the rate of formation of [E·D] is defined as

$$\frac{d[E·D]}{dt} = k_1[E][D] - k_2[E·D] - k_3[E·D] \tag{5.20}$$

At steady state,

$$\frac{d[E·D]}{dt} = 0 \tag{5.21}$$

Therefore,

$$[E\cdot D] = \frac{k_1[E][D]}{k_2 + k_3} \tag{5.22}$$

Substituting Equation 5.14 in Equation 5.22 and K_M for $(k_2 + k_3)/k_1$ yields

$$[E\cdot D] = \frac{[E_t][D] - [E\cdot D][D]}{K_M} \tag{5.23}$$

Therefore,

$$[E\cdot D] = \frac{[E_t][D]}{K_M + [D]} \tag{5.24}$$

$$k_3[E\cdot D] = v = \frac{V_{max} \times C_D}{K_M + C_D} \tag{5.25}$$

As the rate of metabolism is $k_3[E\cdot D]$, Equation 5.25 is the same as Equation 5.19. The difference between the two assumptions is the definition of K_M. Under certain in vitro conditions when equilibrium is achieved the meaning of K_M is as described for Equation 5.19. For in vivo conditions K_M has the same meaning as described for Equation 5.25.

Equation 5.19 or 5.25 is known as the Michaelis–Menten equation and it defines the relationship between the rate of metabolism and the concentration of drug (Figure 5.2).

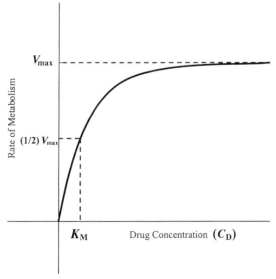

FIGURE 5.2 Hyperbolic curve of Michaelis–Menten equation. The plateau rate corresponds to the maximum rate of metabolism, and the concentration at half-maximum rate represents K_M, the Michaelis–Menten constant.

The equation predicts a hyperbolic curve that represents the capacity-limited nature of drug metabolism.

K_M is known as the Michaelis–Menten constant and corresponds to the concentration of drug at half-maximum rate of metabolism, that is, when $v = V_{max}/2$, $K_M = C_D$:

$$\frac{V_{max}}{2} = \frac{V_{max} \times C_D}{K_M + C_D}$$

Therefore,

$$2C_D = K_M + C_D$$

$$K_M = C_D \tag{5.26}$$

K_M and V_{max} are useful parameters for a number of purposes, for example, estimation of intrinsic clearance, quantitative comparison of different drugs, comparison of different isozymes from different tissues or different species. When the concentration of drug, C_D, is much smaller than K_M, the rate of metabolism follows first-order kinetics:

$$v = \frac{V_{max}}{K_M} C_D \qquad K_M > C_D \tag{5.27}$$

When C_D is much greater than K_M, the rate follows zero-order kinetics:

$$v = V_{max} \qquad K_M < C_D \tag{5.28}$$

K_M and V_{max} are usually estimated by measuring the rate of metabolism at a series of different concentrations of drug. Various approaches to determining K_M and V_{max} are based on rearranging the Michaelis–Menten equation into a straight-line relationship.

5.6.3.1 Lineweaver–Burk Plot or Double-Reciprocal Plot: This graphic method is based on plotting the reciprocal of the rate of metabolism against the reciprocal of drug concentration (Figure 5.3). The corresponding equation is

$$\frac{1}{v} = \frac{K_M}{V_{max}} \frac{1}{C_D} + \frac{1}{V_{max}} \tag{5.29}$$

5.6.3.2 Hanes Plot: The Hanes plot (Figure 5.4) is constructed on the basis of an equation that is derived by multiplication of the Lineweaver–Burk equation by C_D:

$$\frac{C_D}{v} = \frac{K_M}{V_{max}} + \frac{C_D}{V_{max}} \tag{5.30}$$

5.6.3.3 Eadie–Hofstee Plot: Multiplication of the Lineweaver-Burk equation by $V_{max} \times v$ provides a different rearrangement of the Michaelis–Menten equation (Figure 5.5):

$$v = V_{max} - K_M \frac{v}{C_D} \tag{5.31}$$

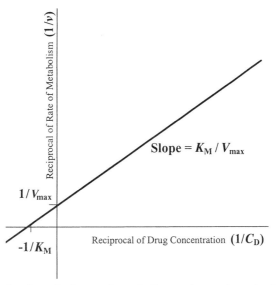

FIGURE 5.3 Plot of reciprocal of rate of metabolism against reciprocal of drug concentration, known as Lineweaver–Burk or double reciprocal plot.

5.6.3.4 Direct Linear Plot: In this method the rate of metabolism, v, is plotted on the y axis and the corresponding concentration of drug, C_D, is multiplied by -1 and plotted on the x axis. The two points ($+v$ and $-C_D$) are connected together and extrapolated into the positive quadrant ($+v$ and $+C_D$). Therefore, for each pair of data a line is generated. The point of intersection of the lines in the positive quadrant has the coordinates K_M and V_{max}

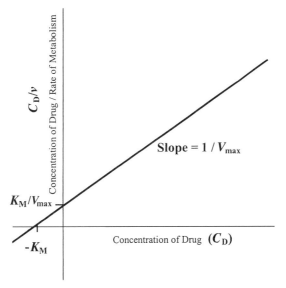

FIGURE 5.4 Hanes plot.

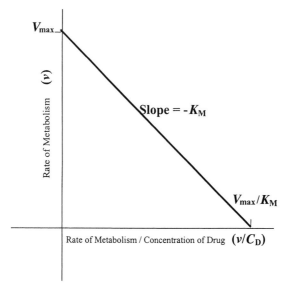

FIGURE 5.5 Eadie–Hofstee plot.

(Figure 5.6). If the lines form more than one point of intersection the median of coordinates of intersections is selected for estimation of the parameters of the Michaelis–Menten equation (Figure 5.7).

5.6.3.5 Advantages and Disadvantages of Graphic Methods for Estimation of K_M and V_{max}

LINEWEAVER–BURK PLOT

Although it provides the best straight line, this method suffers from the distortion of the errors associated with the measurements. Reciprocals of small errors appear as large de-

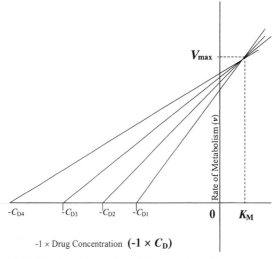

FIGURE 5.6 Direct plot with one point of intersection.

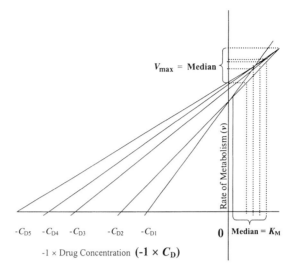

FIGURE 5.7 Direct plot with more than one point of intersection.

viations and reciprocals of large errors appear as small deviations. Therefore, the estimates of K_M and V_{max} from the slope and y intercept of the unweighted data are likely to contain significant error.

HANES PLOT
The errors in measurements of the rate of metabolism (v) contribute to the uncertainty in the precision of the y intercept (K_M/V_{max}); however, V_{max}, estimated from the slope of the line ($1/V_{max}$), is more precise than the Lineweaver–Burk plot.

EADIE–HOFSTEE PLOT
The rate of metabolism, v, is associated with both the x and y axes of this plot. Therefore, errors in measurements of the rate of metabolism can influence both coordinates. The advantage is that values of K_M and V_{max} can be estimated directly from the graph.

DIRECT LINEAR PLOT
No transformation of v or C_D is needed. Estimation of the parameters does not require regression analysis. The disadvantage is that if the relationship between the rate of metabolism and the drug concentration depart from the simple Michaelis–Menten hyperbolic relationship, it would not be apparent in the direct linear plot.

5.6.4 Hill Plot

The relationship between the rate of metabolism and drug concentration for some drugs is sigmoidal and does not exhibit the classic hyperbolic curve of Michaelis–Menten kinetics. This may indicate that the enzyme responsible for the metabolism has more than one binding site for the drug and the binding of one molecule may help (positive cooperativity) or delay (negative cooperativity) the binding of other molecules. Under this condition the rate of metabolism is governed by the following equation known as the Hill equation:

$$v = \frac{V_{max} \times C_D{}^n}{K + C_D{}^n} \tag{5.32}$$

where K and n are the Hill coefficients.

Equation 5.32 can also be transformed into a straight-line equation:

$$V_{max}C_D{}^n = vK + vC_D{}^n \tag{5.33}$$

$$K = \frac{C_D{}^n(V_{max} - v)}{v} \tag{5.34}$$

$$\log \frac{v}{V_{max} - v} = n \log C_D - \log K \tag{5.35}$$

Thus, a plot of $\log(v/(V_{max} - v))$ versus $\log C_D$ yields a straight line with slope $= n$ and y intercept $= \log K$ (Figure 5.8). Determination of K and n requires a known value for V_{max}. If we set $v = 1/2V_{max}$, $v/(V_{max} - v)$ would be equal to 1 and $\log 1 = 0$. Therefore,

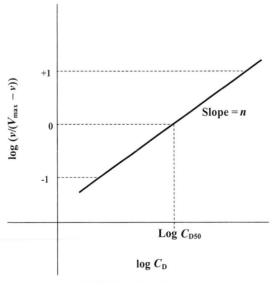

FIGURE 5.8 Hill plot.

the zero on the y axis corresponds to a value on the x axis that represents the logarithm of drug concentration that yields a rate of metabolism equal to $1/2V_{max}$:

$$\log \frac{v}{V_{max} - v} = 0$$

$$n \log C_{D50} = \log K \tag{5.36}$$

Therefore,

$$K = C_{D50}{}^n$$

5.6.5 In Vitro Model Systems for Drug Metabolism Study

In recent years, with the advent of combinatorial chemistry, the synthesis of numerous new chemicals, and the desire for quick screening methods for studying metabolic patterns and toxicity, there has been great expansion of the use of in vitro model systems. These systems can be divided into two major groups:

Group I: Cellular fractions
    1. Microsomal
    2. Cytosol
    3. S-9 (liver homogenate without mitochondria and nuclei)
    4. Purified enzymes

Group II: Organ Fractions
    1. Isolated intact perfused liver
    2. Organ slices (such as liver slices)
    3. Intact cells (such as hepatocytes)

5.6.5.1 Cellular Fractions: The cellular fractions (Group I) require cofactors such as NAD, NADPH, FAD, and FAM during incubation with drugs. Among the cellular fractions microsomal and cytosolic fractions are considered the most valuable and economical in studying drug metabolism under different experimental conditions. The microsomal fraction is prepared by homogenization of liver tissue and centrifugation at $12,000g$ for 1 hour, followed by separation of supernatant and further centrifugation at $110,000g$ for 1 hour. The pellet from the latter centrifugation is the microsomal fraction and its supernatant is called the cytosolic fraction. Both fractions are used in:

1. High-throughput investigation of metabolism of new chemicals.
2. Investigation of the effects of inducers or inhibitors on metabolism of drugs.
3. Determination of metabolic drug–drug interactions.
4. Investigation of metabolic activation and deactivation.
5. Identification of metabolites.
6. Mutagenicity tests.
7. Studies of covalent binding of drugs to proteins or DNA.
8. Comparison of metabolism of drugs in different species.

The major disadvantage of cellular fractions is that they lack cellular control; therefore caution should be exercised in extrapolation of the metabolic data from these systems to in vivo conditions.

5.6.5.2 Organ Fractions: Among the organ fractions (Group II) the isolated intact perfused liver, because of the intact tissue and vascular systems, is an excellent in vitro model for metabolic investigation of drugs; however, the methodology is expensive and somewhat time consuming, and the organ cannot be maintained viable over a long period. Therefore, it is not considered an ideal system with which to screen new chemicals.

Liver slices are less desirable. Many cells are damaged and the availability of oxygen is limited.

Among cultured cells, hepatocytes offer a novel tool in metabolic investigation of drugs. Hepatocytes are multitask parenchymal cells of the liver that are responsible for metabolism of drugs. Hepatocytes, isolated from the liver of all species including humans, are prepared by infusing the liver with a medium that lacks calcium to separate the cells from each other and then infusing with a proteolytic enzyme such as collagenase to digest the extracellular proteins. The procedure for separation and culture of hepatocytes requires special care to prepare cells without bacterial contamination and free from damaged cells. Various techniques are also used to preserve the integrity and viability of the cells. Incubation of hepatocytes with drugs is a good in vitro procedure for evaluation of drug metabolites. The major advantage of using hepatocytes is that the cells are intact and the metabolism mimics the in vivo conditions. Quantitative extrapolation of data from this in vitro metabolism to in vivo situations, however, suffers from similar shortcomings of cellular fractions.

5.6.6 In Vivo Samples for Drug Metabolism Study

The major site of metabolism is the liver. In intact in vivo systems (ie, whole animals) the metabolites are determined in urine, blood, bile, and portal vein blood. Collection of urine and plasma is more practical in humans. Generally, the concentrations of metabolites in plasma for most drugs are below the sensitivity of detection, and urine usually contains mostly Phase II metabolites.

Bile duct cannulation and portal vein cannulation are useful technique but invasive for humans. Substituting the measurement of metabolites in the feces for bile duct cannulation is neither accurate nor practical. Therefore, intact animals such as rats are often used as the animal model for determination of the metabolic profile of a drug in the portal vein and bile.

5.6.6.1 Portal Vein Concentration: The portal vein is one of the blood vessels that bring blood to the liver. It carries venous blood from the gut, spleen, pancreas, and gallbladder to the liver. By comparing the drug concentration of this vein before entering the liver with blood levels in systemic circulation we can obtain important information about the absorption of drug and the first-pass effect in the liver.

5.6.6.2 Bile Cannulation: A major function of the liver is the production of bile at a rate of about 600 to 1200 mL/d. Bile is formed at canaliculi, which represent specialized extracellular spaces between hepatocytes. The canaliculi unite to form bile preductules that lead to bile ductules and finally the hepatic duct. The hepatic duct joins with the gall-bladder duct to form the bile duct, which connects through the sphincter of Oddi to the duodenum. An important physiologic role of bile is the metabolism of fats. For the physiologic and biochemical roles of bile in the body, physiology and biochemistry textbooks should be consulted. Like urine, bile is a valuable biological sample for evaluation of metabolism and elimination of xenobiotics. Most drugs undergo Phase II metabolism before excretion into bile. There are, however, compounds such as anthracyclines whose major route of elimination is the bile; in addition to Phase II metabolites, significant amounts of unchanged drug and Phase I metabolites are also excreted into the bile. The drug and its metabolites in the bile, on entry into the duodenum, are available for reabsorption, which is known as enterohepatic recirculation. The enterohepatic recirculation of drugs often masks the biliary elimination of drugs. It is important to note that without the biliary elimination of drugs and their metabolites, no enterohepatic recirculation can take place.

As a general rule polarity and molecular weight influence the biliary excretion of drugs. Polar and ionizable molecules increase the biliary excretion of drugs. These molecules can be Phase II metabolites and/or parent compounds and/or Phase I metabolites. It is worth noting that protein-bound drugs may undergo spontaneous dissociation in the liver, and the unbound drug undergoes metabolism and/or excretion in the bile. A number of biologic factors such as sex, age, fasting, and pregnancy influence the biliary excretion of drugs.

APPLICATION

5.1 The initial rates of metabolism of a new drug evaluated at different initial concentrations are reported in Table 5.1. Calculate the following:

1. Michaelis–Menten constant: According to the observed data $V_{max} = 150$ μmol L^{-1} min^{-1}.

$$v = (V_{max} \times C_D)/(K_M + C_D)$$

or $$v/V_{max} = C_D/(K_M + C_D)$$

$$120/150 = (2 \times 10^{-4})/(K_M + 2 \times 10^{-4})$$

$$K_M = 5 \times 10^{-5} \text{ M}$$

TABLE 5.1 Data Related to Application 5.1: Initial Rates of Metabolism of the Drug at Different Initial Concentrations

Initial Concentration of Drug (M)	Initial Rate of Metabolism (μmol L^{-1} min^{-1})
2×10^{-2}	150
2×10^{-3}	150
2×10^{-4}	120
1.5×10^{-4}	112.5
1.25×10^{-5}	30.0

2. Initial rate of metabolism at concentration of 0.02 M: As a general rule we may assume that when $C_D \geq 100K_M$ the rate of metabolism follows zero-order kinetics.

$$C_D/K_M = 0.02/(5 \times 10^{-5}) = 400$$

thus

$$v = V_{max} = 150 \ \mu\text{mol L}^{-1} \ \text{min}^{-1}$$

3. Rate of metabolism at initial concentrations of (i) 5×10^{-5} M and (ii) 2.5×10^{-5} M: The concentration of 5×10^{-5} M is equal to K_M, that is, $C_D = K_M$. Therefore, $v = V_{max}/2 = 75 \ \mu\text{mol L}^{-1} \ \text{min}^{-1}$. When $C_D = 2.5 \times 10^{-5}$ M,

$$v = (V_{max} \times C_D)/(K_M + C_D) = (150 \times 2.5 \times 10^{-5})/(5 \times 10^{-5} + 2.5 \times 10^{-5})$$

$$v = 50 \ \mu\text{mol L}^{-1} \ \text{min}^{-1}$$

4. Concentration of metabolite 6 minutes after addition of 0.08 and 0.1 M parent drug: As $C_D/K_M = 0.08/(5 \times 10^{-5}) = 1600$ and $0.1/(5 \times 10^{-5}) = 2000$, the rate of metabolism at these two concentrations would follow zero-order kinetics, that is, $v - V_{max}$. Therefore,

$$[\text{metabolite}] = V_{max} \times \text{time} = 150 \times 6 = 900 \ \mu\text{mol L}^{-1}$$

$$= 900 \times 10^{-6} \ \text{M} = 9 \times 10^{-4} \ \text{M}$$

5. Initial rate of metabolism at 2×10^{-4} M if the concentration of the enzyme system is doubled: The rate of metabolism is directly proportional to the concentration of the protein. If we double the enzyme concentration, the initial rate would double. Therefore, at $C_D = 2 \times 10^{-4}$ with doubling of the protein concentration,

$$v = 120 \times 2 = 240 \ \mu\text{mol L}^{-1} \ \text{min}^{-1}$$

5.2 The rate of metabolism of a drug at a concentration of 0.02 M is 70 μmol L^{-1} min^{-1}. If the K_M for this drug is 4×10^{-5} M, what would be the initial rate of metabolism at the concentrations reported in Table 5.2.

1. Because the C_D/K_M ratio at 0.02 M is greater than $100K_M$ $(0.02/(4 \times 10^{-5}) = 500)$ the corresponding rate of metabolism would equal V_{max}. Therefore, $v = V_{max} = 70 \ \mu\text{mol}$ L^{-1} min^{-1}.

TABLE 5.2 Data Related to Application 5.2

C_D	7×10^{-3} M	8×10^{-4} M	4×10^{-4} M	4×10^{-6} M	2.4×10^{-6} M

2. The C_D/K_M ratio at 7×10^{-3} M is also greater than $100K_M$ ((7×10^{-3})/(4×10^{-5}) = 175). Therefore, $v = V_{max} = 70$ μmol L^{-1} min^{-1}

3. The ratio at 8×10^{-4} M is less than $100K_M$ ((8×10^{-4})/(4×10^{-5}) = 20). Therefore,

$$v = \frac{V_{max} \times 20K_M}{K_M + 20K_M} = \frac{20}{21} V_{max} = 66.7 \ \mu\text{mol L}^{-1} \text{ min}^{-1}$$

4. At 4×10^{-4} M, the ratio is equal to 10. Therefore,

$$v = \frac{V_{max} \times 10K_M}{K_M + 10K_M} = \frac{10}{11} V_{max} = 63.7 \ \mu\text{mol L}^{-1} \text{ min}^{-1}$$

5. At 4×10^{-6} M, the ratio is 0.1. Thus,

$$v = \frac{V_{max} \times 0.1K_M}{K_M + 0.1K_M} = \frac{0.1}{1.1} V_{max} = 6.37 \ \mu\text{mol L}^{-1} \text{ min}^{-1}$$

6. For $C_D = 2.4 \times 10^{-6}$ M, the ratio is 0.06. Therefore,

$$v = \frac{V_{max} \times 0.06K_M}{K_M + 0.06K_M} = 3.96 \ \mu\text{mol L}^{-1} \text{ min}^{-1}$$

5.3 The data presented in Table 5.3 are the results of an in vitro drug metabolism study. Calculate K_M and V_{max} by the Lineweaver–Burk, Hanes, and Eadie–Hofstee methods:

1. Lineweaver–Burk method: The reciprocals of the data are listed in Table 5.4. Regression analysis of $1/v$ versus $1/C_D$ yields the equation

$$1/v = 0.0104 + 0.498 \ (1/C_D)$$

TABLE 5.3 Data Related to Application 5.3

Drug Concentration μmol/L	Initial Rate of Metabolism (μmol L^{-1} min^{-1})
10.00	16.56
12.00	19.20
15.00	22.92
20.00	28.56
24.00	32.04
30.00	36.96
39.60	43.44
60.00	53.40
120.00	68.64
240.00	80.04

TABLE 5.4 Lineweaver–Burk (Double-reciprocal) Data for Application 5.3

$1/v$ (μmol^{-1} L min)	$1/C_D$ (L/μmol)
0.060	0.1
0.052	0.0833
0.044	0.0667
0.035	0.0500
0.031	0.0416
0.027	0.0333
0.023	0.0252
0.0187	0.0166
0.0145	0.0083
0.0125	0.0041

Therefore,

$$\text{slope} = 0.498 \text{ minute}$$

$$y \text{ intercept} = 0.0104 \ \mu mol^{-1} \text{ L min}$$

$$V_{max} = 1/0.0104 = 96.15 \ \mu mol \ L^{-1} \ min^{-1}$$

$$K_M = 0.498 \times 96.15 = 47.88 \ \mu mol \ L^{-1}$$

2. Hanes method: The y and x values according to this method are listed in Table 5.5. The regression equation of C_D/v versus C_D is

$$C_D/v = 0.497 + 0.0104 C_D$$

TABLE 5.5 y and x Values for Application 5.3 According to Hanes Method

C_D/v (min)	C_D ($\mu mol/L$)
0.600	10.00
0.624	12.00
0.660	15.00
0.700	20.00
0.744	24.00
0.810	30.00
0.911	39.60
1.123	60.00
1.747	120.00
3.00	240.00

TABLE 5.6 Data for Application 5.3 According to Eadie–Hofstee Plot

v (μmol L^{-1} min^{-1})	v/C_D (min^{-1})
16.56	1.656
19.20	1.600
22.92	1.528
28.56	1.428
32.04	1.335
36.96	1.232
43.44	1.096
53.40	0.890
68.64	0.572
80.04	0.333

Therefore,

$$\text{slope} = 0.0104 \ \mu\text{mol}^{-1} \ \text{L min}$$

$$y \text{ intercept} = 0.497 \text{ minute}$$

$$V_{\max} = 1/0.0104 = 96.15 \ \mu\text{mol L}^{-1} \ \text{min}^{-1}$$

$$K_M = 0.498 \times 96.15 = 47.88 \ \mu\text{mol L}^{-1}$$

3. Eadie–Hofstee plot: The data for this method are summarized in Table 5.6. The regression equation is

$$v = 96.00 - 47.8 \ (v/C_D)$$

Therefore,

$$\text{slope} = K_M = 47.80 \ \mu\text{mol L}^{-1}$$

$$y \text{ intercept} = V_{\max} = 96 \ \mu\text{mol L}^{-1} \ \text{min}^{-1}$$

5.4 The direct linear plot of a set of data with more than one intersection provided the estimates of K_M and $V_{\max}$ listed in Table 5.7. What pair of data would you select as the ac-

TABLE 5.7 Estimated Pairs of K_M and $V_{\max}$ from the Direct Linear Plot (Application 5.4)

K_M (μmol/L)	22.0	21.6	20.2	22.5	22.8	23.1	24.4	20.5	22.8
$V_{\max}$ (μmol/L min)	54.9	54.0	50.8	56.2	56.7	57.5	63.8	51.2	56.7

TABLE 5.8 Data of Table 5.7 in Ascending Order

K_M (μmol/L)	20.2	20.5	21.6	22.0	22.5	22.8	22.8	23.1	24.4
V_{max} (μmol/L min)	50.8	51.2	54.0	54.9	56.2	56.7	56.7	57.5	63.0

tual values of these parameters. First the data are organized according to their ascending or descending order (Table 5.8). Then the median K_M value and its corresponding V_{max} are determined. The actual values of K_M and V_{max} are 22.6 and 56.2, respectively.

ASSIGNMENT

5.1 For the following data determine K_M and V_{max} by using Lineweaver–Burk, Hanes, and Eadie–Hofstee plots. The data are not ideal and require regression analysis (Table 5.9).

5.2 Determine the Michaelis–Menten parameters of the following equations:
   5.2.1 $1/v = 0.035$ μmol^{-1} L min $+ (0.673$ min$)/C_D$
   5.2.2 $v = 54$ μmol^{-1} L min $- (54\mu$mol L^{-1}) (v/C_D)
   5.2.3 $1/v = 0.01$ μmol^{-1} L min $+ (0.2$ min$)/C_D$
   5.2.4 $C_D/v - 0.23$ min $+ (0.05$ μmol^{-1} L min$)$ C_D
   5.2.5 $v = 110$ μmol L^{-1} min^{-1} $- (29$ μmol L^{-1}) (v/C_D)
   5.2.6 $C_D/v = 0.096$ min $+ (0.075\mu$mol^{-1} L min$)$ C_D

ASSIGNMENT (EXTRA CREDIT)

EC-5.1 Review the following article and answer the following questions:

Esteban A, Calvo R, Peres-Mateo. Paracetamol metabolism in two ethnically different Spanish populations. *Eur J Drug Metab Pharmacokinet* 1996;23:233–9.

■ Which of the metabolic pathways showed significant interindividual variation. Name the enzyme system involved in the pathway.

TABLE 5.9 Data for Assignment 5.1

Drug Concentration (μmol/L)	Rate of Metabolism (μmol/L)
1.613	2.671
1.935	3.096
2.420	3.696
3.225	4.606
3.871	5.167
4.839	5.813
6.387	7.006
9.677	8.613
19.354	11.071
38.710	12.910

■ There were no significant differemnces found in sulfate conjugation of paracetamol at the dose level used in the investigation. Why? Would you expect a similar observation for other drugs?

■ Explain the enhancement of glucuronidation of paracetamol in smokers.

EC-5.2 Answer the following questions based on the article by Coleman et al.

Coleman S, Liu S, Linderman R, Hodgson E, Rose RL. In vitro metabolism of alachlor by human liver microsomes and human cytochrome P450 isoforms. *Chemico-Biol Interact* 1999;122:27–39.

■ Summarize the method of preparation of microsomes.

■ What isoform of CYP450 is responsible for metabolism of alachlor to CHEEPA and CDPA in humans?

■ Discuss the major differences in metabolism of alachlor in humans, rats, and primates.

BIBLIOGRAPHY

1. Arber N, Zajicek G, Ariel I. The streaming liver. II The hepatocyte life history. *Liver* 1988;8:80.
2. Behnia K, Boroujerdi M. Inhibition of aldo–keto reductases by phenobarbital alters metabolism, pharmacokinetics and toxicity of doxorubicin. *J Pharm Pharmacol* 1999;51:1275.
3. Behnia K, Boroujerdi M. Investigation of the enterohepatic recirculation of Adriamycin and its metabolites by linked-rat model. *Cancer Chemother Pharmacol* 1998;41:370.
4. Billings RE, Mcmahon RE, Ashmore J, Wagle SR. The metabolism of drugs in isolated rat hepatocytes. *Drug Metab Dispos* 1977;5:518.
5. Birkett DJ, Mackenzie PI, Veronese ME, Miners JO. *In vitro* approaches can predict human drug metabolism. *Trends Pharmacol Sci* 1993;14:292.
6. Booth CL, Pollack GM, Brouwer KL. Hepatobiliary disposition of valproic acid and valproate glucuronide: use of a pharmacokinetic model to examine the rate-limiting steps and potential sites of drug interaction. *Hepatology* 1996;23:771.
7. Boroujerdi M, Wilson AGE, Kung HC, Anderson MW. Metabolism and DNA binding of benzo(a)pyrene *in vivo* in the rat. *Cancer Res* 1981;4:951.
8. Brierley CH, Buchell B. Human UDP-glucuronosyltransferases chemical defence, jaundice and gene therapy. *Bioessays* 1993;15:749.
9. Cox JW, Dring G, Ginsberg LC, Larson PG, Constable DA, Ultrich RG. Distribution and disposition of trospectomycin sulfate in the *in vivo* rat, perfused liver and cultured hepatocytes. *Drug Metab Dispos* 1990;18:726.
10. Cummings AJ, Martin BK. Excretion and accrual of drug metabolites. Nature 1963;200:1296.
11. Dallner G. Isolation of microsomal subfractions by use of density gradient. *Methods Enzymol* 1978;52:71.
12. Dutton GJ. *Glucuronidation of Drugs and Other Compounds,* Boca Raton, FL: CRC Press, 1980.
13. Ekins S. Past, present, and future applications of precision-cut liver slices for *in vitro* xenobiotic metabolism. *Drug Metab Rev* 1996;28:591.
14. Fabre G, Combalbert J, Berger Y, Cano J-P. Human hepatocytes as a key *in vitro* model to improve preclinical drug development. *Eur J Drug Metab Pharmacol* 1990;15:165.
15. Guengerich FP. *Mammalian Cytochromes* P-450, vol 2. Boca Raton, FL: CRC Press, 1987.
16. Guyton AC, Hall JE. Textbook of Medical Physiology. Philadelphia: WB Saunders, 1996:315.
17. Henderson PJF. Statistical analysis of enzyme kinetic data. In: Eisenthal R, Danson MJ, editors. Enzyme Assays: A Practical Approach. Oxford: IRL Press/Oxford University Press, 1992:284.

18. Keppler D, Arias IM. Hepatic canalicular membrane. Introduction: Transport across the hepatic canalicular membrane. *FASEB J* 1997;11:15.

19. Kroemer HK, Klotz U. Glucuronidation of drugs: a reevaluation of the pharmacological significance of the conjugates and modulating factors. *Clin Pharmacokinet* 1992;23:292.

20. Lake BG, Eaver MJ, Esclangon F, Beamand JA, Price RJ, Walters DG. Metabolism of coumarin by precision-cut calf liver slices and calf livernmicrosomes. *Xenobiotica* 1995;25:133.

21. McLaughlin WJ, Boroujerdi M. BHA (2(3)-*tert*-butyl-4-hydroxyanisole)-mediated modulation of acetaminophen Phase II metabolism *in vivo* in Fisher 344 rats. *Res Commun Chem Pathol Pharmacol* 1987;56:321.

22. Nebert DW, Nelson DR, Conn MJ, Estrabrook RW, Feyerseisen R, Fujuiikuriyama Y, Gonzalez FJ, Guengerich FP, Gunsalus IC, Johnson EF, Loper JC, Sato R, Waterman MR, Waxman DJ. The P450 superfamily: update on new sequences gene mapping, and recommended nomenclature. *DNA Cell Biol* 1991;10:1.

23. Nemoto N, Gelboin HV. Enzymatic conjugation of benzo(a)pyrene oxides, phenols and dihydrodiols with UDP-glucuronic acid. *Biochem Pharmacol* 1976;25:1221.

24. Porter TD, Coon MJ. Cytochrome P-450: multiplicity of isoforms, substrates, catalytic and regulatory mechanisms. *J Biol Chem* 1991;266:13469.

25. Poulsen LL, Ziegler DM. The liver microsomal FAD-containing monooxygenase. *J Biol Chem* 1979;254:6449.

26. Suchy FJ, Buscuvalas JC, Novak DA. Determinants of bile formation during development: ontogeny of hepatic bile acid metabolism and transport. *Liver Dis* 1987;7:77.

27. Vaidyanathan S, Boroujerdi M. Interaction of dexrazoxane with red blood cells and hemoglobin alters pharmacokinetics of doxorubicin. *Cancer Chemother Pharmacol* 2000;46:93.

28. Wrighton SA, Vanden Branden M, Stevens JC, Shipley LA, Ring BJ, Rettie AE, Cashman JR. *In vitro* methods for assessing human hepatic drug metabolism: their use in drug development. *Drug Metab Rev* 1993;25:453.

29. Wrighton SA, Ring BJ, Vanden Branden M. The use of *in vitro* metabolism techniques in the planning and interpretation of drug safety studies. *Toxicol Pathol* 1995;23:199.

CHAPTER 6

LINEAR ONE-COMPARTMENT MODEL WITH INSTANTANEOUS INPUT AND FIRST-ORDER OUTPUT

The natural path is to start from what is better known and more perspicuous to us, and to advance to what is more perspicuous and better known by nature; for what is better known to us is not the same as what is better known without qualification. We must advance in this way, then, from what is less perspicuous by nature but more perspicuous to us, to what is more perspicuous and better known by nature.

ARISTOTLE (BOOK I—PHYSICS)

OBJECTIVES

■ To review the general principles, assumptions, and basic terms and definitions of the linear one-compartment model.

■ To develop the equations of the model based on the plasma concentration of unchanged drug.

■ To present the practical aspects of the model.

6.1 INTRODUCTION

The purpose of pharmacokinetic models, in general, is to describe mathematically the complex biologic processes of absorption, distribution, metabolism, and excretion (ADME) of drugs in relation to their therapeutic outcome. The mathematical equations of the models in their abstract form enable us to understand the behavior of a drug in the body or the way the body handles a drug. One approach to developing the relevant mathematical relationships is based on compartmental analysis. The description and assumptions of compartmental models are the same as described in Chapter 2. Briefly, we assume the body is made up of one, two, or more compartments that have no physiologic or anatomic significance. Each compartment represents an amount of drug, which kinetically behaves as it would in a well-mixed, homogeneous, and distinct volume. When a compartmental model has input (dose) and output (elimination) it is referred to as an *open compartment*. When it has no exit rate it is referred to as a *closed compartment*. All compartmental models used to describe the fate of exogenous compounds in the body, such as therapeutic agents, are open compartments. Closed compartmental models are more relevant to endogenous compounds that may participate in the formation of other endogenous compounds in the body.

6.2 LINEAR ONE-COMPARTMENT OPEN MODEL

The one-compartment open model assumes that the input in the body is mixed and exchanged very rapidly between the plasma and tissues, which behave collectively as a single well-mixed and homogeneous volume. Plasma or serum and urine are then the reference samples of this well-mixed volume. Therefore, any change in the concentration or amount of drug in the reference samples reflects equivalent changes in the compartments. Another assumption of the model is that the elimination (ie, metabolism and excretion) is governed by first-order kinetics.

The instantaneous input in Figure 6.1 refers to any kind of drug input without a definable rate; that is, at time zero the drug is outside of the compartment and at no time (ie, at $t = 0$) is the drug in the body. A good example of instantaneous input is intravenous bolus injection. The first-order overall elimination rate constant K represents renal excretion, hepatic metabolism, and other significant elimination rate constants.

$$K = k_e + k_m + k_n \tag{6.1}$$

In Equation 6.1, k_e is the first-order excretion (ie, renal) rate constant; k_m is the first-order metabolic (ie, hepatic) rate constant and k_n represents the other first-order rate con-

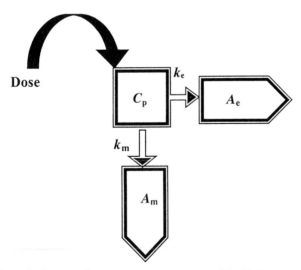

FIGURE 6.1 Schematic diagram of one-compartment open model with instantaneous input (eg, intravenous bolus injection) and first-order elimination through excretion of unchanged drug via the kidney (A_e) and metabolism via the liver (A_m). k_e and k_m are the first-order rate constants of excretion and metabolism, respectively.

stants of elimination such as those for elimination through sweat glands, milk, exhaled air, etc. For most drugs k_n is considered negligible and Equation 6.1 is simplified to

$$K = k_e + k_m \tag{6.2}$$

In Figure 6.1 C_p is the plasma concentration of free drug at time t and V_d is the apparent volume of distribution. The product of $C_p \times V_d$ is the total amount of free drug in the compartment at time t, A_t.

$$A_t = C_{p_t} \times V_d \tag{6.3}$$

C_p and A are variables and their magnitude is dependent on time and dose. On the other hand, K and V_d are considered constant for a given compound in linear pharmacokinetics.

The overall rate of elimination from the compartment, which represents the body, according to first-order kinetics, is defined by the differential equation

$$dA/dt = -KA \tag{6.4}$$

According to Equation 6.4 the rate of elimination of a drug (ie, dA/dt) at time t is proportional to the amount of drug in the body. Therefore, the rate of elimination is a variable and decreases as the amount or concentration of drug in the body declines. The negative sign reflects the reduction of drug in the body as a result of metabolism and excretion. The rate constant of elimination, K, remains constant during the elimination process. Therefore, the "rate of elimination" is a variable equal to KA, and the "rate constant of elimination" is a constant at all times. An analogy can be made between first-order elimination and a simple physical hydrodynamic model to make a better distinction between the rate and rate constant of elimination. Consider two tanks of water with a drain outlet at the bottom (Figure 6.2). The diameter of one opening is twice that of the other. Assume

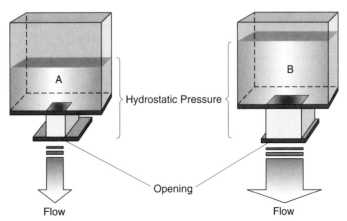

FIGURE 6.2 Representation of hydrodynamic models. The higher the level of fluid in the tank and the larger the opening of the outlet, the greater is the exit flow rate. Obviously, a larger volume of fluid but smaller opening would result in a lower flow rate and it would take longer for the fluid to leave the tank (an analogy for renal or hepatic impairment).

that the flow of water from the tanks via the outlet per unit of time is analogous to the rate of elimination of drug from the body. It is obvious that the flow rate of water from the tank depends on the volume of water and its hydrostatic pressure. As the volume of water declines, the pressure declines. This hydrostatic pressure of water is analogous to the amount of drug in the body. As the amount of drug in the body declines, so does the rate of elimination. The diameter of the outlets, which remains unchanged during removal of water from the tanks, is analogous to K. A smaller diameter tends to lower the flow rate, which is analogous to reduction of K in disease states such as renal impairment and hepatic failure.

6.3 EQUATIONS OF THE MODEL

An important assumption of one-compartment models discussed in this chapter is that only free and unchanged drug can interact with receptor sites to provide the desirable pharmacologic response. As was discussed in Chapter 2, the measurement of drug concentration at the receptor site for most drugs may not be achievable or practical. Furthermore, the therapeutic outcome for most drugs may or may not be a measurable variable. For instance, to optimize the therapeutic outcome of a drug that lowers blood sugar we can measure the concentration of sugar in blood as a biomarker and optimize the dosing regimen accordingly. For most drugs, however, the outcome is not so easily attainable. For example, in infectious diseases or in cancer chemotherapy no direct biomarker yet exists to correlate directly with the outcome of therapy. Therefore, we assume that the concentration of free drug in plasma or serum is proportional to the concentration of free drug at its receptor site, which is in equilibrium with the concentration of drug bound to the receptor site:

$$\text{free drug + receptor} \;\rightleftharpoons\; \text{drug–receptor complex} \longrightarrow \text{response}$$

Hence, based on the above assumption it can be emphasized that the equation of the model based on plasma/serum concentration of free drug is useful not only for defining the time course of a drug in the body but also for optimizing the therapeutic outcome of the drug.

Equation 6.4 can be integrated to yield the following equations based on the amount of free drug in the compartment:

$$\ln A = \ln A^0 - Kt \tag{6.5}$$

$$\log A = \log A^0 - Kt/2.303 \tag{6.6}$$

$$A = A^0 e^{-Kt} \tag{6.7}$$

where A is the amount of free drug in the body at time t and A^0 is the initial amount or dose at time zero.

Equations 6.5 to 6.7 may also be written in terms of the plasma or serum concentration of free drug:

$$\ln C_p = \ln C_p^0 - Kt \tag{6.8}$$

$$\log C_p = \log C_p^0 - Kt/2.303 \tag{6.9}$$

$$C_p = C_p^0 e^{-Kt} \tag{6.10}$$

C_p and C_p^0 are the plasma concentration of free drug at time t and the initial concentration ($t = 0$), respectively.

6.3.1 Half-life of Elimination

A useful pharmacokinetic constant of the model is the half-life of elimination. It is the time required for 50% of the drug at any initial level to be eliminated from the compartment:

At $\quad\quad\quad\quad\quad t = T_{1/2},\ C_{p_2} = \frac{1}{2}C_{p_1},\ \text{or}\ A_2 = \frac{1}{2}A_1.$

Therefore,

$$\log \tfrac{1}{2}C_{p_1} = \log C_{p_1} - K(T_{1/2})/2.303$$

$$2.303 \log (C_{p_1}/(\tfrac{1}{2}C_{p1})) = KT_{1/2}$$

$$2.303 \log 2 = KT_{1/2}$$

$$0.693 = KT_{1/2}$$

$$T_{1/2} = 0.693/K, \quad \text{or } T_{1/2} = \ln 2/K, \quad \text{or } T_{1/2} = 2.303 \log 2/K \tag{6.11}$$

Equation 6.11 indicates that the half-life of elimination of a drug that follows linear pharmacokinetics is independent of the amount or concentration and inversely proportional to the overall elimination rate constant.

6.3.2 Time Constant

Occasionally it is more convenient to use the time constant rather than the half-life. The time constant is the reciprocal of the first-order rate constant. The relationship between the time constant and the half-life is

$$\text{time constant} = 1/K \tag{6.12}$$

$$1/K = 1/(0.693/T_{1/2}) = 1.44T_{1/2} \tag{6.13}$$

The time constant is also known as turnover time, and in noncompartmental analysis of an intravenous bolus, $1/K$ is referred to as mean residence time (MRT). Noncompartmental analysis is discussed in Chapter 17. The time constant or MRT represents the time for 63% of an intravenous bolus dose to be eliminated from the body. The relationship between MRT and $T_{1/2}$ is

$$MRT_{iv} = 1/K = T_{1/2}/0.693 \qquad (6.14)$$

$$T_{1/2} = 0.693(MRT)_{iv\ bolus} \qquad (6.15)$$

6.3.3 Apparent Volume of Distribution

Another useful constant of the one-compartment model is the apparent volume of distribution (V_d). This constant, although referred to as the volume of distribution, has no relationship with total body water. It should be considered only as a constant of conversion of concentration to total amount of free drug in the compartment. A large volume of distribution indicates that the concentration of free drug in plasma is low and the drug is localized and associated with regions that are not easily accessible or are a part of the sampling compartment. The apparent volume of distribution is determined by dividing the amount of free drug by plasma concentration:

$$V_d = A_t/C_{p_t} \qquad (6.16)$$

As the amount of free drug is only known at time zero, a more practical equation would be

$$V_d = Dose/C_p^0 \qquad (6.17)$$

6.3.4 Total Body Clearance

Total body clearance (Cl_t), as was discussed in Chapter 5, is the rate of elimination of drug from the body per unit of concentration:

$$Cl_t = \frac{rate}{concentration} = \frac{KA_t}{A_t/V_d} = K \times V_d \qquad (6.18)$$

Therefore, total body clearance is the product of the apparent volume of distribution and the first-order overall elimination rate constant, and according to the following equations, it is also the sum of metabolic and renal clearances:

$$Cl_t = V_d \times K = V_d\ (k_e + k_m) = Cl_r + Cl_m \qquad (6.19)$$

6.3.5 Duration of Action

The duration of action is the time the plasma concentration remains within the therapeutic range of a drug. When the concentration falls below the minimum effective level no effective response should be expected. For a single-dose intravenous bolus injection, the duration of action may be estimated as

$$t_d = \frac{2.303}{K} \log \frac{C_p^0}{C_{P_{MEC}}} = 3.3 T_{1/2} \log \frac{C_p^0}{C_{P_{MEC}}} \tag{6.20}$$

where $C_{P_{MEC}}$ is the minimum effective concentration of drug.

According to Equation 6.20, the duration of action is inversely proportional to K and directly proportional to the half-life of elimination. This indicates that the duration of action of a drug in patients with renal impairment or hepatic failure is longer than normal. The duration of action is not directly proportional to the administered dose or initial concentration. For example, if the dose is doubled, C_p^0 doubles, but the duration of action increases by one half-life:

$$t_{d1} = 3.3 T_{1/2} \log \frac{C_{p_1}^0}{C_{P_{MEC}}} \tag{6.21}$$

$$t_{d2} = 3.3 T_{1/2} \log \frac{2 C_{p_1}^0}{C_{P_{MEC}}} \tag{6.22}$$

$$t_{d2} - t_{d1} = 3.3 T_{1/2} \left(\log \frac{2 C_p^0}{C_{P_{MEC}}} - \log \frac{C_p^0}{C_{P_{MEC}}} \right) = 1 T_{1/2} \tag{6.23}$$

Thus, if the dose is quadrupled, the duration of action increases by two half-lives.

6.3.6 Fraction of Dose Remaining in the Body at Time t

If Equation 6.10 is normalized with respect to C_p^0 (ie, dividing both sides of the equation by C_p^0) the following equations, which represent the fraction of dose in the body (f_b) at time t, are obtained:

$$f_b = \frac{C_p}{C_p^0} = e^{-Kt} = e^{-(0.693/T_{1/2})t} = (0.5)^{t/T_{1/2}} \tag{6.24}$$

Equation 6.24 indicates that at $t = 1 T_{1/2}$, $f_b = 0.5$; at $t = 2 T_{1/2}$, $f_b = 0.25$; at $t = 3.3 T_{1/2}$, $f_b = 0.1$; at $t = 4.3 T_{1/2}$, $f_b = 0.05$; at $t = 6.6 T_{1/2}$, $f_b = 0.01$; and at $t = 7 T_{1/2}$, $f_b \approx 0$.

6.3.7 Fraction of Dose Eliminated by All Routes of Elimination at Time t

At time zero the fraction of dose in the body is equal to one. As the fraction of dose in the body declines with time the fraction of dose eliminated by all routes of elimination increases. Therefore the sum of fraction in the body and fraction eliminated at any time is 1. Based on this concept of mass balance the following equations define the fraction of dose eliminated (f_{el}) from the body by all routes of elimination at time t:

$$f_{el} = 1 - f_b = 1 - \frac{C_p}{C_p^0} = 1 - e^{-Kt} = 1 - e^{(0.693/T_{1/2})t} = 1 - (0.5)^{t/T_{1/2}} \tag{6.25}$$

6.3.8 Area under Plasma Concentration–Time Curve after Intravenous Bolus

The area under the plot of plasma concentration of free drug versus time (AUC) is a useful parameter in determining the extent of availability of a drug in the body after any route of administration. This parameter is also useful in calculating other parameters and constants of a model. AUC can be estimated by the model-dependent method of integration or by the model-independent trapezoidal rule (consult Chapter 1 for more information). Integration of Equation 6.10 provides the following relationship for the AUC of a one-compartment model:

$$\left.\mathrm{AUC}\right|_0^\infty = \int_0^0 C_\mathrm{p}^0 e^{-Kt} = \left. C_\mathrm{p}^0 \frac{e^{-Kt}}{-K}\right|_0^\infty = \frac{C_\mathrm{p}^0}{K} \tag{6.26}$$

AUC may also be calculated by using the trapezoidal rule:

$$\left.\mathrm{AUC}\right|_0^\infty = \sum_{i=0}^n \frac{C_{\mathrm{p}_i} + C_{\mathrm{p}_{i+1}}}{2} (t_{i+1} - t_i) + \frac{C_{\mathrm{p}_\mathrm{last}}}{K} \tag{6.27}$$

Multiplying the numerator and denominator of the left side of Equation 6.26 by the apparent volume of distribution yields the relationship

$$\left.\mathrm{AUC}\right|_0^\infty = \frac{\mathrm{dose}}{\mathrm{Cl}_\mathrm{t}} \tag{6.28}$$

Equations 6.26 and 6.28 indicate that in linear pharmacokinetics (ie, dose-independent pharmacokinetics), the AUC is directly proportional to the initial plasma concentration or dose and inversely proportional to the overall elimination rate constant and clearance. This means that if we double the dose, the area under the curve is doubled. Figures 6.3 and 6.4 demonstrate this linear relationship. The plot of AUC versus dose is used to determine the dose dependency of the pharmacokinetics of a drug. A nonlinear relationship as presented in Figure 6.5 indicates that the rate of elimination of drug from the body is no longer first-order kinetics and the equations of linear pharmacokinetics as described in this chapter are not applicable. A nonlinear relationship between dose and AUC exists when saturable processes govern the excretion and/or metabolism. As demonstrated in Figure 6.5, in a nonlinear relationship, if the dose is doubled the AUC increases significantly more than double.

6.3.9 Other Useful Equations

The following equations are some useful equations for a one-compartment model derived on the basis of AUC, Cl_t, and dose:

$$\mathrm{Cl}_\mathrm{t} = K \times V_\mathrm{d} = K\,(\mathrm{dose}/C_\mathrm{p}^0) = \mathrm{dose}/\mathrm{AUC} \tag{6.29}$$

$$\mathrm{AUC} = \mathrm{dose}/\mathrm{Cl}_\mathrm{t} = D/V_\mathrm{d}K = C_\mathrm{p}^0/K \tag{6.30}$$

$$\mathrm{dose} = \mathrm{Cl}_\mathrm{t} \times \mathrm{AUC} = K \times V_\mathrm{d} \times C_\mathrm{p}^0/K = C_\mathrm{p}^0 \times V_\mathrm{d} \tag{6.31}$$

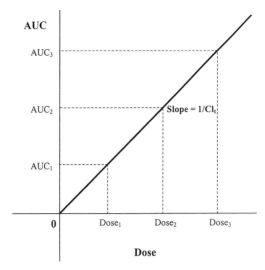

FIGURE 6.3 Relationship between the administered dose and related area under the plasma concentration–time curve in linear pharmacokinetics. $Dose_3 = 3 \times Dose_1 = Dose_2 + Dose_1$. $AUC_3 = 3 \times AUC_1 = AUC_2 + AUC_1$.

APPLICATION

6.1 An adult male patient was given the first dose of an antibiotic at 6:00 AM. At 12:00 noon the plasma level of the drug was measured and reported as 5 μg/mL. The drug is known to follow the one-compartment model with a half-life of 6 hours. The recommended dosage regimen of this drug is 250 mg q.i.d. The minimum inhibitory concentration is 3 μg/mL. Calculate the following:

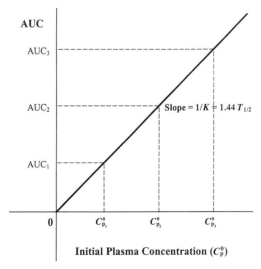

FIGURE 6.4 Linear relationship between AUC and CP^0 in dose-independent pharmacokinetics. $C_{p_3}^0 = 3 \times C_{p_1}^0 = C_{p_2}^0 + C_{p_1}^0$. $AUC_3 = 3 \times AUC_1 = AUC_2 + AUC_1$.

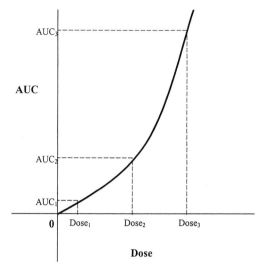

FIGURE 6.5 Profile of nonlinear relationship between AUC and dose in dose-dependent pharmacoknietics. $Dose_3 = 3 \times Dose_1 = Dose_2 + Dose_1$. $AUC_3 > 3 \times AUC_1 > AUC_2 + AUC_1$ and $AUC_2 > 2AUC_1$.

1. Apparent volume of distribution

Equation: $V_d = dose/C_p^0$

$$K = 0.693/6 = 0.1155 \text{ h}^{-1}$$

$$C_p^0 = 5/e^{-0.1155(6)} = 10 \ \mu g/mL$$

Or, because 6:00 AM to 12:00 noon is equal to one half-life

$$C_p^0 = 2 \times 5 = 10 \ \mu g/mL$$

Therefore,

$$V_d = 250 \text{ mg}/10 \ \mu g/mL = 25 \text{ L}$$

2. Expected plasma concentration at 10 AM

Equation: $C_p = C_p^0 e^{-Kt}$

$$C_p = 10e^{-0.1155 \times 4} = 6.30 \ \mu g/mL$$

3. Total amount in the body immediately after injection of the second dose at 12:00 noon

Equation: $A_{12 \text{ noon}} = 2\text{nd dose} + (C_{p_{12 \text{ noon of 1st dose}}} \times V_d)$

$$A_{12 \text{ noon}} = 250 + (5 \text{ mg/L} \times 25 \text{ L}) = 375 \text{ mg}$$

4. Duration of action of the first dose only

Equation: $t_d = (2.303/K)\log(C_p^0/C_{p_{MEC}})$

$t_d = (2.303/0.1155)\log(10/3) = 10.42$

5. Total body clearance

Equation: $Cl_t = \text{dose/AUC}$ or $Cl_t = K\,V_d$

$AUC = 10/0.1155 = 86.58$ mg h/L

$Cl_t = 250/86.58 = 2.88$ L/h $= 48.125$ mL/min

or $Cl_t = (0.1155\ h^{-1})(25\ L) = 2.88$ L/h

6. Fraction of dose in the body 5 hours after injection

Equation: $f_b = e^{-Kt}$

$f_b = e^{-0.1155(5)} = 0.56$, ie, 56% of the dose

7. Total amount in the body 5 hours after injection

Equation: $A = A^0\,e - Kt$

$A_{7\,h} = 250(0.56) = 140$ mg

8. Exponential and logarithmic equation of pharmacokinetic model

$$C_p = 10e^{-0.1155t}$$

$$\log C_p = 2.845 - 0.0215t$$

(C_p^0 is expressed in $\mu g/mL$ and K in h^{-1})

9. Rate of elimination at $t = 5$ h

Equation: rate $= Cl_t C_p$ or rate $= KA$

rate $= (2.88\ L/h)(140/25)$ mg/L $= 16.14$ mg/h

or rate $= 0.1155\ h^{-1} \times 140 = 16.17$ mg/h

10. Duration of action of first dose only if dose administered at 6:00 AM was 500 mg

Equation: $t_{d500} = t_{d250} + 1T_{1/2}$

$t_{d500} = 10.42$ h $+ 6$ h $= 16.42$ h

6.2 The ideal data presented in Table 6.1 are plasma concentrations of a new drug at different time points after an intravenous bolus injection of 50 mg to a 70-kg patient. Calculate the following:

1. Overall elimination rate constant: The regression equation of log C_p versus time is

$$\log C_p = 0.602 - 0.401t$$

As the data are ideal the following conventional relationship can also be used to determine the slope of the line:

$$\text{slope} = (\log C_{p_2} - \log C_{p_1})/(t_2 - t_1)$$

$$\text{slope} = (0.401 - (-0.599))/(0.5 - 3.0) = -0.4$$

$$K = (0.4)(2.303) = 0.921 \text{ h}^{-1} = 0.0154 \text{ min}^{-1}$$

2. Half-life of elimination

$$T_{1/2} - 0.693/K$$

$$T_{1/2} = 0.693/K = 0.693/0.921 = 0.752 \text{ h} = 45 \text{ min}$$

3. Initial plasma concentration

$$C_p^0 = \text{antilog } 0.602 = 4 \text{ mg/L}$$

4. Exponential and logarithmic equations of pharmacokinetic model

$$C_p = 4e^{-0.921t}$$

$$\log C_p = 0.602 - 0.4t$$

$$(C_p^0 \text{ is expressed in } \mu g/mL \text{ and } K \text{ in h}^{-1})$$

TABLE 6.1 Data for Application 6.2

Time (h)	Plasma concentration (mg/L)	Log Plasma Concentration
0.5	2.52	0.401
1.0	1.59	0.201
1.5	1.00	0.000
2.0	0.64	−0.194
2.5	0.40	−0.398
3.0	0.25	−0.600

5. Plasma concentration 5 minutes after injection

$$C_{p5 \text{ min}} = 4 \text{ (mg/L)} \, e^{-0.0154(5)} = 3.7 \text{ mg/L}$$

6. Apparent volume of distribution and total body clearance

$$V_d = 50 \text{ mg/4 mg/L} = 12.5 \text{ L}$$

$$\text{TBC} = (12.5) \, (0.924) = 11.55 \text{ L/h} = 192.5 \text{ ml/min}$$

7. Rate of elimination at $t = 5$ min

$$\text{rate} = (11.55) \, (3.7) = 42.73 \text{ mg/h} = 712 \text{ } \mu\text{g/min}$$

8. Fraction of dose remaining in the body at $t = 5$ min

$$f_b = 3.7/4 = 0.925 \quad \text{or} \quad f_b = e^{-(0.0154)(5)} = 0.925$$

$$f_b = (1/2)^{0.11} = 0.925$$

9. Fraction of dose eliminated from body at $t = 5$ min

$$f_{el} = 1 - 0.925 = 0.075$$

10. Fraction of dose remaining in body at $t = 1.5$ h

$$1.5 \text{ h} = 2T_{1/2}, \quad \text{therefore} \quad f_b = 0.25$$

11. Area under plasma concentration–time curve from time zero to ∞

$$\text{AUC}\Big|_0^\infty = 4 \text{ mg/L}/0.0154 \text{ min}^{-1} = 259.7 \text{ mg min/L} = 4.33 \text{ mg h/L}$$

12. Total amount of drug in body at $t = 5$ min

$$A_t = 0.925 \times 50 \text{ mg} = 46.25 \text{ mg}$$

13. Total amount eliminated from body at $t = 5$ min

$$A_{el_5 \text{ min}} = (0.075) \, (50 \text{ mg}) = 3.75 \text{ mg}$$

or

$$\text{AUC}_t = \int_0^t C_p^0 e^{-Kt} = (C_p^0/K)(1 - e^{-Kt})$$

$$\text{AUC}_{5 \text{ min}} = (4.33 \text{ mg h/L}) \, (0.075) = 0.325 \text{ mg h/L}$$

$$A_{el_5 \text{ min}} = (11.55 \text{ L/h}) \, (0.325 \text{ mg h/L}) = 3.75 \text{ mg}$$

6.3 The following equation is based on regression analysis of the free concentration of a drug after the intravenous injection of 1 g. The concentrations were measured in units of milligrams per liter and time in hours:

$$\log C_p = 2 - 0.1t$$

Calculate the following:

1. Minimum effective concentration of the drug if duration of action is 6 hours

$$\log C_p = 2 - 0.1(6) = 1.4$$

$$C_{P_{MEC}} = \text{antilog } 1.4 = 25.12 \text{ mg/L}$$

2. Area under plasma concentration–time curve

$$AUC = \text{antilog } 2/(2.303 \times 0.1) = 434.21 \text{ mg h/L}$$

3. Total body clearance

$$Cl_t = (1000 \text{ mg/antilog } 2)(0.1 \times 2.303) = 2.303 \text{ L/h}$$

4. Time required for 63.3% of dose to be eliminated

$$MRT = 1/K = 1/(2.303 \times 0.1) = 4.34 \text{ h}$$

5. Area under plasma concentration–time curve if dose is reduced to 500 mg

$$AUC = 434.21/2 = 217.1 \text{ mg h/L}$$

6.4 The data in Table 6.2 are reported for two drugs (A and P) following intravenous bolus injections of 4 g each to a group of six volunteers. The study was carried out in crossover design and plasma data for each subject were analyzed individually according to a one-compartment model. The values in Table 6.2 represent the means of the calculated parameters and constants. The minimum effective/inhibitory concentration of both drugs is 4.50 mg/L. Calculate the following for both drugs:

TABLE 6.2 Data for Application 6.4

Drug	Half-life (h)	Cl_t (mL/min)	AUC (mg h/L)
A	6.00	95.00	780.00
P	4.00	99.00	670.00

1. Exponential equation of the one-compartmental model

$$K_A = 0.693/6 = 0.1155 \text{ h}^{-1}, \quad K_B = 0.695/4 = 0.173 \text{ h}^{-1}$$

Drug A: $C_p = (780 \times 0.1155) \, e^{-0.1155t}$

   $C_p = 90 \, e^{-0.1155t}$

Drug P: $C_p = (670 \times 0.173) \, e^{-0.173t}$

   $C_p = 116 \, e^{-0.173t}$

2. Duration of action

Drug A: $C_{p_{MEC}} = 5\% \, C_p^0$

   $\therefore t_d = 4.3 T_{1/2} = 4.3 \times 6 = 25.8 \text{ h}$

Drug P: $t_d = (3.3 \times 4) \log (116/4.5) = 18.63 \text{ h}$

3. Percent of the dose eliminated during t_d:

Drug A: $f_{el} = 0.95$ (ie, 95%)

Drug P: $f_{el} = 1 - e^{-0.173 \times 18.63} = 0.96$ (ie, 96%)

ASSIGNMENT

6.1 Acylampicillin is eliminated primarily by glomerular filtration and tubular secretion and is not absorbed from the GI tract when given orally. Its minimum effective plasma concentration is 64 mg/L. Probenecid is a uricosuric and renal tubular transport-blocking agent. It inhibits the tubular secretion of most penicillins. In Part One of the assignment you evaluate the effect of probenecid on the pharmacokinetics of this acylampicilin, and in Part Two, the effect of renal impairment.

   Part One   Twenty patients with normal renal function and no known allergies to penicillin were administered 2 g of the drug intravenously (treatment A). Venous blood samples were collected at different times after the injection. After a 3-day washout period, they were crossed over to receive a regimen consisting of the oral administration of 1 g probenecid followed by intravenous injection of 2 g of acylampicillin (treatment B). The plasma portions of blood samples from both treatments were assayed for free acylampicilin. Table 6.3 summarizes a typical set of data from one patient.

   6.1.1 The data for both treatments can be fitted to a one- or two-compartment model. Assume the data for both treatments follow a one-compartment model. Plot both sets of data semilogarithmically with their trend lines and report the regression equations.

TABLE 6.3 Data for Assignment 6.1

Time (h)	Treatment A (μg/mL)	Treatment B (mg/L)
0.3	230	300
0.4	190	247
0.5	150	195
1.0	110	145
2.0	44	58
3.0	20	26
4.0	11	15
5.0	5	7
6.0	2	3
7.0	1	1.40

6.1.2 Calculate and compare the following parameters and constants for both treatments:

a. Half-life and overall elimination rate constants

b. Area under plasma concentration–time curve

c. Total body clearance

d. Duration of action

e. Fraction of dose in the compartment 1 hour after injection.

6.1.3 Compare the half-life, total body clearance, and AUC in a table and briefly comment on the effect of probenecid on these constants and parameters.

Part Two Twelve patients with renal impairment (GFR < 30 mL/min) were injected with 2 g of acylampicillin. The plasma samples were collected and assayed as in Part One. The data were analyzed by regression analysis and the mean values of the measurements are reported in Table 6.4. Thus, the data can be considered ideal and you may use the conventional slope relationship of $(y_2 - y_1)/(x_2 - x_1)$.

6.1.4 Calculate the half-life and overall elimination rate constant.

6.1.5 Calculate the initial plasma concentration and apparent volume of distribution.

6.1.6 Calculate the area under the plasma concentration–time curve and total body clearance.

TABLE 6.4 Data for Assignment 6.1, Part Two

Time (h)	Plasma Concentration (mg/L)
1	340
2	244
3	172
4	124
5	88
7	44

6.1.7 Calculate the plasma concentration 10 hours after injection.

6.1.8 Because in Part Two the patients received only the drug without probenecid, the effect of renal impairment on the pharmacokinetics of the drug should be compared with treatment A. Compare the half-life, Cl_t, AUC, and MRT of Part Two with those of the control group of Part One.

6.2 The initial plasma concentrations of two different drugs A and B following intravenous bolus injection of equal doses in a crossover design to a patient are 300 mg/L and 150 μg/mL, respectively. The half-life of drug B is twice that of drug A, the plasma concentration of drug B four hours after injection is 75 mg/L, and the minimum effective concentration of both drugs is 15 mg/L.

6.2.1 Calculate the duration of action of each drug.

6.2.2 How long would it take for 95% of drug A to be eliminated?

6.2.3 What would be the duration of action of drug B if the dose were doubled?

6.2.4 If the apparent volume of distribution of drug A is 10% of body weight (ie, 10 L/100 kg body wt), how much (in mg) of drug B would be eliminated from the body in $2T_{1/2B}$.

6.2.5 Calculate the area under the plasma concentration–time curve for each drug.

6.3 Answer the following short questions without the use of a calculator. Assume a one-compartment open model with intravenous bolus input:

6.3.1 What percentage of a dose of a drug with a half-life of 3 hours is eliminated in 9.9 hours?

6.3.2 What fraction of a dose of a drug with a half-life of 3 hours is eliminated by all routes of elimination in 6 hours?

6.3.3 What is the half-life of a drug if 25% of the dose remains in the body 10 hours after injection?

6.3.4 What fraction of an intravenous bolus dose of a drug with a mean residence time of 24 hours remains in the body 2 hours after injection?

6.3.5 What is the initial rate of elimination of a 200-mg dose of a drug with total body clearance of 12 L/h and apparent volume of distribution of 10 L?

6.3.6 What is the overall elimination rate constant of a drug if the durations of action after injection of 250 and 1000 mg are 2 and 14 hours, respectively?

6.3.7 What is the dose of a drug with a half-life of 2 hours if 1500 mg is eliminated by all routes of elimination in 4 hours?

6.3.8 What dose of a drug with a half-life of 1 hour provides an initial rate of elimination of 69.3 mg/h (ie, at $t = 0$)?

6.3.9 What is the half-life of a drug if its durations of action after injection of 500 and 4000 mg are 4 and 10 hours, respectively?

6.3.10 What is the overall elimination of a drug if 475 mg of an intravenously injected dose of 500 mg is eliminated in 43 hours?

6.3.11 What is the total body clearance of a drug if its area under the plasma concentration–time curve following an intravenous bolus injection of 1500 mg is 50 mg h/L?

6.3.12 How long does it take for 450 mg of a drug with a half-life of 3 hours to be eliminated after injection of 500 mg?

6.4 A 70-kg patient with normal renal function (patient A) and a 60-kg patient with chronic renal failure (patient B) receive 500 mg of a new antimicrobial drug twice daily. The plasma concentration of the drug after the first dose was assayed at different time intervals for both patients. Patient B, however, undergoes hemodiaysis twice a week and the time course of the drug in this patient was evaluated both between dialyses and during dialysis. The dialysis started 10 min after the injection of the drug, and the plasma samples were collected during dialysis. The plasma concentrations of free drug in all three cases are reported in Table 6.5. Assume the drug follows a one-compartment model and complete the following for all three cases:

6.4.1 Formulale the logarithmic equation of the one-compartment model.
6.4.2 Calculate the initial plasma concentration.
6.4.3 Calculate the AUC.
6.4.4 Calculate total body clearance.
6.4.5 Calculate turnover time.
6.4.6 Calculate the fraction of dose eliminated during 6 hours.
6.4.7 How long would it take for 375 mg of the drug to be eliminated from the body?
6.4.8 Briefly discuss which of the parameters and constants are affected by renal impairment and dialysis.

6.5 Different doses of two different drugs (A and B) are administered in a crossover design to a 60-kg patient by bolus intravenous injection. Both drugs follow a linear one-compartment model with initial plasma concentration of 60 mg/L. The half-life and total body clearance of drug B are twice those of drug A and the total amount of drug A eliminated in $2T_{1/2}$ is 675 mg. The minimum effective concentration of drug A is 15 mg/L and the duration of action with the administered dose is 6 hours. Calculate the following for both drugs:

6.5.1 Total body clearance.
6.5.2 Dose.
6.5.3 Area under plasma concentration–time curve from 0 to ∞.
6.5.4 Total amount eliminated in 6 hours.

TABLE 6.5 Data for Assignment 6.4

Time (h)	Cp (mg/L)		
	Patient A	Patient B (between dialyses)	Patient B (during dialysis)
1	59	70	47
2	48	65	41
4	37	57	32
6	29	50	25
8	23	44	—
12	15	33	—
16	10	—[a]	—
24	5	—	—

[a]—, No sample was collected.

TABLE 6.6 Data for Assignment 6.7

Time (h)	0.25	0.50	1.00	3.00	6.00	10.00	14.00
C_p (μg/mL)	46.00	43.50	38.00	23.00	10.50	3.70	1.30

6.6 The preliminary calculations of regression analysis of a set of plasma concentration–time data yielded the following information:

$$n = 20$$

$$\sum t = 40 \text{ h} \qquad \sum dt^2 = 110 \qquad \sum C_p = 763 \text{ mg/L}$$

$$\sum \log C_p = 52 \qquad \sum dtd \log C_p = -22 \qquad \sum dtdC_p = 220$$

$$\sum d \log C_p^2 \qquad \sum dC_p^2 = 24800 \qquad \sum d \log t^2 = 36$$

Write the exponential equation of the model.

6.7 A 50-kg patient was given a single intravenous bolus dose of 10 mg/kg of a drug. The concentration of unchanged drug in plasma was measured at different time intervals as reported in Table 6.6. Determine the following according to a one-compartment model:

    6.7.1 Half-life.
    6.7.2 Apparent volume of distribution.
    6.7.3 Total body clearance.
    6.7.4 Total amount eliminated in $2T_{1/2}$.
    6.7.5 Time required for 60% of the dose to be eliminated.

6.8 In a clinical trial of two new drugs (A and B) 12 volunteers with normal renal function received 4 g of each drug in a crossover design. The plasma concentration of free drug was measured and analyzed according to a linear one-compartment model and the following equations of the model were reported:

    Drug A: $\log C_p = 2.477 - 0.1t$. Drug B: $C_p = 200e^{-0.462t}$. (Plasma concentrations and time points were measured in units of milligrams per liter and hours, respectively.)

    Fill in the blanks of Table 6.7.

TABLE 6.7 Table for Assignment 6.8

Parameter/Constant	Drug A	Drug B
Fraction of dose in the body at $t = 3$ h		
AUC (mg h/L)		
Mean residence time (h)		
Total body clearance (mL/min)		
Rate of elimination (mg/h) at $t = 3$ h		

6.9 Following an intravenous bolus injection of 500 mg of a new drug the following data were reported: $T_{1/2} = 2$ hours, $C_p^0 = 25$ μg/mL. Calculate the following:

   6.9.1 Plasma concentration 4 hours after injection.

   6.9.2 Total body clearance.

   6.9.3 Fraction of dose remaining in the body 6.6 hours after injection.

   6.9.4 Total amount of drug eliminated by all routes of elimination 4 hours after injection.

6.10 The following data were reported after intravenous bolus injection of 1 g of a drug that follows a one-compartment model:

MRT = 2.89 hours, AUC = 250 mg h/L.

Calculate the minimum effective concentration if the duration of action is 4 hours.

6.11 The therapeutic range of a drug is 50 to 300 mg/L. After an intravenous bolus injection of 2 g followed by regression analysis of the concentration of free drug in plasma (in units of milligrams per liter) versus time (in units of hours), the following linear equation was obtained: $\log C_p = 2 - 0.1t$. Calculate the following:

   6.11.1 Duration of action.

   6.11.2 Total body clearance.

   6.11.3 Total amount eliminated in 6 hours.

   6.11.4 Rate of elimination at $t = 3$ hours.

   6.11.5 Area under plasma concentration–time curve.

6.12 Answer the following short questions without the use of a calculator. Assume a one-compartment open model with intravenous bolus input:

   6.12.1 The initial rate of elimination of a drug (ie, at $t = 0$) after an intravenous injection is 69.30 mg/h and its half-life is 1 hour. What is the dose?

   6.12.2 The durations of action of a drug after intravenous injection of 100 and 800 mg are 4 and 10 hours, respectively. What is the half-life of the drug?

   6.12.3 The total amount of a drug eliminated 43 hours after an intravenous dose of 500 mg is 475 mg. What is the half-life of the drug?

BIBLIOGRAPHY

1. Gibaldi M, Perrier D. *Pharmacokinetics.* 2nd ed. New York: Marcel Dekker, 1982:1.
2. Gibaldi M, Nagashima R, Levy G. Relationship between drug concentration in plasma or serum and amount of drug in the body. *J Pharm Sci* 1969;58:193.
3. Rescigno A, Seger G. *Drug and Tracer Kinetics.* Waltham, MA: Blaisdell, 1966:10.
4. Riegleman S, Loo Jack, Rowland M. Shortcomings in pharmacokinetic analysis by conceiving the body to exhibit properties of a single compartment. *J Pharm Sci* 1968;57:117.
5. Rowland M, Benet LZ, Graham GG. Clearance concept in pharmacokinetics. *J Pharmacokinet Biopharm* 1973;1:123.
6. Wagner G. *Clinical Pharmacokinetics.* Hamilton, IL: Drug Intelligence, 1975:57.

CHAPTER 7

LINEAR ONE-COMPARTMENT MODEL WITH ZERO-ORDER INPUT AND FIRST-ORDER OUTPUT

Motions seems to be continuous, and the first thing discerned in the continuous is the infinite. That is why those who define the continuous often turn out to be relying on the account of the infinite as well, since they assume that what is infinitely divisible is continuous.

ARISTOTLE (BOOK III—PHYSICS)

OBJECTIVES

■ To review the general principles of steady state.

■ To develop the equations of the model based on the plasma concentration of unchanged drug.

■ To demonstrate the practical aspects of the model.

■ To demonstrate the differences between intravenous bolus injection and continuous infusion.

■ To review the effect of inaccuracies of the rate of infusion on the plasma concentration and biological disturbances.

7.1 INTRODUCTION

The assumptions of the model in this chapter are the same as discussed in Chapters 2 and 6. The input, however, into the compartment, contrary to the instantaneous bolus injection, is constant and continuous. This model can be used for various applications:

■ Zero-order absorption of drugs from any site such as the gastrointestinal tract.

■ Intravenous infusion of drugs given by infusion pump or intravenous drip.

■ Direct and constant rate of input into the systemic circulation by implanted delivery devices.

Among these applications the intravenous infusion of drugs and fluids has become an important part of treatment in hospitals, ambulatory infusion centers, home infusion therapies, home tele-infusion and telecare industries, and so on.

The intravenous infusion is used often for one or more of the following reasons:

■ To ensure a constant supply of drug such that the drug accumulates in the body and ultimately reaches a constant steady-state level within the therapeutic range.
■ To achieve a consistent pharmacologic response and therapeutic outcome over a period. For drugs with a narrow therapeutic range and short half-life, the intravenous infusion is considered the method of choice for administration.
■ To avoid certain side effects associated with bolus injection, such as precipitation or crystallization of drug at the site of administration and speed shock. The objective here is no longer to achieve the steady-state level but, rather, to deliver the drug safely.
■ To avoid fluctuations of plasma concentration caused by the multiple dosing regimen.
■ To determine an accurate assessment of the total body clearance of drugs.

EXAMPLES OF THE APPLICATION OF CONTINUOUS INFUSION
■ Total parenteral nutrition (TPN) or peripheral parenteral nutrition (PPN) therapy.
■ Antineoplastic therapy.
■ Pain management.
■ Chelation therapy (eg, removal of high levels of aluminum from the plasma of patients on dialysis).
■ Chemotherapy with low-therapeutic-index drugs.
■ Antiinfective infusion therapy in geriatric patients.
■ Lifetime immunosuppressive therapy.
■ Hydration therapy.
■ Adjunctive therapies (eg, simultaneous intravenous therapy with antiemetic, antidiarrheal, anticonvulsant, and antiinflammatory agents in AIDS patients to control the symptoms of disease and/or the side effects of medications.

7.2 RATE EQUATIONS OF THE MODEL

A diagram of the model is presented in Figure 7.1. Drug is introduced into the systemic circulation by a constant zero-order rate of input with units of mass/time. The administered drug is then eliminated from the body by first-order elimination at a rate that depends on the amount or concentration of the drug in the body. At the start, the amount of drug in the compartment is low and consequently the rate of elimination is lower than the rate of input ($k_0 > KA$). As the administration of drug continues the amount in the body

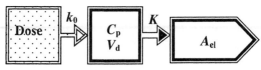

FIGURE 7.1 One-compartment open model with zero-order input (k_0) and first-order elimination ($K \times C_p \times V_d$).

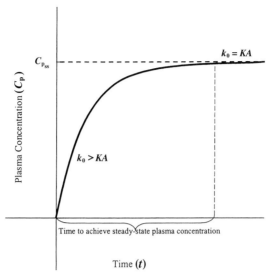

FIGURE 7.2 Plasma concentration–time profile of an intravenously infused drug over a period long enough to attain the steady-state plasma concentration ($C_{p_{ss}}$).

increases gradually and the rate of elimination increases accordingly. As the rate of output cannot exceed the rate of input these rates eventually become equal; that is the total amount introduced into the body per unit of time is equal to the total amount eliminated from the body by all routes of elimination per unit of time. Therefore, the amount or concentration of drug in the body remains constant. This plateau concentration is the steady-state level and represents the maximum accumulation of drug in the body that can be achieved with the selected zero-order rate of input (Figure 7.2).

The steady-state level remains constant as long as we continue with the same rate of infusion. The following differential equation defines the rate of change or rate of accumulation of drug in the body during a single infusion with constant rate:

$$dA/dt = \text{rate of input } (k_0) - \text{rate of output } (KA)$$

$$dA/dt = k_0 - KA \qquad (7.1)$$

Equation 7.1 can also be written as

$$dA/dt = k_0 - (Cl_t \times C_p)$$

Because at steady state there is no change in plasma concentration and accumulation of drug in the body remains constant, the rate of change in concentration as presented in Equation 7.1 would be equal to zero and rate of input = rate of output.

$$dA/dt = 0 \qquad (7.2)$$

Therefore,

$$k_0 = KA$$

7.3 INTEGRATED EQUATIONS OF THE MODEL

The integrated form of Equation 7.1 using the Laplace transform and Table 1.7 (conversion 11) is

$$A = \frac{k_0}{K} (1 - e^{-Kt})$$ (7.3)

A is the amount in the body at time t, k_0 is the zero-order rate of infusion, and K is the overall elimination rate constant. In terms of plasma concentration,

$$C_p = \frac{k_0}{KV_d} (1 - e^{-Kt})$$ (7.4)

As infusion proceeds, t becomes larger, e^{-Kt} becomes negligible, and plasma concentration is converted into a constant that is equal to the plateau or steady-state level.

$$C_{p_{ss}} = \frac{k_0}{Cl_t}$$ (7.5)

Equation 7.5 indicates that the steady-state level is directly proportional to the rate of infusion and inversely proportional to the total body clearance or half-life of a drug. It also confirms that at steady state the rate of input, k_0, is equal to the rate of output, $Cl_t \times C_{p_{ss}}$. Substitution of Equation 7.5 into Equation 7.4 yields the relationship

$$C_p = C_{p_{ss}}(1 - e^{-Kt})$$ (7.6)

or

$$C_p = C_{p_{ss}}(1 - (1/2)^{t/T_{1/2}})$$ (7.7)

where t is the time of infusion.

Equation 7.5 is also useful in estimating the total body clearance:

$$Cl_t = k_0/C_{p_{ss}}$$

The zero-order infusion rate is determined either by dividing the total amount intended for infusion by the interval of infusion, that is,

$$k_0 = dA/dt = \text{mass/time}$$

or by multiplying the desired target concentration of steady state by the total body clearance, that is,

$$k_0 = C_{p_{ss}} \times Cl_t$$

7.4 REQUIRED TIME FOR ACHIEVING STEADY-STATE CONCENTRATION

According to Equation 7.7, at $t = 0$, C_p is equal to zero. (*Note:* Any number raised to the power of zero would be equal to one.) When the time of infusion is equal to one half-life of the drug (ie, $t = T_{1/2}$) the plasma concentration is at 50% of the targeted steady-state level. If the time of infusion is twice the half-life (ie, $t = 2T_{1/2}$) the plasma concentration is 75% of the steady-state level. At $3.3T_{1/2}$, $C_p = 90\%$ of C_{pss}; at $4.3T_{1/2}$, $C_p = 95\%$ of C_{pss}; and at $6.6T_{1/2}$, $C_p = 99\%$ of C_{pss}. The reverse of this concept is also useful. For example, if the ratio C_{p_t}/C_{pss} is 0.75, the time of infusion is twice the half-life:

$$f_{ss} = \frac{C_{p_t}}{C_{pss}} = (1 - e^{-Kt}) \qquad (7.8)$$

In Equation 7.8, 1 represents 100% of steady-state level, e^{-Kt} is the fraction left to reach the steady-state level, and $1 - e^{-Kt}$ (ie, f_{ss}) is the fraction of steady-state level (Figure 7.3).

In clinical practice after infusion of a drug for about four to five half-lives it is assumed that the steady-state level has been achieved. This is a practical assumption because 95 to 97% of the steady-state level is close enough to be considered 100%. In this chapter, however, for Applications and Assignments, we assume that seven half-lives are needed to achieve approximately 99 to 100% of a targeted steady-state level.

If the duration of an infusion is less than seven half-lives of a drug, the plasma concentration at any time during the infusion can be estimated by using Equation 7.4, 7.6, or 7.7. When the duration of infusion reaches seven half-lives of the drug, a steady-state level is achieved. The magnitude of the steady-state level depends on the rate of infu-

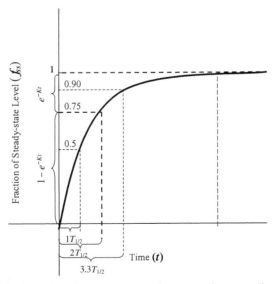

FIGURE 7.3 Plot of fraction of steady-state concentration versus time according to Equation 7.8. For example, when the fraction remaining to reach to steady state (ie, e^{-Kt}) is equal to 0.25 or 0.1, the fraction of steady state (ie, $1 - e^{-Kt}$) is 0.75 or 0.9, respectively, representing 75 and 90% of C_{pss}.

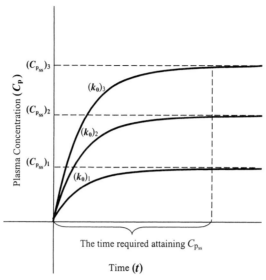

FIGURE 7.4 The magnitude of steady-state concentration depends on the zero-order rate of infusion; that is, for $(k_0)_3 > (k_0)_2 > (k_0)_1$ we attain plasma concentrations that are $(C_{p_{ss}})_3 > (C_{p_{ss}})_2 > (Cp_{ss})_1$. The time required for attaining these plateau levels, however, would remain the same.

sion; however, the time required to achieve any level of steady state with any rate of infusion depends only on the half-life of the drug. In other words, by increasing the rate of infusion we do not reduce the time needed to achieve the steady state level; we only form a new steady-state level that would require the same length of time to be reached (Figure 7.4).

Consider the following equation that defines the plasma concentration at steady state and is derived from Equation 7.5:

$$C_{p_{ss}} = \frac{k_0}{KV_d} = \frac{1.44 T_{1/2} k_0}{V_d} \tag{7.9}$$

In Equation 7.9, as K or $T_{1/2}$ and V_d are constant, the steady-state plasma concentration is proportional only to k_0. In disease states, however, when the half-life is longer or K is smaller, if treatment of a patient is continued at a rate that is designed for normal patients, a higher steady-state level is achieved.

7.5 SIMULTANEOUS INTRAVENOUS BOLUS AND INTRAVENOUS INFUSION

One approach to reaching the steady-state level of a drug immediately is to give a loading intravenous bolus dose with simultaneous intravenous infusion. To determine the

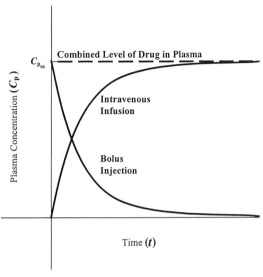

FIGURE 7.5 Simultaneous intravenous bolus injection (ie, loading dose equal to $C_{p_{ss}}V_d$) and intravenous infusion (ie, maintenance dose $= C_{p_{ss}}Cl_t$) produce the desired steady-state plasma level immediately.

loading dose we assume the steady-state level is equal to the initial plasma concentration of the loading dose; that is, set $C_{p_{ss}} = C_p^0$. The loading dose is equal to

$$D_L = V_d C_{p_{ss}} \tag{7.10}$$

The combination of intravenous bolus and infusion can be represented as

$$C_{p_{total}} = C_{p_{ss}}e^{-Kt} + C_{p_{ss}}(1 - e^{-Kt}) = C_{p_{ss}} \tag{7.11}$$

Therefore, when a drug follows a one-compartment model this combination provides an immediate steady-state level (Figure 7.5).

7.6 PLASMA CONCENTRATION AFTER TERMINATION OF INFUSION

The plasma concentration of a drug after discontinuation of infusion would decline exponentially, similar to that of an intravenous bolus injection. The appropriate equation for estimation of plasma concentration after the end of infusion is

$$C_{p_{t'}} = [C_{p_{ss}}(1 - e^{-Kt_{inf}})]e^{-Kt'} \tag{7.12}$$

$$C_{p_{t'}} = C_{p_{end}}e^{-Kt} \tag{7.13}$$

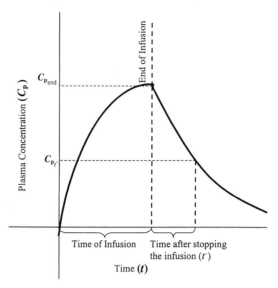

FIGURE 7.6 Profile of plasma concentration–time curve after stopping the infusion, t' represents any time point after the end of infusion.

where t' is any time after the termination of infusion and t_{inf} is the period of infusion (Figure 7.6).

Similarly if the infusion is discontinued after the steady-state level is reached, the plasma concentration at any time t' after the termination of infusion is calculated as

$$C_{p_{t'}} = C_{p_{ss}} e^{-Kt'} \tag{7.13}$$

7.7 CONSECUTIVE FAST INFUSION FOLLOWED BY SLOW INFUSION

There are circumstances in which administration of an intravenous bolus loading dose for reasons such as speed shock or precipitation and/or crystallization of drug at the site of injection may not be possible. In such circumstances the loading dose is given by fast infusion to achieve accumulation of a specific amount of drug in the body, followed by a slower infusion to maintain the level of the drug. It is important to remember that any change in the rate of infusion has a direct influence on the plasma concentration of the drug. Thus, terminating one infusion at one rate and starting a second infusion at a different rate at the time of discontinuation of the first infusion create a temporary fluctuation in plasma concentration (Figure 7.7). The equation of plasma concentration of the combined infusions is

$$C_{p_{total}} = C_{p_{end}} e^{-Kt'} + \frac{k_{0_{slow}}}{Cl_t} (1 - e^{-Kt'}) \tag{7.14}$$

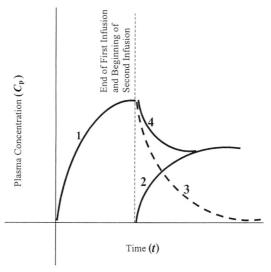

FIGURE 7.7 Theoretical profile of plasma concentration of a drug following administration of a fast infusion followed by slow infusion. Curves 1 and 2 represent the plasma concentration–time of fast and slow infusions, respectively. Curve 3 is the decline in plasma concentration of the fast infusion after starting the second infusion, and curve 4 is the combined concentration of fast and slow infusions.

As t' increases, $e^{-Kt'}$ approaches zero and $C_{p_{total}}$ becomes the steady-state concentration of the slow infusion:

$$C_{p_{total}} = \frac{k_{0_{slow}}}{Cl_t} \qquad (7.15)$$

7.8 DURATION OF ACTION

Duration of action of a drug during an infusion is the time that the plasma concentration is above the minimum effective concentration. If an infusion is initiated without a loading dose the interval during which the concentration is below the therapeutic range should be subtracted from the duration of infusion. This interval can be identified as the time to onset of action (t_{onset}). In addition, after termination of infusion the plasma concentration may remain above the minimum effective concentration for some time. This postinfusion period (t_{post}) should be added to the duration of action of infusion. The following stepwise calculations may be used to determine the duration of action of a drug during infusion.

Step 1 Define the minimum effective concentration in terms of fraction of steady-state plasma concentration.

$$(f_{ss})_{MEC} = \frac{C_{p_{MEC}}}{C_{p_{ss}}} \qquad (7.16)$$

Step 2 Determine the time to onset of action by presenting Equation 7.8 as

$$t_{\text{onset}} = \frac{\ln(1 - f_{\text{ss}})}{K} \qquad (7.17)$$

Step 3 Subtract t_{onset} from the time of infusion to determine the interval in which the concentration is above the minimum effective level while the infusion is running.

$$(t_d)_{\text{infusion}} = t_{\text{infusion}} - t_{\text{onset}} \qquad (7.18)$$

Step 4 Determine the time, after discontinuation of infusion, that the plasma concentration of drug remains above the minimum effective level.

$$t_{\text{post}} = \frac{2.303}{K} \log \frac{C_{\text{p}_{\text{ss}}}}{C_{\text{p}_{\text{MEC}}}} \qquad (7.19)$$

or

$$t_{\text{post}} = \frac{2.303}{K} \log \frac{C_{\text{p}_{\text{end}}}}{C_{\text{p}_{\text{MEC}}}} \qquad (7.20)$$

Step 5 Calculate the actual duration of action:

$$t_d = (t_d)_{\text{infusion}} + t_{\text{post}} \qquad (7.21)$$

When the loading dose is given simultaneously with infusion the time to onset of action is zero ($t_{\text{onset}} = 0$).

APPLICATION

7.1 A 20-year-old male patient with ideal body weight of 60 kg is receiving 950 mg of a cephalosporin infused intravenously over 15 minutes. The half-life of the drug is 45 minutes and the apparent volume of distribution is 0.8 L/kg. Calculate the following:

1. Rate of infusion

$$\text{rate of input} = k_0 = dA/dt$$

$$k_0 = 950 \text{ mg/15 min} = 63.3 \text{ mg/min} = 3800 \text{ mg/h} = 3.8 \text{ g/h}$$

2. If the drug were supplied in 100-mL solution with a concentration of 10 mg/mL, at what rate in milliliters per hour (volume/time) would you infuse the solution for 15 minutes to obtain an infusion rate of 3.8 g/h (mass/time)?

$$\text{rate(volume/time)} = \text{rate(mass/time)/concentration(mass/volume)}$$

$$\text{rate (volume/time)} = (3800 \text{ mg/h})/(10 \text{ mg/mL}) = 6.34 \text{ ml/min}$$

(Note: 6.34 ml/min $\times$ 15 min $\times$ 10 mg/ml = 950 mg)

3. Plasma concentration at the end of 15-minute infusion

$$V_d = (0.8)(60) = 48 \text{ L}$$

$$K = 0.693/0.75 \text{ h} = 0.924 \text{ h}^{-1} = 0.0154 \text{ min}^{-1}$$

$$C_{p_{15 \text{ min}}} = \frac{3800 \text{ mg/h}}{0.924 \text{ h}^{-1} \times 48 \text{ L}} (1 - e^{-0.0154 \times 15}) = 17.633 \text{ mg/L}$$

4. Total amount of drug in the body at the end of 15-minute infusion

$$A_{15} = (17.633 \text{ mg/L})(48 \text{ L}) = 846.384 \text{ mg}$$

5. Total amount of drug eliminated during the 15-minute infusion

$$A_{\text{eliminated}} = 950 - 846.384 = 103.616 = 104 \text{ mg}$$

6. Peak plasma concentration if the dose is administered as an intravenous bolus:

$$C_p^0 = 950/48 = 19.8 \text{ mg/L}$$

Note that the total amount eliminated during the infusion can also be calculated as

$$(19.8 - 17.633) V_d = 104 \text{ mg}$$

7. If the minimum effective concentration of the drug is 10 mg/L, would the plasma concentration 5 minutes after the start of infusion be therapeutically effective?

$$C_{p_{5 \text{ min}}} = \frac{3800 \text{ mg/h}}{0.924 \text{ h}^{-1} \times 48 \text{ L}} (1 - e^{-0.0154 \text{ min}^{-1} \times 5 \text{ min}}) = 6.35 \text{ mg/L}$$

Answer: NO.

8. Steady-state plasma concentration that can be achieved with the rate calculated in part 1

$$Cl_t = (0.924)(48) = 44.35 \text{ L/h}$$

$$C_{p_{ss}} = (3800 \text{ mg/h})/(44.35 \text{ L/h}) = 85.7 \text{ mg/L}$$

9. Rate for a single infusion to achieve a plateau concentration of 150 mg/L for the drug

$$k_0 = (150 \text{ mg/L})(44.35 \text{ L/h})$$

$$k_0 = 6652.5 \text{ mg/h} = 6.65 \text{ g/h}$$

10. Rate of elimination of the drug after achieving the steady-state level of part 9

$$\text{rate of elimination at steady state} = C_{p_{ss}}Cl_t = KA_{ss} = k_0$$

That is,

$$\text{rate of input} = \text{rate of output}$$

Therefore,

$$C_{p_{ss}} \times Cl_t = 6.65 \text{ g/h} = k_0$$

11. Time required to reach 90% of the steady-state plasma concentration of 85.7 mg/L or 150 mg/L:

$$(T_{95\%})C_{p_{ss}} = 3.3T_{1/2} = 3.3 \times 0.75 \text{ h} = 2.475 \text{ h}$$

12. Bolus loading dose and zero-order maintenance dose to attain and maintain plateau concentration of 10 mg/L

$$D_L = 10 \text{ mg/L} \times 48 \text{ L} = 480 \text{ mg} \cong 0.5 \text{ g}$$

$$k_0 = 0.924 \text{ h}^{-1} \times 48 \text{ L} \times 10 \text{ mg/L} = 443.52 \text{ mg/h}$$

7.2 A 40-year-old female patient with ideal body weight of 70 kg and complicated urinary tract infection is to be treated with 1 gram of a third-generation cephalosporin infused over 1 hour, given every 8 hours for 10 consecutive days. The half-life of the drug is 2 hours and the total body clearance is 110 mL/min.

1. If we start the first infusion at 8:00 AM and stop at 9.00 AM what would be the plasma concentration of the drug at 1:00 PM?

$$k_0 = 1000 \text{ mg/h}$$

$$Cl_t = 110 \text{ mL/min} = 6.6 \text{ L/h}$$

$$C_{p_{9 \text{ AM}}} = \frac{1000 \text{ mg/h}}{6.6 \text{ L/h}} (1 - e^{-0.3465 \text{ h}^{-1} \times 1 \text{ h}}) = 44.37 \text{ mg/L}$$

$$C_{p_{1 \text{ PM}}} = 44.37e^{-0.3465 \text{ h}^{-1}(4h)} = 11.1 \text{ mg/L}$$

or

$$4h = 2T_{1/2}$$

Therefore,

$$C_{p_{1\ PM}} = 0.25 \times 44.37 = 11.1 \text{ mg/L}$$

2. What would be the plasma concentration just before the second infusion at 4:00 PM?

$$C_{p_{4\ PM}} = 44.37e^{-0.3465 \text{ h}^{-1} \times 7 \text{ h}} = 3.92 \text{ mg/L}$$

or

$$C_{p_{4\ PM}} = 11.1e^{-0.3465 \text{ h}^{-1} \times 3 \text{ h}} = 3.92 \text{ mg/L}$$

3. What would be the total amount in the body at the end of the second infusion (ie, 5 PM)?

$$C_{p_{5\ PM}} = 44.37 \text{ mg/L} + 3.92e^{-0.3465 \text{ h}^{-1} \times 1 \text{ h}} = 47.14 \text{ mg/L}$$

$$\text{total amount} = 47.14 \text{ mg/L}(6.6 \text{ L/h})/0.3465 \text{ h}^{-1} = 897.9 \text{ mg}$$

ASSIGNMENT

7.1 Three grams of ticarcillin and 100 mg of clavulanic acid, a potent inhibitor of β-lactamase, were reconstituted in 100 mL of sterile water for injection. The solution was infused over 30 minutes to a male patient with ideal body weight of 70 kg. The pharmacokinetic data of the two drugs are summarized in Table 7.1. Calculate the following:

7.1.1 Plasma concentration of ticarcillin at the end of the 30-minute infusion.
7.1.2 Plasma level of clavulanic acid at the end of the 30-minute infusion.
7.1.3 Plasma level of ticarcillin 140 minutes after termination of the infusion.
7.1.4 Plasma concentration of clavulanic acid 1 hour after termination of the infusion.
7.1.5 Volume of distribution of clavulanic acid.
7.1.6 Total amount of ticarcillin eliminated during the 30-minute infusion.
7.1.7 Metabolic clearance of clavulanic acid.
7.1.8 Duration of action if the minimum inhibitory concentration of ticarcillin is 60 mg/L.

7.2 Continuous intravenous infusion of a potent analgesic is recommended for a patient with inoperable colon cancer and a body weight of 110 pounds. The dose is prepared by

TABLE 7.1 Data Related to Assignment 7.1

Constant	Units	Ticarcillin	Clavulanic Acid
Total body clearance	mL/min	100	200
Renal clearance	mL/min	80	100
Half-life	min	70	60

dissolving 200 mg of the drug in 500 mL of 5% dextrose in water. The solution is infused over 24 hours. The drug has a half-life of 2 hours and an apparent volume of distribution of 3 L/kg. Calculate the following:

    7.2.1 Plasma concentration 20 hours after the start of therapy.

    7.2.2 Rate of infusion in milliliters per minute.

    7.2.3 Plasma concentration 6 hours after the start of infusion.

    7.2.4 Rate of elimination at $t = 21$ hours.

    7.2.5 Total amount of drug in the body 15 hours after the start of infusion.

    7.2.6 Loading dose.

7.3 The therapeutic plasma concentration of a drug is 4 to 15 mg/L. You have decided to attain a target concentration of 10 mg/L immediately and maintain this concentration over 12 hours. The drug has a half-life of 6 hours with renal and metabolic clearances of 5 and 6.55 L/h, respectively. The patient has an ideal body weight of 65 kg.

    7.3.1 Calculate the loading dose (bolus) and maintenance dose (rate of infusion in units of mass/time).

    7.3.2 Calculate the volume and concentration of the infusion solution (maintenance dose) if the rate of input is decided at 1 mL/min.

    7.3.3 Calculate the time taken to reach the 5 mg/L level.

    7.3.4 Calculate the time needed to reach 80% of the steady-state plasma concentration.

    7.3.5 Plasma concentrations 1, 6, and 12 hours after the infusion was stopped at the plateau level of 10 mg/L.

    7.3.6 If the patient develops acute renal failure and the renal clearance is reduced to 2 L/h, what bolus loading dose and maintenance infusion rate would you recommend to achieve the steady-state level of 10 mg/L? Assume metabolic clearance and the apparent volume of distribution remain constant.

7.4 A 40-year old, 80-kg, hospitalized urology patient suffering from painful urination demonstrates symptoms consistent with urinary tract infection. The infection was confirmed by the presence of bacteria in urine, an alkaline urinary pH, and epithelial cells. An antibiotic was recommended with following characteristics: half-life of elimination = 1 hour, apparent volume of distribution = 0.3 L/kg. The first dose (4 g in 50 mL of 5% glucose) was infused at 6:00 AM and ended at 6:30 AM. The second dose was infused at 12:00 noon and ended at 12:30 PM. The therapy continued with four short infusions around the clock every 6 hours for 3 days. Determine the following for the first day of therapy:

    7.4.1 Plasma concentration at 6:30 AM.

    7.4.2 Plasma concentration at 12:00 noon.

    7.4.3 Total amount in the body at 12:00 noon.

    7.4.4 Total amount in the body at 12:30 PM.

7.5 If the total amount of a drug infused over 1 hour were 1000 mg and the plasma concentration at the end of infusion were 50 mg/L, what would be the total amount eliminated during the infusion if the apparent volume of distribution of the drug is 15 L?

7.6 If 1200 mg of a drug were diluted in 500 mL normal saline and infused over 10 hours, what would be the rate of infusion in milliliters per minute?

7.7 If the desired steady-state plasma concentration of a drug is 20 mg/L, its total body clearance is 10 L/h, and its half-life is 2 hours, what is the plasma concentration 4 hours after the start of infusion?

7.8 If the steady-state plasma concentration of 25 mg/L for a drug were achieved with an infusion rate of 10 mg/h, what would be the steady state level with an infusion rate of 30 mg/h for the same drug?

7.9 If an infusion rate of 20 mg/h has achieved a steady-state plasma concentration of 10 mg/L, what is the rate of elimination at steady state?

7.10 A female patient (70 years old, 176 pounds) is receiving 500 mg of a low-therapeutic-index drug to control cardiac arrythmia. The drug is scheduled for 1-hour infusion q.i.d. for 3 consecutive days. On the first day of treatment the first infusion started at 6:00 AM and ended at 7:00 AM. The second infusion started at 12:00 noon and ended at 1:00 PM. The third and fourth infusions were carried out at 6:00 to 7:00 PM and 12:00 to 1:00 AM. The drug is known to have a half-life of 90 minutes, an apparent volume of distribution of 40% body weight, and a therapeutic range of 10 to 20 mg/L. Calculate the following:

   7.10.1 Plasma concentration at 7 AM.

   7.10.2 Plasma concentration at 12 noon.

   7.10.3 Plasma concentration at 1:00 PM.

   7.10.4 Loading dose and maintenance dose if it is desired to achieve and maintain a steady-state plasma concentration of 15 mg/L for 3 days.

ASSIGNMENT (EXTRA CREDIT)

EC-7.1 Prepare a brief summary of the following article:

Sultan E, Richard C, Pezzano M, Auzepy P, Singlas E. Pharmacokinetics of pefloxacin and amikacin administered simultaneously to intensive care patients. *Eur J Clin Pharmacol* 1988;43:637–43.

- Calculate the rate of infusion of amikacin.
- Calculate the plasma concentration at the end of the first infusion.
- Calculate the plasma concentration before the start of the second infusion.
- Calculate the total amount eliminated during the first infusion.
- Explain why the difference between accumulation indexes of the first and last infusions is as low as 0.2.
- Recommend a single infusion rate to achieve a steady-state level equal to the plasma concentration of the end of the first infusion.

BIBLIOGRAPHY

1. Chiou WL, Gadalla MA, Peng GW. Method for the rapid estimation of the total body drug clearance and adjustment of dosage regimen in patients during a constant-rate intravenous infusion. *J Pharmacokinet Biopharm* 1978;6:135.

2. Gibaldi M, Perrier D. *Pharmacokinetics.* 2nd ed. New York: Marcel Dekker, 1982:63.

3. Krüger-Thiemer E. Continuous intravenous infusion and multicompartment accumulation. *Eur J Pharmacol* 1968;4:317.

4. Loo JCL, Riegelman S. Assessment of pharmacokinetic constants from postinfusion blood curves obtained after i.v. infusion. *J Pharm Sci* 1970;59:53.

5. Raymond K, Morgan DJ. The effect of infusion time on the time course of drug concentration in blood. *J Pharmacokinet Biopharm* 1980;8:573.

6. Rescigno A, Seger G. *Drug and Tracer Kinetics.* Waltham, MA: Blaisdell, 1966:86.

7. Rowland M, Tozer TN. *Clinical Pharmacokinetics.* 3rd ed. Media, PA: Williams & Wilkins, 1994:66.

8. Tsuei SE, Nation R, Thomas J. Design of infusion regimens to achieve and maintain a predetermined plasma level range. *Clin Pharmacol Ther* 1980;28:289.

9. Sawchuck RJ, Zaske DE. Pharmacokinetics of dosing regimens which utilize multiple intravenous infusion: gentamicin in burn patients. *J Pharmacokinet Biopharm* 1976;4:1983.

10. Wagner JG. Clinical Pharmacokinetics. Hamilton, IL: Drug Intelligence, 1975:97.

CHAPTER 8

LINEAR ONE-COMPARTMENT MODEL WITH FIRST-ORDER INPUT AND FIRST-ORDER OUTPUT

In every sort of study and line of inquiry, more humble and more honorable alike, there appear to be two sorts of competence. One of these is rightly called scientific knowledge of the subject, and the other is a certain type of education; for it is characteristic of an educated person to be able to reach to a judgment based on a sound estimate of what people expound their conclusion in the right or wrong way.
ARISTOTLE (BOOK I—PARTS OR ANIMALS)

OBJECTIVES

- To discuss the pharmacokinetics of drugs given by extravascular routes of administration.
- To interpret the plasma concentration–time curves of drugs given orally or intramuscularly.
- To discuss various methods of determining the absorption rate constant.
- To estimate important parameters of oral absorption such as T_{max}, $C_{p_{max}}$, AUC, and fraction of dose absorbed.

8.1 INTRODUCTION

Drugs that are administered by extravascular routes must pass through a barrier to reach the systemic circulation. The barrier that separates a drug at its site of administration from the vascular system can be as complex as the gastrointestinal wall in oral absorption or as simple as the capillary wall in intramuscular, rectal, or sublingual administration. When the drug ultimately reaches the vascular system it is subjected to metabolism and excretion. Therefore, two biological processes of absorption and elimination influence the plasma concentration–time profile of a drug that is administered by an extravascular route.

8.2 FACTORS AFFECTING THE RATE OF ABSORPTION

The absorption from extravascular routes can be limited by a number of factors. These factors are studied more extensively for the oral route of administration affect the rate of absorption, the plasma concentration–time profile, and the area under the plasma concentration–time curve:

■ Physiochemical characteristics of drug molecule.
■ Formulation factors of dosage forms such as:
  —solutions, suspensions, syrups
  —solid dosage forms (capsule, tablet, controlled release, etc)
  —semisolid dosage forms
■ Physiochemical properties of the dosage form.
■ Degree of complexity of membrane.

8.2.1 Physiochemical Characteristics of Drug Molecule: Rule of Five

In addition to the physicochemical factors affecting the absorption of drugs that were discussed in Chapter 3, the following criteria known as the Rule of Five, are also recommended for prediction of absorption of new drugs. These criteria are used mostly by the pharmaceutical industry to screen new drug molecules during the discovery stage for selection of the best orally absorbed drug. This type of quick decision making or high-throughput screening methods for prediction of absorption of new drugs are economical and necessary to keep up with the output of the automated combinatorial chemistry.

   The physicochemical criteria that may influence the absorption of a drug molecule (Rule of Five) are:

■ Numbers of NH bonds and OH bonds in the molecule of a drug. These types of bonds reflect the hydrogen bond-donating ability of the molecule. If a drug molecule has fewer than five H-bond donors of types OH and NH collectively, the permeability of the drug is enhanced; if there are more than five H-bond donors, permeability is reduced.
■ Numbers of oxygen (Os) and nitrogen (Ns) groups in the molecule of a drug. These represent the hydrogen bond-accepting ability of the molecule. If a drug molecule has more than 10 H-bond acceptors of types Os and Ns altogether, the permeability of the molecule is retarded.
■ Molecular weight of a drug. If the molecular weight of a drug is above 500, the drug is less likely to permeate the barrier and be absorbed.
■ Logarithm of partition coefficient ($\log P$) of drug molecule, which corresponds to the logarithm of the equilibrium constant of a drug distribution between 1-octanol and water in a test tube. This parameter reflects the degree of lipid solubility of a drug. If $\log P$ exceeds 5, the permeability of the molecule is poor.

8.2.2 Types of Dosage Forms

In general, the rate of absorption of a drug is dependent on the availability of the drug at the site of absorption. If a drug were administered in solution, suspension, or emulsions, its absorption, under normal conditions, would be faster than if it were given in solid or semisolid dosage forms. The slower rate of release of drug from a solid dosage form slows down the rate of absorption and thus the release of drug from dosage form can become a rate-limiting factor for absorption.

8.2.3 Physiochemical Properties of Active and Inactive Ingredients of Dosage Form

Some important physicochemical characteristics affect the rate of absorption:

- Drug solubility controls the dissolution of solid dosage forms. The low aqueous solubility of a drug at the site of absorption reduces its rate of absorption and bioavailability. This type of absorption is known as solubility-limited absorption.
- Particle size affects the solubility and absorption of a drug. An increase in surface area of a dosage form enhances the wettability and, thus, the release and solubility of drug molecules.
- Salt formation is also an effective technique to increase drug solubility. As a general rule the solubility of salts is greater than that of free acids.
- Polymorphic forms of a drug may contribute to different aqueous solubilities and different rates of absorption. Crystal polymorphism is a common characteristic of a number of therapeutic agents such as novobiocin, methylprednisolone, phenylbutazone, and sulfathiazole. To achieve reproducibility in the absorption and bioavailability of these types of drugs, the same crystal form must always be selected for manufacture.
- State of hydration and solvation influence the solubility of a drug and the rate of absorption. In general, the anhydrous form of drugs is more soluble than the hydrated form (monohydrate, dihydrate, trihydrate, etc).
- Amorphicity as opposed to crystallinity also has an effect on the solubility of drugs. Normally, an amorphous drug is more soluble than the crystal form.

8.2.4 Formulation Factors

Manufacturing and formulation factors are also important in the solubility and absorption of a drug.

- Addition of an optimum amount of disintegrant with strong swelling capacity can facilitate the dissolution, solubility, and absorption of a drug.
- Selection of appropriate diluents, the inert fillers that are added to provide an acceptable size for a solid dosage form, is also important for the dissolution and solubility of drugs.
- Other manufacturing factors such as granulating agents, lubricants, surfactants, coloring agents, coating ingredients, methods of granulation, compression force, types of capsules and tablets, and factors related to polymeric delivery systems (eg, type of polymer and type of release) can influence the absorption and bioavailability of a drug.

8.2.5 Degree of Complexity of Membrane

As was discussed earlier in Chapter 3, although the absorption and onset of action of drugs administered by various extravascular routes are somewhat different, their most prominent underlying mechanism, namely, passive diffusion, is the same. The most complex among these routes is gastrointestinal administration. With the diversity of physiologic factors that affect the absorption of drugs such as pH, gastric emptying rate, intestinal motility, liver first-pass effect, active routes of absorption, and presence of Pgp and metabolic enzymes such as CYP3A, the GI route is the most interesting and extensively studied extravascular route.

In this chapter we consider the pharmacokinetics of an orally administered single dose of a drug. The equations, with minor modifications, may also be used to define the pharmacokinetics of drugs administered by other extravascular routes.

8.3 RATE EQUATIONS OF THE MODEL

A diagram of the model is presented in Figure 8.1. The assumptions of the model can be summarized as follows: The total dose of drug is administered orally as a single dose at time zero. The dose at the site of absorption is gradually absorbed into the systemic circulation, and declines exponentially with time. The driving force for transfer of drug from the GI tract to the systemic circulation is the concentration gradient. The transfer or absorption of drug is thus governed by passive diffusion and follows first-order kinetics. Therefore, the rate of absorption from the GI tract to the systemic circulation (rate of input) can be defined as

$$\text{rate of absorption} = k_a A_D$$

where k_a is the absorption rate constant and A_D is the absorbable amount of drug at the site of absorption. As both processes of absorption and elimination follow first-order kinetics, their rates are variable and a function of the amount. The rate of absorption is higher at the early time points when the amount of drug is larger at the site of absorption. The rate of elimination (rate of output), on the other hand, at the early time points, because of the smaller amount of drug in the body, is low and gradually increases as more drug is absorbed until a point is reached when the rate of elimination is equal to the rate

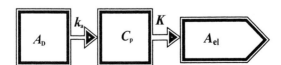

FIGURE 8.1 One-compartment open model with first-order absorption and first-order elimination. A_D represents the amount at the site of absorption, C_p is the plasma concentration of unchanged drug in the body, A_e is the amount of drug excreted unchanged, and k_a and K are the rate constants of absorption and elimination, respectively.

of absorption. The plasma concentration at that point, T_{max}, reaches its maximum, $C_{p_{max}}$. Thus, at T_{max},

$$Cl_t\, C_{p_{max}} = k_a A_D$$

After T_{max}, the rate of elimination gradually becomes greater than the rate of absorption until no more drug is absorbed. The time required for the absorption of drug to be completed is approximately equal to $7(T_{1/2})_{k_a}$. After completion of absorption the terminal portion of the plasma concentration–time curve is a function of only the elimination process. The combination of the changing rates of input and output influences the shape of the plasma concentration–time curve, which, as presented in Figure 8.2, resembles a skewed bell-shaped curve. Hence, the rate of change of plasma concentration of a drug can be written as

$$\text{rate of change of plasma concentration} = \text{rate of absorption} - \text{rate of elimination} \quad (8.1)$$

that is,

$$\frac{dA}{dt} = k_a A_D - KA \quad (8.2)$$

At maximum plasma concentration, the rates are equal and the rate of change of drug concentration in plasma is zero.

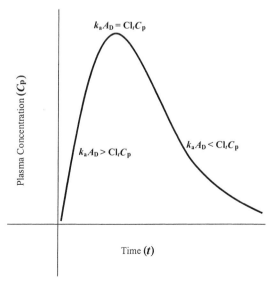

FIGURE 8.2 Profile of the plasma concentration–time curve of an orally administered dose. The changes in the rate of absorption ($k_a A_D$) and elimination ($Cl_t C_p$, or KA) throughout the absorption process contribute to the formation of the skewed bell-shaped curve representing the rise and fall of plasma concentration.

8.4 Integrated Equations of the Model

The integration of Equation 8.2 by Laplace transform, as was developed in Chapter 1 (Equation 1.38), yields the relationship

$$A = \frac{(A_D{}^0)(k_a)}{K - k_a} (e^{-Kt} - e^{-k_a t})$$

where A is the amount of drug in the body at time t, and $A_D{}^0$ represents the total amount of absorbable drug at the site of absorption at $t = 0$. In oral absorption, because of the many factors discussed earlier in this chapter, only a portion of the administered dose may reach the systemic circulation. Thus, it would be more realistic to use the total amount absorbed, FD, in the equation rather than the administered dose. F corresponds to the fraction of dose absorbed, a value that is equal to or less than one, and is known as *absolute bioavailability*, and the product FD represents the total amount absorbed or total amount of absorbable drug.

Equation 1.38 can be presented in terms of plasma concentration, which is the mathematical relationship for the one-compartment model with first-order input and first-order output:

$$C_p = \frac{FDk_a}{V_d(k_a - K)} (e^{-Kt} - e^{-k_a t}) \tag{8.3}$$

The equation represents the two biological processes of absorption and elimination:

$$C_p = \underbrace{\frac{FDk_a}{V_d(k_a - K)} e^{-Kt}}_{\text{elimination}} - \underbrace{\frac{FDk_a}{V_d(k_a - K)} e^{-k_a t}}_{\text{absorption}}$$

Equation 8.3 also indicates that plot of log C_p versus time, t, will have a linear terminal portion, as shown in Figure 8.3. The slope of this linear portion is a function of the smallest rate constant.

- When $k_a > K$, the slope of the terminal portion of the curve is equal to $-2.303/K$. The majority of drugs fall into this category and follow Equation 8.3.
- When $K > k_a$, the slope of the terminal linear segment of the curve equals $-k_a/2.303$ and the equation is modified to

$$C_p = \frac{FDk_a}{V_d(K - k_a)} (e^{-k_a t} - e^{-Kt}) \tag{8.4}$$

- When the two rate constants are equal ($K = k_a$), Equations 8.3 and 8.4 do not apply and it would be difficult to demarcate a terminal linear slope from the logarithmic plot. Under this condition, the appropriate equation for plasma concentration is

$$C_p = \frac{\lambda FD}{V_d} t e^{-\lambda t} \tag{8.5}$$

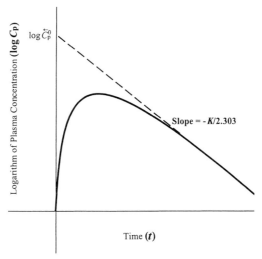

FIGURE 8.3 A plot of logarithm of plasma concentration versus time according to Equation 8.3, assuming that $k_a > K$, yields a curve with a linear terminal portion with slope of $-K/2.303$.

where $\lambda = K = k_a$ and the logarithmic form of the equation is

$$\log C_p = \log \frac{\lambda F D}{V_d} + \log t - \frac{\lambda t}{2.303} \qquad (8.6)$$

An absorption rate constant significantly greater than the elimination rate constant (ie, $k_a > K$) would indicate that the absorption is very fast and the plasma concentration–time curve may resemble that for an intravenous bolus injection. Under this condition $e^{-k_a t}$ would approach zero, K would become negligible in comparison to k_a, and the relationship would be simplified to

$$C_p = \frac{F D}{V_d} (e^{-K t}) \qquad (8.7)$$

8.5 CALCULATION OF INITIAL ESTIMATES OF K and k_a

Commercially available pharmacokinetic software packages can be used to determine more accurate values of K and k_a. Discussion of the use of these packages is beyond the scope of this textbook; however, the Sections 8.5.1 and 8.5.2 present some of the classic methods of determination of initial estimates of the rate constants of elimination and absorption under the assumption $k_a > K$.

8.5.1 Estimation of Overall Elimination Rate Constant, K

When the measurements of plasma concentration of a drug following oral administration at different time points are presented as ideal data (ie, a hypothetical set of data with no random error), the slope of the linear terminal portion can be determined by using the last two data points in the slope relationship:

$$\text{slope} = \frac{\log C_{p_{n-1}} - \log C_{p_n}}{t_{n-1} - t_n} = -\frac{K}{2.303} \tag{8.8}$$

Therefore

$$K = 2.303 \times \text{slope} \tag{8.9}$$

In Equation 8.8, n corresponds to the last data point and $n - 1$ to the data point before the last one. Extrapolating the linear terminal portion of the curve with the slope calculated by Equation 8.8 to the y axis gives the y intercept of this extrapolated line, which is identified as $\overleftarrow{C}_p^0$. The extrapolated line with the slope $-K/2.303$ and y intercept $\overleftarrow{C}_p^0$ represents the elimination component of Equation 8.3 (Figure 8.3). The y intercept, $\overleftarrow{C}_p^0$, which is equal to the coefficient of Equation 8.3, can be estimated for an ideal set of data as

$$\overleftarrow{C}_p^0 = \frac{C_{p_n}}{e^{-Kt_n}} = \frac{FDk_a}{V_d(k_a - K)} \tag{8.10}$$

Therefore, the equation of the extrapolated line is

$$\overleftarrow{C}_p = \overleftarrow{C}_p^0 e^{-Kt} \quad \text{or} \quad \log \overleftarrow{C}_p = \log \overleftarrow{C}_p^0 - \frac{Kt}{2.303} \tag{8.11}$$

When the plasma concentrations are presented as real data (usually scattered due to the presence of random error), a better estimate of K is made by using regression analysis on the last data points located on the linear terminal portion of the curve. The y intercept and slope are then determined as described in Chapter 1 Section 1.5,

$$\text{slope} = \frac{\sum dxdy}{\sum dx^2} = -\frac{K}{2.303} \tag{8.12}$$

where $x = t$ and $y = \log C_p$

By substituting the numerical value of slope and mean values of the variables x and y in the following equation, the y intercept, $\overleftarrow{C}_p^0$, can be estimated:

$$y = \bar{y} + m(x - \bar{x})$$

The above equation can also be presented as the summary of the regression calculations,

$$\log C_p = \underbrace{\frac{\sum\limits_{i=1}^{n} \log C_p}{n} + \frac{\sum\limits_{i=1}^{n} (dt \times d\log C_p)}{\sum\limits_{i=1}^{n} (dt)^2}\left(t - \frac{\sum\limits_{i=1}^{n} t}{n}\right)}_{\text{known values} \qquad \text{known values}} \tag{8.13}$$

where n represents the number of data points located on the linear terminal portion of the curve. Substitution of the known values in Equation 8.13 gives rise to Equation 8.11.

The parameter $\overleftarrow{C}_p^0$ is a virtual value that cannot be measured directly. It can be interpreted as the hypothetical y intercept of an intravenous dose equal to FD.

8.5.2 Estimation of Absorption Rate Constant, k_a

8.5.2.1 Method of Residuals (Also Known as "Feathering" or "Peeling"): If we subtract Equation 8.11, the elimination part, from Equation 8.3, which represents both elimination and absorption, we obtain the following equation that represents the absorption component of Equation 8.3:

$$(\overleftarrow{C}_p - C_p) = \frac{FDk_a}{V_d(k_a - K)} e^{-k_a t} \quad \text{or} \quad (\overleftarrow{C}_p - C_p) = \overleftarrow{C}_p^0 e^{-k_a t} \tag{8.14}$$

Plotting $\log(\overleftarrow{C}_p - C_p)$ versus time on the same graph on which $\log C_p$ versus time was plotted gives the residual line with slope $-k_a/2.303$ (Figure 8.4). The manual calculation of the line of residuals is according to the following stepwise procedure:

1. Substitute the early time points, that is, the time points before the maximum plasma concentration, into Equation 8.11 to determine the calculated values of $\overleftarrow{C}_p$ that are located on the early part of the extrapolated line.
2. Subtract the corresponding plasma concentrations of the early part of the curve from the calculated values of $\overleftarrow{C}_p$ (step 1).

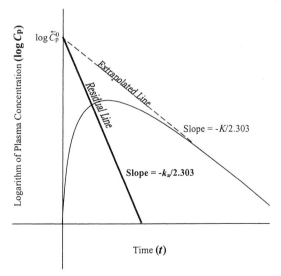

FIGURE 8.4 The line of residuals, calculated by subtraction of observed plasma concentration from calculated extrapolated line, represents the absorption part of the plasma concentration–time curve of an orally administered drug. The slope of the line is used to determine the absorption rate constant, k_a.

TABLE 8.1 Summary of Required Steps for Estimation of Residual Line

Time	$C_{p_n} = C_{poe}^{-Kt}$	C_p	$\tilde{C}_p - C_p$	$\log(\tilde{C}_p - C_p)$
t_1	$\tilde{C}_{p_1}$	C_{p_1}	$\tilde{C}_{p_1} - C_{p_1}$	$\log(\tilde{C}_{p_1} - C_{p_1})$
t_2	$\tilde{C}_{p_2}$	C_{p_2}	$\tilde{C}_{p_2} - C_{p_2}$	$\log(\tilde{C}_{p_2} - C_{p_2})$
t_3	$\tilde{C}_{p_3}$	C_{p_3}	$\tilde{C}_p - C_{p_3}$	$\log(\tilde{C}_{p_3} - C_{p_3})$
$\vdots$	$\vdots$	$\vdots$	$\vdots$	$\vdots$

3. Use regression analysis or the slope relationship to estimate the slope of $\log(C_p - \overleftarrow{C}_p^0)$ versus time. The slope is equal to $-k_a/2.303$.

Table 8.1 summarizes the steps required to estimate the residual line. The method of residuals is applicable when there are enough early data points.

8.5.2.2 Lag Time of Absorption: A y intercept of the residual line greater than the y intercept of the extrapolated line would indicate that the absorption starts after a delay, which is known as the lag time of absorption. There are various reasons for the delay, for example, the physicochemical characteristics of a drug, such as being a weak base, and formulation factors, such as coated tablets. The lag time of absorption can be estimated graphically (Figure 8.5) or calculated from Equations 8.11 and 8.14. Setting the equations of the lines equal each other and solving for lag time provide the calculated value of lag time (Equation 8.15)

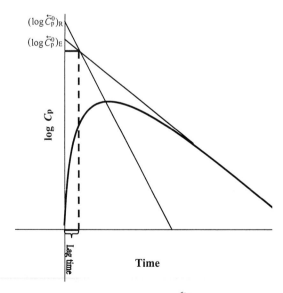

FIGURE 8.5 When the y intercept of the residual line, $(\overleftarrow{C}_p^0)_R$, is greater than the y intercept of the extrapolated line, $(\overleftarrow{C}_p^0)_E$, the two lines intersect at a late time point that corresponds to the lag time of absorption. (Abbreviation: R for residual line and E for extrapolated line)

$$(\log \overleftarrow{C}_p^0)_R - \frac{k_a t_1}{2.303} = (\log \overleftarrow{C}_p^0)_E - \frac{K t_1}{2.303}$$

$$(\log \overleftarrow{C}_p^0)_R - (\log \overleftarrow{C}_p^0)_E = t\left(\frac{k_a - K}{2.303}\right)$$

Therefore,

$$t_1 = \frac{2.303}{k_a - K} \log \frac{(\overleftarrow{C}_p^0)_R}{(\overleftarrow{C}_p^0)_E} \tag{8.15}$$

8.5.2.3, Krüger–Thiemer Method of Calculation of k_a: The absorption rate constant of a drug can also be estimated from the y intercept of the extrapolated line, $\overleftarrow{C}_p^0$; however, the method requires that equal doses of drug be given both intravenously and orally in a crossover design. By substituting the C_p^0 of the intravenous dose into Equation 8.10 the following relationship can be developed for estimation of k_a:

$$\overleftarrow{C}_p^0 = \frac{F C_p^0 k_a}{k_a - K} \tag{8.16}$$

Therefore,

$$\frac{k_a - K}{k_a} = \frac{F C_p^0}{\overleftarrow{C}_p^0}$$

$$k_a = \frac{K}{1 - (F C_p^0 / \overleftarrow{C}_p^0)} \tag{8.17}$$

This method is applicable when a drug can be given both orally and intravenously.

8.5.2.4 Wagner–Nelson Method of Calculation of k_a Using the Linear Plot of Percentage Remaining to be Absorbed versus Time: This method is based on the principle of mass balance for total amount of drug absorbed at any time, that is,

total amount absorbed up to time t = total amount in the body + total amount eliminated

total amount absorbed up to time $t = (A_D)_{abs}$

total amount in the body $= V_d C_p$

total amount eliminated $= Cl_t \times AUC_0^t$

Therefore,

$$(A_D)_{abs} = (V_d C_p) + (Cl_t \times AUC_0^t) \tag{8.18}$$

Dividing both sides of Equation 8.18 by the apparent volume of distribution provides a different form of the same equation:

$$\frac{(A_D)_{abs}}{V_d} = C_p + (K \times AUC_0^t) \tag{8.19}$$

where the quantity $(A_D)_{abs}/V_d$ is the amount of drug absorbed per unit of volume of distribution. A plot of this quantity versus time results in a curve that may have a linear portion. As this quantity represents the cumulative amount absorbed, curve reaches a plateau level that represents the total amount absorbed at $t \Rightarrow \infty$ (Figure 8.6).

Dividing $(A_D)_{abs}/V_d$ values on the linear segment of the curve by their average values on the plateau level results in fractional values of the points on the linear segment. These fractions, after multiplying by 100, can also be plotted as percentage amount absorbed per unit of volume; that is, $\%(A_D)_{abs}/V_d$, or as $100 - \%(A_D)_{abs}/V_d$, which corresponds to percentage amount remaining to be absorbed. All calculations are done according to the steps outlined in Table 8.2.

Subtracting $\%(A_D)_{abs}/V_d$ from 100 gives the percentage of drug remaining to be absorbed (ie, $100 - \%(A_D)_{abs}/V_d$). A semilogarithmic plot of $100 - \%(A_D)_{abs}/V_d$ versus time provides a straight line with slope $-k_a/2.303$ (Figure 8.7).

The Wagner–Nelson method of determining the absorption rate constant works under the assumptions that the drug follows a one-compartment model and the absorption is sufficiently fast so that the K value can be approximated from the terminal portion of the curve.

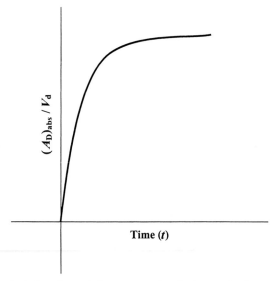

FIGURE 8.6 Theoretical plot of cumulative amount absorbed per unit of concentration versus time.

TABLE 8.2 Stepwise Calculations of Wagner–Nelson Method of Estimation of Absorption Rate Constant for One-compartment Model, Oral Absorption

t	C_p	$AUC_{t_{n-1}}^{t_n}$	AUC_0^t	$\dfrac{(A_D)abs}{V_d} = C_p + (K + AUC_0^t)$	$\% \dfrac{(A_D)abs}{V_d} \times \dfrac{100}{p}$
t_1	C_{p_1}	$((0 + C_{p_1})/2)(t_1 - 0) = AUC_1$	$AUC_0^1 = AUC_1$	$\dfrac{(A_{D_1})abs}{V_d} = C_{p_1} + (K \times AUC_0^1)$	$\dfrac{(A_{D_1})abs}{V_d} \times \dfrac{100}{p}$
t_2	C_{p_2}	$((C_{p_1} + C_{p_2})/2)(t_2 - t_1) = AUC_2$	$AUC_0^2 = AUC_0^1 + AUC_2$	$\dfrac{(A_{D_2})abs}{V_d} = C_{p_2} + (K \times AUC_0^2)$	$\dfrac{(A_{D_2})abs}{V_d} \times \dfrac{100}{p}$
t_3	C_{p_3}	$((C_{p_2} + C_{p_3})/2)(t_3 - t_2) = AUC_3$	$AUC_0^3 = AUC_0^2 + AUC_3$	$\dfrac{(A_{D_3})abs}{V_d} = C_{p_3} + (K \times AUC_0^3)$	$\dfrac{(A_{D_3})abs}{V_d} \times \dfrac{100}{p}$
t_4	C_{p_4}	$((C_{p_3} + C_{p_4})/2)(t_4 - t_3) = AUC_4$	$AUC_0^4 = AUC_0^3 + AUC_4$	$\dfrac{(A_{D_4})abs}{V_d} = C_{p_4} + (K \times AUC_0^4)$	$\dfrac{(A_{D_4})abs}{V_d} \times \dfrac{100}{p}$
t_5	C_{p_5}	$((C_{p_4} + C_{p_5})/2)(t_5 - t_4) = AUC_5$	$AUC_0^5 = AUC_0^4 + AUC_5$	$\dfrac{(A_{D_5})abs}{V_d} = C_{p_5} + (K \times AUC_0^5)$	$\dfrac{(A_{D_5})abs}{V_d} \times \dfrac{100}{p}$
t_6	C_{p_6}	$((C_{p_5} + C_{p_6})/2)(t_6 - t_5) = AUC_6$	$AUC_0^6 = AUC_0^5 + AUC_6$	$\dfrac{(A_{D_6})abs}{V_d} = C_{p_6} + (K \times AUC_0^6)$	$\dfrac{(A_{D_6})abs}{V_d} \times \dfrac{100}{p}$
...	...	...	...	...	
t_n	C_{p_n}	$((C_{p_{n-1}} + C_{p_n})/2)(t_n - t_{n-1}) = AUC_n$	AUC_0^n	$\dfrac{(A_{D_n})abs}{V_d} = C_{p_n} + (K \times AUC_0^n)$	Plateau (p)

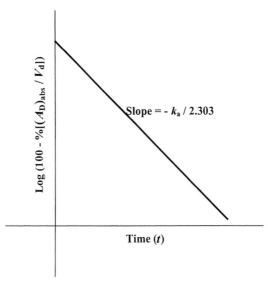

FIGURE 8.7 Graph of percentage remaining to be absorbed versus time according to Wagner–Nelson method yields a straight line with a slope of $-k_a/2.303$.

8.6 ESTIMATION OF T_{max}, $C_{p_{max}}$, AND AUC

The three important parameters of the model that are used to evaluate the formulation of a dosage form, comparison of different dosage forms, and evaluation of bioavailability and bioequivalence of drugs are T_{max} (peak time), $C_{p_{max}}$, and AUC. T_{max} is an indicator of how fast a drug is absorbed. If the rate of absorption is fast, T_{max} is short. If the rate of absorption is slow, the peak concentration occurs after a longer T_{max}. The maximum plasma concentration represents the highest concentration that can be achieved with a single dose. Obviously it is preferable to achieve this concentration within the therapeutic range. Therefore, $C_{p_{max}}$ and T_{max} describe the plasma concentration–time profile of a drug administered orally only by identifying one point over the entire period of sampling and data collection. AUC, on the other hand, is a parameter that covers the entire observation period. It represents the extent of absorption and how complete is the absorption. These and other parameters of oral absorption are presented graphically in Figure 8.8.

8.6.1 T_{max}

The equation of T_{max} is derived from the first derivative of Equation 8.3. At T_{max} the rate of absorption equals the rate of elimination; thus the rate of change of plasma concentration in the body with respect to time at this particular point is equal to zero (see also Chapter 1, Section 1.14). The function is

$$C_p = \tilde{C}_p^0(e^{-Kt} - e^{-k_a t}) \tag{8.20}$$

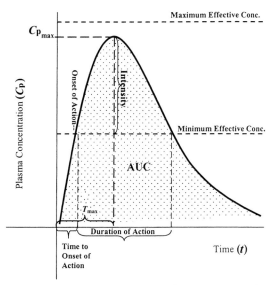

FIGURE 8.8 Principal parameters of plasma concentration–time curve of an orally administered drug that are important in drug development and bioavailability assessment.

The first derivative of the function is

$$\frac{dCp}{dt} = -K\overleftarrow{C}_p^0 e^{-Kt} + k_a \overleftarrow{C}_p^0 e^{-k_a t} = 0 \tag{8.21}$$

Therefore,

$$Ke^{-KT_{max}} = k_a e^{-k_a T_{max}} \tag{8.22}$$

By dividing both sides of Equation 8.22 by K, taking the natural logarithm of both sides, and rearranging the resulting equation we obtain

$$T_{max}(k_a - K) = \ln \frac{k_a}{K} \tag{8.23}$$

$$T_{max} = \frac{1}{k_a - K} \ln \frac{k_a}{K} \tag{8.24}$$

$$T_{max} = \frac{2.303}{k_a - K} \log \frac{k_a}{K} \tag{8.25}$$

8.6.2 $C_{p_{max}}$

By using Equations 8.22 and 8.3 we derive the equation of maximum plasma concentration. From Equation 8.22

$$e^{-k_a t} = \frac{K}{k_a} e^{-KT_{max}} \qquad (8.26)$$

By substituting Equation 8.26 into Equation 8.3 we obtain

$$C_{p_{max}} = \frac{FDk_a}{V_d(k_a - K)} \left(e^{-KT_{max}} - \frac{K}{k_a} e^{-KT_{max}} \right) \qquad (8.27)$$

Therefore,

$$C_{p_{max}} = \frac{FD}{V_d} (e^{-KT_{max}}) \qquad (8.28)$$

According to Equation 8.28, the maximum plasma concentration is directly proportional to the total amount absorbed, FD, and the fraction of dose in the body at T_{max} (ie, $f_{b_{max}} = e^{-KT_{max}}$). Thus, the maximum amount of drug in the body is

$$A_{max} = FDf_{b_{max}} \qquad (8.29)$$

8.6.3 AUC

The area under the plasma concentration–time curve is another important parameter of oral absorption and is considered a sensitive indicator of the amount of drug that ultimately reaches the systemic circulation. Its magnitude is directly proportional to the total amount absorbed. Therefore, equal doses of a drug should provide equal AUCs. This parameter is very useful in determining the bioavailability and bioequivalence of therapeutic agents (see also Chapter 16). AUC can be estimated by one of the following approaches:

For the Area under the Curve Between Zero and Infinity:

1.
$$AUC_0^\infty = \frac{FD}{Cl_t} \qquad (8.30)$$

2. Using the trapezoidal rule,

$$AUC_0^\infty = \sum_{i=0}^{n} [(y_i + y_{i+1})/2](x_{i+1} - x_i) + AUC_n^\infty \qquad (8.31)$$

3. Using the integration method,

$$\mathrm{AUC}_0^\infty = \tilde{C}_p^0 \left(\frac{1}{K} - \frac{1}{k_a} \right) \tag{8.32}$$

For the Area under the Curve Between 0 and a Given Time: The given time can be the length of the observation and sampling or a well-defined time such as T_{max}. Using the trapezoid rule,

$$\mathrm{AUC}_0^t = \sum_{i=0}^{n} \left(\frac{y_i + y_{i+1}}{2} \right)(x_{i+1} - x_i) \tag{8.33}$$

Using the integration method,

$$\mathrm{AUC}_0^t = \int_0^t \tilde{C}_p^0 (e^{-Kt} - e^{-k_a t}) = \tilde{C}_p^0 \left(\frac{e^{-Kt}}{-K} + \frac{e^{-k_a t}}{k_a} \right) = \frac{\tilde{C}_p^0}{K \times k_a} (Ke^{-k_a t} - k_a e^{-Kt}) \tag{8.34}$$

AUC and $C_{p_{max}}$ are dependent on the dose. As the dose increases both AUC and $C_{p_{max}}$ increase proportionately; however, T_{max} remains the same for all doses (Figure 8.9).

If the total amount absorbed remains the same but the rate of absorption changes with each dose, the slower the rate of absorption, the longer T_{max} and the lower $C_{p_{max}}$. The area under the curve, however, may remain the same for three different oral dosage forms with different $C_{p_{max}}$ and T_{max} (Figure 8.10). Therefore, AUC, although considered a sensitive

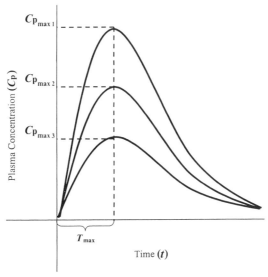

FIGURE 8.9 Oral administrations of different doses of the same drug in the same dosage form (ie, same rate of absorption) increase AUC and $C_{p_{max}}$ proportionately while T_{max} remains the same.

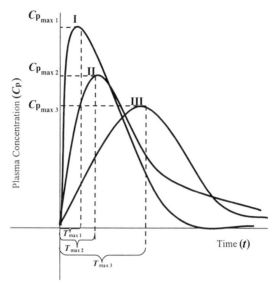

FIGURE 8.10 The rate of absorption influences the plasma concentration–time profile of a drug. A fast rate of absorption (curve I) would increase the maximum plasma concentration and reduce $T_{\max}$. A slow rate of absorption (curve III), on the other hand, would lower the $C_{p_{\max}}$ and extend $T_{\max}$. The AUC may remain the same for all three curves I, II, and III.

indicator of completeness of absorption, provides no information about the rate of absorption, $T_{\max}$ or $C_{p_{\max}}$.

8.7 ESTIMATION OF OTHER
PARAMETERS AND CONSTANTS OF ORAL ABSORPTION

8.7.1 Total Body Clearance and Apparent Volume of Distribution

The definitions of total body clearance and apparent volume of distribution are the same as described in previous chapters. The following are practical methods of estimation of these constants:

$$Cl_t = \frac{F \times \text{dose}}{\text{AUC}_0^\infty} \qquad (8.35)$$

We can also estimate total body clearance from the equation $Cl_t = KV_d$, contingent on knowing the volume of distribution.

Equation 8.35 provides the following equation for the apparent volume of distribution of an orally administered dose:

$$V_d = \frac{F \times \text{dose}}{K \times \text{AUC}_0^\infty} \qquad (8.36)$$

It should be noted that because in most cases $\tilde{C}_p^0 \neq (C_p^0)_{\text{iv bolus}}$ dividing the dose by $\tilde{C}_p^0$ would overestimate the apparent volume of distribution and should be avoided, unless $F = 1$ and $k_a > K$.

8.7.2 Fraction of Dose Absorbed, F

This parameter can be estimated by one of the following approaches:

1. From the y intercept of the extrapolated line,

$$F = \frac{\tilde{C}_p^0 V_d (k_a - K)}{\text{dose} \times k_a} \tag{8.37}$$

2. From Equation 8.35 or 8.36,

$$F = \frac{\text{TBC} \times \text{AUC}_0^\infty}{\text{dose}} \tag{8.38}$$

3. By dividing $(\text{AUC})_{\text{oral}}$ by $(\text{AUC})_{\text{iv}}$, assuming the doses are the same and total body clearance remains the same:

$$F = \frac{(\text{AUC})_{\text{po}}}{(\text{AUC})_{\text{iv}}} \tag{8.39}$$

The methods of estimation of F and its meaning are discussed in Chapter 16.

8.8 DURATION OF ACTION

The equation of an extrapolated line can be used to estimate the duration of action of an orally administered dose as long as it is corrected for the time to the onset of action. As shown in Figure 8.11, the appropriate equation is

$$t_d = \left(\frac{2.303}{K} \log \frac{\tilde{C}_p^0}{C_{P_{\text{MEC}}}} \right) - t_{\text{onset}} \tag{8.40}$$

where t_{onset} is the time to the onset of action. Obviously when the the rate constant of absorption is much greater the rate constant of elimination, $t_{\text{onset}} = 0$.

   The duration of action is therefore the time required for the extrapolated concentration at point O to decline to point M.

APPLICATION
8.1 A 1000-mg single dose of drug X is given orally to a patient. Eighty percent of the drug is absorbed and the balance is eliminated unchanged through fecal elimination. The

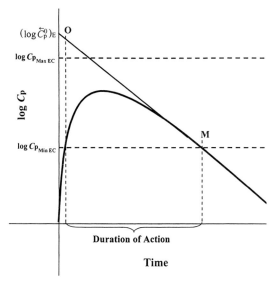

FIGURE 8.11 The duration of action of an orally administered dose can also be assumed as the time required for the extrapolated concentration at point O that corresponds to the onset of action to decline to the minimum effective concentration ($C_{P_{\min EC}}$) at point M.

volume of distribution is 24 L. The half-lives of elimination and absorption are 10 and 0.25 hours, respectively. Determine the following:

1. AUC

$$\mathrm{AUC} = \frac{F \times \text{dose}}{\mathrm{Cl_t}} = \frac{0.8 \times 1000 \text{ mg}}{0.0693 \text{ h}^{-1} \times 24 \text{ L}} = 48 \text{ L}$$

2. $T_{\max}$ and $C_{p_{\max}}$

$$T_{\max} = \frac{2.303}{k_a - K} \log \frac{k_a}{K} = \frac{2.303}{2.77 \text{ h}^{-1} - 0.0693 \text{ h}^{-1}} \log \frac{2.77}{0.0693} = 1.366 \text{ h}$$

$$C_{p_{\max}} = \frac{F \times \text{dose}}{V_d} (e^{-0.0693 \times 1.366}) = 30.32 \text{ mg/L}$$

3. Equation of the model for this drug

$$\tilde{C}_p^0 = \frac{0.8 \times 1000 \times 2.77}{24(2.77 - 0.0693)} = 34.20 \text{ mg/L}$$

Therefore,

$$C_p = 34.20 \text{ mg/L}(e^{-0.0693(\text{h}^{-1})t} - e^{-2.77(\text{h})t^1})$$

The equations of the extrapolated and residual lines are

$$\tilde{C}_p = 34.20e^{-0.0693t} \quad \text{and} \quad (\tilde{C}_p - C_p) = 34.20e^{-2.77t}$$

4. Initial plasma concentration if the dose were administered as an intravenous bolus:

$$(C_p^0)_{\text{iv bolus}} = \frac{1000 \text{ mg}}{24 \text{ L}} = 41.66 \text{ mg/L}$$

5. Plasma concentration 10 hours after administration of oral drug: $10 \text{ h} > 7(T_{1/2})_{k_a}$; therefore, $e^{-k_a t} \Rightarrow 0$

$$C_p = \tilde{C}_p^0 e^{-Kt} = 34.20e^{-0.0693(10)} = 17.10 \text{ mg/L}$$

6. Plasma concentration 2 hours after administration of oral dose

$$C_p = 34.20(e^{-0.0693 \times 2} - e^{-2.77 \times 2}) = 29.64 \text{ mg/L}$$

7. Fraction of dose in the body at $t = 2$ hours

$$f_b = (C_{p_{2h}} V_d)/F \times \text{dose} = (29.64 \times 24)/(0.8 \times 1000) = 0.889$$

8. Total body clearance

$$Cl_t = F \times \text{dose}/\text{AUC} = 800/481 = 1.663 \text{ L/h} = 27.72 \text{ mL/min}$$

or

$$Cl_t = KV_d = 0.0693 \text{ h}^{-1} \times 24 \text{ L} = 1.663 \text{ L/h} = 27.72 \text{ mL/min}$$

9. Rate of elimination at $t = 2$ hours

$$\text{rate} = Cl_t \times C_p = 29.64 \text{ mg/L} \times 1.663 \text{ L/h} = 49.3 \text{ mg/h}$$

8.2 Drug B, an ester of drug A, is absorbed from the GI tract and provides serum levels comparable to those achieved after an equimolar intramuscular injection of drug A. A 9-month-old, 6.5-kg infant receives 10 mg/kg drug B, equimolar to 7 mg/kg drug A, every 4 hours. Blood samples were collected after the first dose and the concentration of drug A was determined in plasma as reported in Table 8.3. Calculate the following:

1. Half-life of elimination: The regression analysis of the last five data points yields the following equation for the extrapolated line:

$$\log \tilde{C}_p = 1.198 - 0.364t$$

TABLE 8.3 Data Related to Application 8.3

Time (h)	C_p of Drug A ($\mu g/mL$)
0.05	0.20
0.10	0.50
0.20	2.00
0.30	7.00
0.50	7.50
1.00	6.50
1.50	4.30
2.00	2.85
2.50	1.95
3.00	1.25
4.00	0.55
5.00	0.25
6.00	0.10

Therefore,

$$\log C_p^0 = 1.198$$

$$\tilde{C}_p^0 = 15.776 \text{ mg/L}$$

$$\text{slope} = -0.364 \text{ h}^{-1} = -\frac{K}{2.303}$$

Therefore,

$$K = 2.303 \times 0.364 = 0.838 \text{ h}^{-1}$$

and

$$T_{1/2} = 0.826 \text{ hours.}$$

2. Absorption rate constant using residual line: The residual line can be estimated on the basis of the first five data points:

$$(\tilde{C}_p - C_p)_1 = (15.776 e^{-0.838(0.05)}) - 0.20 = 14.92 \text{ mg/L}$$

$$(\tilde{C}_p - C_p)_2 = (15.776 e^{-0.838(0.10)}) - 0.50 = 14.00 \text{ mg/L}$$

$$(\tilde{C}_p - C_p)_3 = (15.776 e^{-0.838(0.20)}) - 2.00 = 11.34 \text{ mg/L}$$

$$(\tilde{C}_p - C_p)_4 = (15.776 e^{-0.838(0.30)}) - 7.00 = 5.27 \text{ mg/L}$$

$$(\tilde{C}_p - C_p)_5 = (15.776 e^{-0.838(0.50)}) - 7.50 = 2.87 \text{ mg/L}$$

The regression equation of the residual line is

$$\log(\tilde{C}_p - C_p) = 1.302 - 1.70t$$

TABLE 8.4 Stepwise Calculations of Absorption Rate Constant of Application 8.2 Using Wagner–Nelson Method: Part I

Δt	$(C_{p_n} + C_{p_{n+1}})/2$	$AUC_{t_{n-1}}^{t_n}$	AUC_0^t	$K \times AUC_0^t$	$C_p + (K \times AUC_0^t)^a$
0.05	0.100	0.0050	0.0050	0.0042	0.2042
0.05	0.350	0.0175	0.0225	0.0189	0.5189
0.10	1.250	0.1250	0.1475	0.1236	2.1236
0.10	4.500	0.4500	0.5975	0.5007	7.5007
0.20	7.250	1.4500	2.0475	1.7158	9.2158
0.50	7.000	3.5000	5.5475	4.6488	**11.1488**
0.50	5.400	2.7000	8.2475	6.9114	**11.2114**
0.50	3.575	1.7875	10.0350	8.4093	**11.2593**
0.50	2.400	1.2000	11.2350	9.4149	**11.3649**
0.50	1.600	0.8000	12.0350	10.0853	**11.3353**
1.00	0.900	0.9000	12.9350	10.8395	**11.3895**
1.00	0.400	0.4000	13.3350	11.1747	**11.4247**
1.00	0.175	0.1750	13.5100	11.3214	**11.4214**
				Average =	**11.319**

$^a(A_D)_{abs}/V_d$.

Therefore,

$$k_a = 2.303 \times 1.70 = 3.915$$

3. Absorption rate constant using Wagner–Nelson method: Stepwise calculations of the fraction of dose remaining to be absorbed are presented in Tables 8.4 and 8.5. The regression equation of $\log(100 - \%((A_D)_{abs}/V_d))$, that is, log of percentage remaining to be absorbed, against time is

$$y = 2.137 - 1.747t$$

Therefore, the absorption rate constant, k_a, can be estimated as

$$k_a = 2.303 \times 1.747 = 4.023 \text{ h}^{-1}$$

TABLE 8.5 Stepwise Calculations of Absorption Rate Constant of Application 8.2 Using Wagner–Nelson Method: Part II

$\dfrac{(A_D)_{abs}}{V_d}$	$\left(\left[\dfrac{(A_D)_{abs}}{V_d}\right] \div \text{average}\right) \times 100$	$100 - \% \dfrac{(A_D)_{abs}}{V_d}$	$\log\left(100 - \% \dfrac{(A_D)_{abs}}{V_d}\right)$
0.20419	1.8040	98.1960	1.99209
0.51885	4.5839	95.4161	1.97962
2.12361	18.7614	81.2386	1.90976
7.50071	66.2665	33.7335	1.52806
9.21580	81.4189	18.5811	1.26907

4. Time to maximum plasma concentration, T_{max}

$$T_{max} = \frac{2.303}{4.0 - 0.838} \log \frac{4.0}{0.838} = 0.49 \text{ h}$$

5. AUC_0^∞

$$AUC_0^\infty = \sum_{i=0}^{n} \left(\frac{C_{p_i} + C_{p_{i+1}}}{2} \right)(t_{i+1} - t_i) + AUC_n^\infty$$

The relevant calculations are presented in Table 8.6

$$AUC_0^t = 13.510 \text{ mg h/L}$$

$$AUC_0^\infty = 13.510 + \frac{0.10}{0.838} = 13.630 \text{ mg h/L}$$

6. Apparent V_d of drug A if only 80% of the drug is absorbed

$$V_d = \frac{FD}{K \times AUC} = \frac{0.8 \times 7 \text{ mg/kg} \times 6.5 \text{ kg}}{0.838 \text{ h}^{-1} \times 13.63 \text{ mg h/L}} = 3.187 \text{ L}$$

ASSIGNMENT

8.1 To investigate the influence of clavulanic acid on the pharmacokinetics of amoxicillin, a 30-year-old patient received a single dose of 500 mg of amoxicillin orally on day 1 (treatment A) followed by 500 mg of amoxicillin plus 125 mg clavulanic acid on the sec-

TABLE 8.6 Calculation of Area under Plasma Concentration–Time Curve of Application 8.2

$t_{i+1} - t_i$	$\dfrac{C_{p_i} + C_{p_{i+1}}}{2}$	AUC_i^{i+1}
0.05	0.100	0.0050
0.05	0.350	0.0175
0.10	1.250	0.1250
0.10	4.500	0.4500
0.20	7.250	1.4500
0.50	7.000	3.5000
0.50	5.400	2.7000
0.50	3.575	1.7875
0.50	2.400	1.2000
0.50	1.600	0.8000
1.00	0.900	0.9000
1.00	0.400	0.4000
1.00	0.175	0.1750
Total 13.510		

ond day (treatment B). The serum and urine samples were analyzed for amoxicillin and the data were reported as follows:

Treatment A
   Urine data: Total amount excreted unchanged in the urine = 200 mg.
   Serum data: Concentrations of amoxicillin at different time were determined as reported in Table 8.7

Treatment B
   Urine data: Total amount excreted unchanged in the urine = 290 mg.
   Serum data: The equation of the model based on the serum concentrations of treatment B is

$$C_p = 37(\text{mg/L})(e^{-0.013\ \text{min}^{-1}t} - e^{-0.025\ \text{min}^{-1}t})$$

Determine the following:

8.1.1 Absorption and elimination rate constants for both treatments.
8.1.2 Fraction of the dose absorbed if the volume of distribution of amoxicillin is 19 L.
8.1.3 Maximum plasma concentration.
8.1.4 Renal clearance.

8.2 The effect of high-fat and low-fat meals on the absorption of a new drug was evaluated in a crossover design on six volunteers aged 30 to 44 years. No other drug or alcohol was allowed a week before and during the study.

Treatment A
   A single dose of a 10-mg capsule of the drug with 200 mL water immediately after a low-fat meal consisting of fruit juice, skim milk, cereal, and toast with jelly.

Treatment B
   A single dose of a 10-mg capsule of the drug with 200 mL water immediately after a high-fat meal consisting of whole milk, bacon, egg, sausage, and decaffeinated coffee.

The averages of plasma concentrations of the drug are reported in Table 8.8. Compute the following for both treatments. The apparent volume of distribution of drug is 120 L.
   8.2.1 Calculate the absorption and elimination rate constants.
   8.2.2 Calculate the time of the maximum plasma concentration.
   8.2.3 Calculate the fraction of dose absorbed.
   8.2.4 Calculate the maximum plasma concentration.

TABLE 8.7 Serum Concentration of Amoxicillin at Different Times: Data Related to Assignment 8.1

Time (min)	10	20	40	60	90	120	180	240	350
C_p (mg/L)	0.24	0.60	5.00	7.80	8.20	6.50	3.80	1.90	0.44

TABLE 8.8 Average Plasma Concentration of the New Drug at Different Times: Data Related to Assignment 8.2

Time (h)	C_p (ng/mL)	
	Treatment A	Treatment B
0.10	1.0	0.7
0.20	12.0	4.1
0.30	28.0	11.1
0.40	46.0	32.5
0.6	56.0	42.1
0.75	59.7	42.9
1.00	60.0	39.6
2.00	40.0	31.0
3.00	26.2	21.5
4.00	17.5	14.2
5.00	11.5	9.7
6.00	7.6	6.6

8.2.5 Calculate the area under the plasma concentration–time curve.

8.2.6 Calculate the total body clearance.

8.2.7 Summarize your conclusions about the calculated data (parts 8.2.1 to 8.2.6) in one paragraph.

8.3 Two grams of a new drug was administered orally and intravenously in a crossover design with a washout period of 2 days to a 70-kg healthy volunteer. The concentration of the drug in plasma was measured at different time points and the results are presented in Table 8.9.

8.3.1 Estimate the area under the plasma concentration–time curve from 0 to 7 h (AUC_0^{7h}) and 0 to ∞ (AUC_0^{∞}) using the trapezoidal rule.

8.3.2 Calculate the absorption rate constant according to Wagner–Nelson, Krüger–Thiemer and peeling methods. Compare the results.

8.3.3 Calculate T_{max} and $C_{p_{max}}$ of the oral dose.

8.4 The pharmacokinetics of drug X following oral administration of 1 g is defined by the following biexponential equation. Drug is known to have a total body clearance of 27.72 L/h.

$$C_p = 100(\text{mg/L})(e^{-0.1386 \text{ h}^{-1}t} - e^{-3.465 \text{ h}^{-1}t})$$

Fill in the blanks in (Table 8.10)

8.5 If the half-lives of elimination and absorption of a drug are 1 and 5 hours, respectively, what is the total amount remaining to be absorbed 10 hours after the administration of 500 mg?

TABLE 8.9 Data Related to Assignment 8.3

IV Bolus Injection		Oral Administration	
Time (h)	C_p (mg/L)	Time (h)	C_p (mg/L)
0.10	190.246	0.17	47.702
0.25	176.499	0.25	61.519
0.50	155.760	0.33	71.447
0.75	137.458	0.50	83.350
1.00	121.306	0.75	87.283
1.50	94.473	1.00	83.511
2.00	73.576	1.50	69.188
3.00	44.626	2.00	54.810
4.00	27.067	3.00	33.451
5.00	16.417	4.00	20.299
6.00	9.957	5.00	12.312
7.00	6.039	6.00	7.468
		7.00	4.529

8.6 If the therapeutic range of a drug is 8 to 10 mg/L, what is the duration of action for an orally administered dose with maximum plasma concentration of 8 mg/L and T_{max} of 10 minutes?

8.7 The slope of the terminal portion of the log plasma concentration–time curve of an orally administered drug is 1 h^{-1}, and the slope of the residuals versus time is 2 h^{-1}, what is the absorption rate constant if $K > k_a$?

8.8 What is the lag time of absorption if $k_a = 3$ h^{-1}, $K = 0.3$ h^{-1}, $\overleftarrow{C}_p^0 = 100$ mg/L, and $(\overleftarrow{C}_p - C_p^0) = 150$ mg?

ASSIGNMENT (EXTRA CREDIT)
EC-8.1 Based on the following article and related references discuss the significance of methodologies such as the quantitative structure–bioavailability relationship (QSBR) and Lipinski's Rule of Five. Compare the two methods and highlight the advantages and short-comings of each method:
Webster Andews C, Bennett L, Yu LX. Predicting human oral bioavailability of a compound: develop-
    ment of a novel quantitative structure–bioavailability relationship. *Pharm Res* 2000;17:639–644.

TABLE 8.10 Assignment 8.4

Parameter/Constant	Answer
Plasma concentration at $t = 10$ hours	
T_{max}	
Total amount absorbed	
AUC	

EC-8.2 Based on the following article fill in the blanks in the statements:
Carver PL, Fleisher D, Zhou SY, Kaul D, Kazanjian P, Li C. Meal composition effect on the oral bioavailability of indinavir in HIV-infected patients. *Pharm Res* 1999;16:718–24.

1. The gastric pH was evaluated by _____ meals.
2. _____ meals decrease the plasma concentration of the drug significantly.
3. There were significant differences in the area under the curve of the drug between _____ meals.
4. The greatest variability in the plasma concentration–time curve was observed by coadministration of the drug with _____ meals.
5. The decrease in availability of drug with _____ meals was due to _____ of gastric pH and _____ of indinavir.
6. The noncaloric viscous meal was used to evaluate _____.
7. The delayed T_{max} of _____ meals is attributed to _____.
8. Discuss the reasons for the low bioavailability of the drug coadministered with protein, carbohydrate and fat meals.

BIBLIOGRAPHY

1. Curry SH. Theoretical considerations in calculation of terminal phase half-times following oral doses, illustrated with model data. *Biopharm Drug Dispos* 1981;2:115.
2. Gibaldi M, Perrier D. *Pharmacokinetics*. 2nd ed. New York: Marcel Dekker, 1982:145.
3. Lipinski CA, Lombardo F, Dominy BW, Feeney PJ. Experimental and computational approaches to estimate solubility and permeability in drug discovery and development settings. *Adv Drug Delivery Rev* 1997;23:3.
4. Loo JCK, Riegelman S. New method for calculating the intrinsic absorption rate of drugs. *J Pharm Sci* 1968;57:918.
5. Rescigno A, Segre G. Drugs and Tracer Kinetics. Waltham, MA: Blaisdell, 1966:18.
6. Ronfeld RA, Benet LZ. Interpretation of plasma concentration–time curves after oral dosing. *J Pharm Sci* 1977;66:178.
7. Scheupkin RJ, Shoaf SE, Brown RN. Role of pharmacokinetics in safety evaluation and regulatory consideration. *Annu Rev Pharmacol Toxicol* 1990;30:197.
8. Teorell T. Kinetics of distribution of substances administered to the body. I. The extravascular mode of administration. *Arch Int Pharmacodyn* 1937;57:205.
9. Teorell T. General Physico-chemical Aspects of Drug Distribution. In: Raspè G, editor. Advances in biosciences. Braunschweig: Pergamon Press, 1970:21.
10. Till AE, Benet LZ, Kwan KC. An integrated approach to the pharmacokinetic analysis of drug absorption. *J Pharmacokinet Biopharm* 1974;2:525.
11. Wagner JG. "Absorption rate constant" calculated according to the one-compartment model with first-order absorption: implications in *in vivo–in vitro* correlation. *J Pharm Sci* 1970;59:1049.
12. Wagner JG. Pharmacokinetic absorption plots from oral data or oral/intravenous data and an exact Loo–Riegelman equation. *J Pharm Sci* 1983;72:838.
13. Wagner JG, Nelson E. Kinetic analysis of blood levels and urinary excretion in the absorptive phase after single doses of drug. *J Pharm Sci* 1964;53:1392.

CHAPTER 9

ANALYSIS OF URINARY DATA: LINEAR ONE-COMPARTMENT MODEL

What is opposed brings together; the finest harmony is composed of things at variance, and everything comes to be in accordance with strife.
ARISTOTLE (NICOMACHEAN ETHICS)

OBJECTIVES

■ To discuss methods of data analysis of unchanged drug excreted in urine following intravenous bolus injection, intravenous infusion, and oral absorption.

■ To discuss data analysis of metabolites eliminated via the urine.

■ To estimate the parameters and constants of plasma from urinary data.

9.1 INTRODUCTION

For drugs that are fully or partially eliminated in urine, the analysis of cumulative amount of unchanged drug or metabolites may provide useful information that can be obtained only from urinary data. For example, the percentage of dose excreted unchanged or percentage of dose eliminated as metabolites may not be easily estimated from plasma data. In addition, urine is considered a convenient biologic sample. It can be collected easily and noninvasively. Therefore, it has practical use in evaluation of drugs in pediatrics, assessment of bioavailability in human volunteers, and understanding of mass balance of a drug in the body. The volume of urine is a variable that changes irregularly and is a function of a number of factors, some related to the diet and some related to the state of mind and other physiologic factors. To exclude the effect of volume of urine from analysis of urinary data, the appearance of drugs in urine is expressed in terms of amount and not concentration. The amount of drug in the urine is estimated as the amount excreted per interval of urine collection or as cumulative amount excreted between $t = 0$ and any time t. The method of calculation of amount of drug in urine is presented in Table 9.1. The first and second columns of the table are the time of urine collection and the collected vol-

TABLE 9.1 Stepwise Calculations of Cumulative Amount of Drug Excreted Unchanged in Urine

1 Time	2 Volume of Urine, V	3 Concentration, Ce	4 Amount, $Ce \times V = (\Delta A_e)$	5 Cumulative Amount, A_e
$0-t_1$	V_1	C_{e1}	ΔA_{e1}	$A_{e1} = \Delta A_{e1}$
t_1-t_2	V_2	C_{e2}	ΔA_{e2}	$A_{e2} = A_{e1} + \Delta A_{e2}$
t_2-t_3	V_3	C_{e3}	ΔA_{e3}	$A_{e3} = A_{e2} + \Delta A_{e3}$
t_3-t_4	V_4	C_{e4}	ΔA_{e4}	$A_{e4} = A_{e3} + \Delta A_{e4}$
$\vdots$	$\vdots$	$\vdots$	$\vdots$	$\vdots$
$t_n - t_{n-1}$	V_n	C_{en}	ΔA_{en}	A_{en}
When $t_{n=\infty}$				A_e^∞

umes, respectively. The third and fourth columns are the concentration and amount of drug excreted unchanged per each interval of urine collection. The fifth column represents the cumulative amount of drug excreted in the urine from time zero to any time t. If the total interval of urine collection from 0 to t_n were equal to or greater than $7T_{1/2}$ of the drug, the last value of the cumulative column would represent the total amount excreted unchanged in the urine, and the plot of cumulative amount versus time would yield a hyperbolic curve as shown in Figure 9.1 with a plateau level equal to A_e^∞.

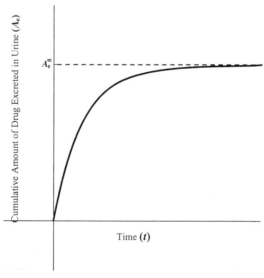

FIGURE 9.1 Plot of cumulative amount of drug excreted unchanged in urine versus time with a plateau level that corresponds to the total amount of drug excreted unchanged in urine, A_e^∞.

9.2 ANALYSIS OF URINARY DATA: UNCHANGED DRUG (I.V. BOLUS)

Consider the model that represents the one-compartment model with instantaneous input and first-order excretion and metabolism (Figure 9.2). The first-order rate of excretion, that is, the rate of emergence of unchanged drug in urine, is directly proportional to the concentration or amount of unchanged drug in the body:

$$\frac{dA_e}{dt} = k_e \times A = k_e \times C_p \times V_d = Cl_r C_p \tag{9.1}$$

Therefore, the rate of excretion after the injection of drug is high and gradually declines as the amount or concentration of drug in the body decreases. This change in the rate of excretion is the reason for the initial rise and plateau level of cumulative amount of unchanged drug in the urine (Figure 9.1). We can develop the computational equation for analysis of urinary data by:

1. Conversion of Equation 9.1 from the differential form dA_e/dt to the difference form $\Delta A_e/\Delta t$. The outcome of the conversion is a semilogarithmic linear equation known as the *rate plot* (Section 9.2.1).
2. Integration of Equation 9.1 to obtain a relationship that defines the amount remaining in the body to be excreted unchanged. This is also a semilogarithmic linear relationship known as the *amount remaining to be excreted* (*ARE*) *plot* or *sigma-minus plot* (Section 9.2.2).

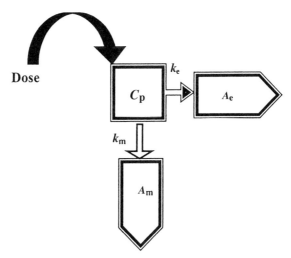

FIGURE 9.2 Diagram of one-compartment open model with intravenous input (instantaneous) and first-order excretion and metabolism.

9.2.1 Rate Plot

Conversion of Equation 9.1 from differential form to difference equation is achieved by the assumption that the amount excreted per interval of urine collection, ΔA_e, represents the amount of drug that is excreted "little by little" (ie, dA_e) in urine per fraction of time (ie, dt). Thus, $\Delta A_e/\Delta t$ can be perceived as a summation of a large number of theoretical quantities of dA_e over a large number of theoretical intervals of time, dt. This indicates that $\Delta A_e/\Delta t$ is an average value of first-order rate of excretion within the interval of urine collection. This average rate does not correspond to the beginning or the end of the interval but rather to the midpoint of the interval of urine collection,

$$\frac{\Delta A_e}{\Delta t} = k_e A \tag{9.2}$$

where ΔA_e is the amount of unchanged drug excreted in urine in interval Δt, and A is the amount of unchanged drug in the body. Because $A = A^0 e^{-Kt}$ Equation 9.2 can be presented as the following equations known as the rate equation:

$$\frac{\Delta A_e}{\Delta t} = k_e A^0 e^{-Kt_{midpoint}} \tag{9.3}$$

or

$$\log \frac{\Delta A_e}{\Delta t} = \log k_e \text{dose} - \frac{Kt_{midpoint}}{2.303} \tag{9.4}$$

The required calculations of the rate plot are presented in Table 9.2 and a plot of $\log(\Delta A_e/\Delta t)$ against $t_{midpoint}$ is shown in Figure 9.3. The rate plot enables us to estimate the values of excretion rate constant, k_e, and overall elimination rate constant, K, from the y intercept and slope, respectively:

$$k_e = \frac{\text{antilog}(y - \text{intercept})}{\text{dose}} \tag{9.5}$$

TABLE 9.2 Stepwise Calculations of Rate Plot

Δt	$t_{midpoint}$	ΔA_e	$\Delta A_e/\Delta t$
$\Delta t_1 = t_1 - 0$	$t_{midpoint\ 1} = (0 + t_1)/2$	ΔA_{e1}	$\Delta A_{e1}/\Delta t_1$
$\Delta t_2 = t_2 - t_1$	$t_{midpoint\ 2} = (t_1 + t_2)/2$	ΔA_{e2}	$\Delta A_{e2}/\Delta t_2$
$\Delta t_3 = t_3 - t_2$	$t_{midpoint\ 3} = (t_2 + t_3)/2$	ΔA_{e3}	$\Delta A_{e3}/\Delta t_3$
$\vdots$	$\vdots$	$\vdots$	$\vdots$
$\Delta t_n = t_{n-1} - t_n$	$t_{midpoint\ n} = (t_{n-1} + t_n)/2$	ΔA_{en}	$\Delta A_{en}/\Delta t_n$

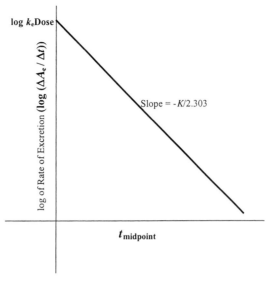

FIGURE 9.3 For a one-compartment model with intravenous bolus injection, a plot of $\log(\Delta A_e/\Delta t)$ versus $t_{midpoint}$, known as a rate plot, is a straight line with slope of $-K/2.303$ and y intercept of log k_e dose.

If the excretion of unchanged drug occurs mainly in the urine, the first-order metabolic rate constant can be estimated as

$$k_m = K - k_e \qquad (9.6)$$

Other equations related to analysis of urinary data, which can be used in rate and ARE plots are reported here as Equations 9.7–9.12

$$\text{fraction of dose excreted unchanged} = f_e = \frac{k_e}{K} = \frac{A_e^\infty}{\text{dose}} \qquad (9.7)$$

$$\text{total amount excreted unchanged} = f_e \times \text{dose} = A_e^\infty \qquad (9.8)$$

$$= \text{antilog of } y \text{ intercept}/K$$

$$\text{fraction of dose eliminated as metabolite(s)} = f_m = \frac{k_m}{K} = \frac{\text{dose} - A_e^\infty}{\text{dose}} \qquad (9.9)$$

$$\text{total amount eliminated as metabolite(s)} = f_m \times \text{dose} = A_m^\infty$$

$$= \text{dose} - A_e^\infty \qquad (9.10)$$

If $K = k_e + k_m$, then $f_e + f_m = 1$ (ie, 100% of the intravenous bolus dose). Also, $f_e = 1 - f_m$ and $f_m = 1 - f_e$. By knowing the apparent volume of distribution from plasma data and the rate constants of excretion and metabolism, the clearance terms can be estimated as

$$\text{renal clearance} = Cl_r = k_e \times V_d = f_e \times Cl_t \qquad (9.11)$$

$$\text{metabolic clearance} = Cl_m = k_m \times V_d = f_m \times Cl_t \qquad (9.12)$$

If a drug were eliminated entirely by metabolism, f_e would be equal to zero, $f_m = 1$, $K = k_m$, and $Cl_t = Cl_m$. When $f_m = 0$, this means that the drug is eliminated without any extrarenal elimination, $K = k_e$, $f_e = 1$, and the renal clearance is equal to total body clearance.

9.2.2 ARE Plot

This approach is based on integration of Equation 9.1. We set the interval of integration between zero, the time of injection, and t, the length of urine collection:

$$\int_0^t dA_e = k_e \int_0^t A\, dt = k_e A^0 \int_0^t e^{-Kt} dt$$

Therefore

$$A_e = \frac{k_e A^0}{K} (1 - e^{-Kt}) = f_e \text{dose}(1 - e^{-Kt}) = A_e^\infty (1 - e^{-Kt}) \qquad (9.13)$$

where A_e represents the cumulative amount excreted up to time t (Table 9.1, column 5; Figure 9.1) and A_e^∞ is the total amount that ultimately will be excreted unchanged.

Equation 9.13 can also be presented as

$$A_e^\infty - A_e = A_e^\infty e^{-Kt} \qquad (9.14)$$

The quantity $A_e^\infty - A_e$ is the amount remaining in the body to be excreted unchanged (ARE) at time t. The logarithmic form of equation 9.14 is

$$\log(A_e^\infty - A_e) = \log A_e^\infty - \frac{Kt}{2.303} \qquad (9.15)$$

The graph of equation 9.15 is presented in Figure 9.4 and the calculations are listed in Table 9.3.

Comparison of the calculation steps of ARE with those of the rate plot (Tables 9.2 and 9.3) indicates that the calculation of ARE data is highly dependent on a correct estimate of A_e^∞. Thus, urine samples should be collected long enough to obtain an accurate assessment of this parameter. The rate plot, however, is independent of A_e^∞, although the data points are usually more scattered than those of the ARE plot.

The information obtained from ARE plots is rather similar to that obtained from rate

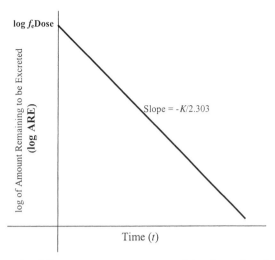

FIGURE 9.4 For drugs that follow a one-compartment model and are given intravenously (bolus), the plot of logarithm of amount remaining to be excreted unchanged against time, known as an ARE plot or sigma-minus plot, is a straight line with slope of $-K/2.303$ and y intercept of A_e^∞.

plots. The slope of the line is equal to $-K/2.303$ but the y intercept is log A_e^∞, that is, log $f_e$dose. Thus,

$$\text{antilog}(y \text{ intercept})_{\text{ARE}} = (\text{antilog}(y \text{ intercept})_{\text{rate}})/K \qquad (9.16)$$

$$k_e = \frac{\text{antilog}(y \text{ intercept})_{\text{ARE}}}{\text{dose}} \times K \qquad (9.17)$$

$$K = 2.303 \times \text{slope}$$

$$\text{total amount excreted unchanged} = A_e^\infty = \text{antilog of } y \text{ intercept} \qquad (9.18)$$

Other relationships are the same as equations 9.6, 9.7 and 9.9–9.12.

TABLE 9.3 Calculations for ARE Plot

Time (h)	Cumulative Amount	ARE
0	0	A_e^∞
t_1	$A_{e1} = \Delta A_{e1}$	$\text{ARE}_1 = A_e^\infty - A_{e1}$
t_2	$A_{e2} = A_{e1} + \Delta A_{e2}$	$\text{ARE}_2 = A_e^\infty - A_{e2}$
t_3	$A_{e3} = A_{e2} + \Delta A_{e3}$	$\text{ARE}_3 = A_e^\infty - A_{e3}$
t_4	$A_{e4} = A_{e3} + \Delta A_{e4}$	$\text{ARE}_4 = A_e^\infty - A_{e4}$
$\vdots$	$\vdots$	$\vdots$
t_n	A_e^{tn}	$\text{ARE}_n = A_e^\infty - A_{en}$
∞	A_e^∞	0

9.3 ANALYSIS OF URINARY DATA: METABOLITES (IV BOLUS)

The appropriate equations describing the formation and elimination of metabolite in the body were developed in Assignment 1.59, Chapter 1. The amount of metabolite in the body as a function of time, A_m, and the cumulative amount of metabolite eliminated from the body up to time t, A_{me}, were expressed in terms of the following equations:

$$A_m = \frac{k_m A_D^{\,0}}{K - k_{me}} \, (e^{-k_{me}t} - e^{-Kt}) \tag{9.19}$$

$$A_{me} = \frac{k_m A_D^{\,0}}{K} \left[1 + \frac{1}{k_{me} - K} \, (K e^{-k_{me}t} - k_{me} e^{-Kt}) \right] \tag{9.20}$$

The first-order rate constants k_m and k_{me} represent the formation and elimination of metabolite, respectively. As $t \to \infty$ the exponential terms of Equation 9.20 become negligible and the total amount eliminated as metabolite can be expressed as

$$A_{me}^{\infty} = \frac{k_m \times \text{dose}}{K} = f_m \, \text{dose} \tag{9.21}$$

Substituting Equation 9.21 into Equation 9.20 gives the following equation that describes the amount of drug remaining to be eliminated as metabolite:

$$A_{me}^{\infty} - A_{me} = \frac{A_{me}^{\infty}}{k_{me} - K} \, (k_{me} e^{-Kt} - K e^{-k_{me}t}) \tag{9.22}$$

The rate plot of elimination of metabolite is determined as

$$dA_{me}/dt = \text{rate of elimination of metabolites} = k_{me} \times A_m$$

Substituting Equation 9.19 for A_m and expressing the rate in terms of $\Delta A_{me}/\Delta t$ give the following rate equation for metabolite:

$$\frac{\Delta A_{me}}{\Delta t} = \frac{k_{me} \times k_m \times \text{dose}}{K - k_{me}} \, (e^{-k_{me}t_{\text{midpoint}}} - e^{-Kt_{\text{midpoint}}}) \tag{9.23}$$

A plot of $\log(A_{me}^{\infty} - A_{me})$ versus time or $\log(\Delta A_{me}/\Delta t)$ versus t_{midpoint} has a linear terminal portion (the extrapolated line) with a slope of $-k_{me}/2.303$. The residual line of the curve has a slope of $-K/2.303$. A typical rate plot for metabolite is presented in Figure 9.5. An estimate of the metabolic rate constant, k_m, can be determined from the y intercept of the extrapolated line of the rate plot of metabolite in urine:

$$k_m = \frac{(y \text{ intercept})(K - k_{me})}{k_{me} \text{dose}} \tag{9.24}$$

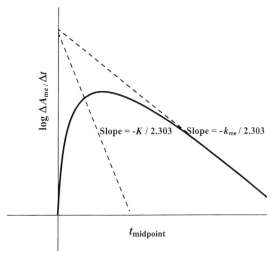

FIGURE 9.5 Rate plot of metabolite(s) eliminated in urine as a function of time. The calculations of y and x axes are the same as described for unchanged drug. Calculation of the residual line was described in Chapter 8.

9.4 ANALYSIS OF URINARY DATA: UNCHANGED DRUG (IV INFUSION)

To demonstrate the basic approaches of rate (Fig. 9.6) and ARE plots for intravenous infusion we start by substituting Equation 7.3, which was developed in Chapter 7, into Equation 9.2:

$$\frac{\Delta A_e}{\Delta t} = \frac{k_e k_0}{K}(1 - e^{-Kt_{\text{midpoint}}}) = k_e A_{ss}(1 - e^{-Kt_{\text{midpoint}}}) = f_e k_0 f_{ss} \tag{9.25}$$

Equation 9.25 indicates that the rate of excretion, so long as the rate of infusion remains constant, is a function of the fraction of steady-state level (f_{ss}). During the infusion and before the steady state level is reached, the rate of excretion changes with changing f_{ss} and time. At steady state $f_{ss} = 1$, the amount of drug in the body is maintained constant, the rate of infusion is equal to the rate of elimination, and thus the first-order rate of excretion, $k_e A_{ss}$, is invariable and equal to $f_e k_0$.

The urinary data of intravenous infusion can also be analyzed by integrating the differential form of Equation 9.25 between zero and time t:

$$\int_0^t \frac{dA_e}{dt} = \int_0^t \frac{k_e k_0}{K} - \int_0^t \frac{k_e k_0}{K} e^{-Kt} \tag{9.26}$$

Therefore,

$$A_e = \frac{k_e k_0}{K} t - \frac{k_e k_0}{K^2}(1 - e^{-Kt}) \tag{9.27}$$

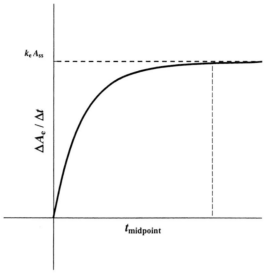

FIGURE 9.6 Rate plot of the urinary excretion of unchanged drug during intravenous infusion. The plateau level corresponds to the constant first-order rate of excretion during the infusion at steady state.

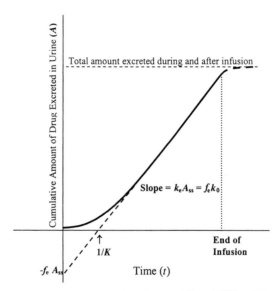

FIGURE 9.7 Plot of amount excreted unchanged in urine during infusion (Equation 9.27). The linear segment of the curve with y intercept $-f_e A_{ss}$ represents Equation 9.28 or 9.29. The plateau level occurs some time after stopping the infusion and represents the total amount excreted unchanged during and after infusion.

As $t \to \infty$, $e^{-Kt} \to 0$; therefore,

$$A_e^\infty = \frac{k_e k_0}{K} t - \frac{k_0 k_e}{K^2}$$ (9.28)

Equation 9.28 indicates that the total amount of drug excreted unchanged in urine, A_e^∞, is a variable that increases with time of infusion. Obviously when the infusion is discontinued, the amount in the body declines gradually and A_e^∞ reaches a plateau that represents total amount excreted during and after infusion. Equation 9.28 is a straight-line relationship with slope $f_e k_0$ or $k_e A_{ss}$ and y intercept $-f_e A_{ss}$ (Figure 9.7). Equation 9.28 may also be written as

$$A_e^\infty = A_{ss}(k_e t - f_e)$$ (9.29)

9.5 ANALYSIS OF URINARY DATA: UNCHANGED DRUG (ORAL ADMINISTRATION)

The rate and ARE equations of drug excreted unchanged in urine following an orally administered dose are similar to the previously described equations in Section 9.3. Substituting Equation 1.38 (Chapter 1) into Equation 9.2 yields the rate equation for an orally administered drug:

$$\frac{\Delta A_e}{\Delta t} = \frac{k_e k_a FD}{k_a - K}(e^{-Kt_{midpoint}} - e^{-k_a t_{midpoint}})$$ (9.30)

We can further revise Equation 9.30 by substituting $V_d \overleftarrow{C}_p^0$ (Equation 8.10) for $k_a FD/k_a - K$ in Equation 9.30:

$$\frac{\Delta A_e}{\Delta t} = k_e \overleftarrow{C}_p^0 V_d (e^{-Kt_{midpoint}} - e^{-k_a t_{midpoint}})$$ (9.31)

According to Equation 9.31, the rate plot of an oral dose is similar to its profile of plasma concentration with a maximum and a linear terminal portion that has a slope of $-K/2.303$. Obviously, as discussed in Chapter 8, depending on how fast is the rate of absorption, the curve can rise sharply or become flatter. When the absorption rate constant is greater than the overall elimination rate constant ($k_a \gg K$) and F is equal to one, the y intercept equals k_e dose.

The equation of the extrapolated line in Figure 9.8 is

$$\log \frac{\Delta A_e}{\Delta t} = k_e \overleftarrow{C}_p^0 V_d (e^{-Kt})$$ (9.32)

Similar to what we discussed in Chapter 8, the extrapolated line enables us to calculate the residual line of the curve which will have a slope of $-ka/2.303$ that provides an esti-

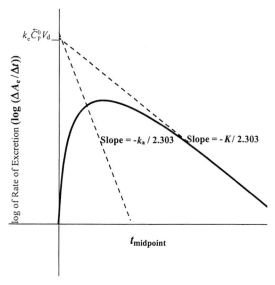

FIGURE 9.8 Theoretical rate plot of unchanged drug excreted in urine following administration of a single dose oral according to Equation 9.30 or 9.31.

mate of the absorption rate constant. Therefore, with knowledge of K, k_a, and FD the excretion rate constant, ke, can be estimated from the y intercept.

The ARE equation of the amount of drug excreted unchanged in urine following an oral dose is developed by integration of the differential form of Equation 9.30.

$$Ae = \frac{keFD}{K} \left[1 + \frac{k_a}{K - k_a} e^{-Kt} - \frac{K}{K - k_a} e^{-k_a t} \right] \tag{9.33}$$

As $t \rightarrow \infty$, the exponential terms become negligible and $A_e = A_e^\infty$:

$$A_e^\infty = f_e FD \tag{9.34}$$

Substitution of Equation 9.34 into Equation 9.33 and solving for the amount remaining to be excreted yield

$$\text{ARE} = (A_e^\infty - A_e) = \frac{A_e^\infty}{k_a - K} (k_a e^{-Kt} - K e^{-k_a t}) \tag{9.35}$$

Equation 9.35 also provides a curve similar to the rate plot (Figure 9.9). Under the condition $k_a > K$, the extrapolated and residual lines provide the estimates of the overall elimination and absorption rate constants, respectively. By multiplication of the y intercept of the extrapolated line by $(k_a - K)/k_a$, the total amount excreted unchanged, A_e^∞, can be estimated:

$$A_e^\infty = \frac{(y \text{ intercept})(k_a - K)}{k_a} \tag{9.36}$$

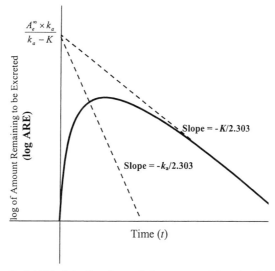

FIGURE 9.9 Theoretical ARE plot of unchanged drug excreted in urine following administration of a single dose orally according to Equation 9.35.

The excretion rate constant, k_e, can then be determined as

$$k_e = \frac{KA_e^\infty}{FD} \tag{9.37}$$

APPLICATION

9.1 After an intravenous bolus injection of 400 mg of an antibiotic with apparent volume of distribution of 20 L, the urinary data reported in Table 9.4 were obtained.

I. Determine the linear equation of $\log(\Delta A_e / \Delta t)$ versus t_{midpoint} (the rate plot). The calculations for $\Delta A_e / \Delta t$ and t_{midpoint} are presented in Table 9.5. The regression equation of $\log(\Delta A_e / \Delta t)$ versus t_{midpoint} is

$$\log \frac{\Delta A_e}{\Delta t} = 1.5 - 0.05 t_{\text{midpoint}}, \quad r^2 = 99.8\%$$

$$\frac{\Delta A_e}{\Delta t} = 31.62 e^{-0.12 t_{\text{midpoint}}}$$

TABLE 9.4 Data Related to Application 9.1

Time (h)	0	0.5	1.0	2.0	4.0	8.0	12.0	24.0	48.0	96.0
Cumulative Amount Excreted unchanged (mg)	0	16.9	32.7	61.1	107.2	168.5	203.4	241.3	249.7	250

TABLE 9.5 Calculations of Rate Plot: Application 9.1 (Part I)

ΔA_e (mg)	Δt (h)	$\Delta A_e / \Delta t$ (mg/h)	$T_{midpoint}$ (h)
16.9	0.5	33.8	(0.0 + 0.5)/2 = 0.25
15.8	0.5	31.6	(1.0 + 0.5)/2 = 0.75
28.4	1.0	28.4	(2.0 + 1.0)/2 = 1.50
46.1	2.0	23.0	(4.0 + 2.0)/2 = 3.00
61.3	4.0	15.3	(8.0 + 4.0)/2 = 6.00
34.9	4.0	8.7	(12.0 + 8.0)/2 = 10.0
37.9	12.0	3.15	(24.0 + 12.0)/2 = 18.0
8.4	24.0	0.35	(48.0 + 24.0)/2 = 36.0
0.3	48.0	0.006	(96.0 + 48.0)/2 = 72.0

Based on the regression equation, calculate the following:

1. Total body clearance

$$Cl_t = (0.12 \text{ h}^{-1})\,(20 \text{ L}) = 2.4 \text{ L/h} = 40 \text{ mL/min}$$

2. Renal and metabolic clearances

$$k_e = 31.623/400 = 0.079 \text{ h}^{-1}$$

$$Cl_r = (20 \text{ L})\,(0.079) = 1.58 \text{ L/h} = 26.33 \text{ mL/min}$$

$$Cl_m = 40 \text{ mL/min} - 26.33 = 13.67 \text{ mL/min}$$

3. Area under plasma concentration–time curve

$$AUC = (400/20)/0.12 = 166.66 \text{ mg h/L}$$

4. Plasma concentration 10 hours after injection

$$C_p^0 = 400/20 = 20 \text{ mg/L}$$

$$C_p^{10 \text{ h}} = 20 \text{ (mg/L)}\, e^{-0.12t}$$

$$C_p^{10 \text{ h}} = 20e^{-1.2} = 6.024 \text{ mg/L}$$

5. Fraction of dose excreted unchanged

$$f_e = 0.079/0.12 = 0.66$$

$$f_e = Cl_r/Cl_t = 1.58/2.4 = 0.66$$

6. Fraction of dose eliminated as metabolites

$$f_m = 0.041/0.12 = 0.34$$

or

$$f_m = Cl_m/Cl_t = 13.6/40 = 0.34$$

or

$$f_m = 1 - 0.66 = 0.34$$

II. Determine the regression equation of log ARE versus t (ARE plot) The calculations for the ARE plot are presented in Table 9.6.

The regression equation of log ARE versus time is

$$\log ARE = 2.398 - 0.055t, \quad r^2 = 100\%$$

$$ARE = 250e^{-0.126t}$$

Based on the above ARE equation calculate the following:

1. Fraction of dose excreted unchanged

$$f_e = A_e^\infty/\text{dose} \quad \text{or} \quad f_e = k_e/K$$

$$f_e = 250/400 = 0.625$$

2. Fraction of dose eliminated as metabolites

$$f_m = (\text{dose} - A_e^\infty)/\text{dose}$$

$$f_m = (400 - 250)/400 = 0.37$$

9.2 Four grams of an antibiotic with a half-life of 0.9 hours was administered intravenously to a patient with normal renal function. The total amount of unchanged drug recovered in the urine 24 hours after the injection was 2471 mg. The initial plasma concentration was estimated as 215 mg/L. Calculate the following parameters and constants.

TABLE 9.6 ARE Data: Application 9.1 (Part II)

Time (h)	0	0.5	1.0	2.0	4.0	8.0	12.0	24.0
ARE (mg)	250.00	223.10	217.30	188.90	142.80	81.50	46.60	8.70

1. Metabolic rate constant:

Because $24\ h > 7T_{1/2}$,

$$A_e^\infty = 2471\ mg$$

$$f_e = 2471\ mg/4000\ mg = 0.6177$$

$$K = 0.693/T_{1/2} = 0.693/0.9\ h = 0.77\ h^{-1}$$

$$f_m = 1 - f_e = 1 - 0.62 = 0.38$$

$$k_m = f_m \times K = (0.38)(0.77) = 0.29\ h^{-1}$$

2. Excretion rate constant

$$k_e = 0.77 - 0.29 = 0.48\ h^{-1}$$

or

$$k_e = (0.62)\ (0.77) = 0.48\ h^{-1}$$

3. Metabolic clearance

$$V_d = 4000\ mg/215\ mg\ L^{-1} = 18.6\ L$$

$$Cl_m = (0.29)\ (18.6) = 5.4\ L/h = 93\ mL/min$$

or

$$Cl_m = (0.38)\ (0.77)\ (18.6) = 5.4\ L/h$$

4. Renal clearance

$$Cl_r = (0.47)\ (18.6) = 8.74\ L/h = 145.7\ mL/min$$

or

$$Cl_r = 0.62\ (14.3) = 8.8\ L/h$$

5. Fraction of dose excreted unchanged in the urine

$$f_e = 0.62$$

6. Fraction of dose remaining in the body 3 hours after injection

$$f_b = e^{-0.77(3)} = 0.1$$

or

$$f_b = (\tfrac{1}{2})^n = (\tfrac{1}{2})^{3.334} = 0.1$$

or

$$3 \text{ h} \cong 3.3T_{1/2}, \quad \text{that is, } f_b = 0.1$$

7. Fraction of dose eliminated from the body 3 hours after injection

$$f_{el} = 1 - 0.1 = 0.9$$

8. Rate of elimination at $t = 3$ h

$$(\text{rate})_{3 \text{ h}} = KA = (0.1)\,(4 \text{ g})\,(0.77) = 0.308 \text{ g/h} = 308 \text{ mg/h}$$

9.3 Following intravenous bolus injection of 1000 mg of a new cephalosporin derivative, urine was collected at various intervals and analyzed for unchanged drug. Ultimately a total of 850 mg of the drug was excreted unchanged. The plasma concentration of free drug 4 hours after injection was measured as 17.5 mg/L. The amount of drug excreted unchanged in urine during each interval of urine collection is reported in Table 9.7. Determine the equation of log $\Delta A_e/\Delta t$ versus t_{midpoint} (rate plot). The calculations for the rate plot are presented in Table 9.8. The regression equation of log $(\Delta A_e/\Delta t)$ versus t_{midpoint} is

$$\log(\Delta A_e/\Delta t) = 2.25 - 0.0905 t_{\text{midpoint}}$$

Calculate the following.

1. First-order rate constants of elimination, excretion, and metabolism

$$K = (0.905)(2.303) = 0.208 \text{ h}^{-1} = 0.21 \text{ h}^{-1}$$

$$k_e = \text{antilog } 2.25/1000 \text{ mg} = 0.178 \text{ h}^{-1}$$

$$k_m = 0.21 - 0.178 = 0.032 \text{ h}^{-1}$$

TABLE 9.7 Data Related to Application 9.3

Time Interval (h)	Amount of Unchanged Drug Excreted during Interval
0–2	295
2–4	189
4–6	126
6–10	135
10–14	59

TABLE 9.8 Calculations of Rate Plot: Application 9.3

Δt	ΔA_e	$\Delta A_e/\Delta t$	$t_{midpoint}$
2	295	147.50	1
2	189	94.50	3
2	126	63.00	5
4	135	33.75	8
4	59	14.75	12

2. Renal clearance in units of mL/min and L/h

$$C_p^0 = C_p/e^{-Kt} = 17.5/e^{-0.21(4)} = 40.5 \text{ mg/L}$$

$$V_d = 1000 \text{ mg}/40.5 \text{ mg/L} = 24.7 \text{ L}$$

$$Cl_r = (0.178 \text{ h}^{-1})(24.7 \text{ L}) = 4.4 \text{ L/h} = 73.3 \text{ mL/min}$$

3. Fraction of dose excreted unchanged in urine

$$f_e = 0.178/0.21 = 0.847$$

9.4 A 75-kg hospitalized urology patient was given 4 g of an antibiotic intravenously by bolus injection. The half-life of the drug is 65 minutes and the apparent volume of distribution is 0.3 L/kg. The total amount of drug excreted unchanged in the 24-hour urine specimen of this patient was 3.65 g. Determine the following:

1. First-order excretion rate constant:

Because 24 h $> 7T_{1/2}$

$$A_e^\infty = 3.65 \text{ g}$$

$$f_e = 3.65 \text{ g}/4 \text{ g} = 0.91$$

$$k_e = (0.91)(0.693/65 \text{ min}) = 0.0097 \text{ min}^{-1} = 0.58 \text{ h}^{-1}$$

2. Rate and ARE equations of the drug for this patient

$$\frac{\Delta A_e}{\Delta t} = 2.32(\text{g/L})e^{-0.64(\text{h}^{-1})t_{midpoint}}$$

$$ARE = 3.65(\text{g})e^{-0.64(\text{h}^{-1})t}$$

9.5 A female patient (55 years old, 80 kg) with normal renal function receives an antibiotic by intravenous infusion at the rate of 15 mg/h. The urine was collected by catheter from the start of infusion and the cumulative amount of drug was determined as reported in Table 9.9. Calculate the following:

TABLE 9.9 Cumulative Amount of Antibiotic Excreted Unchanged in Urine: Application 9.5

Time (h)	0.25	0.50	0.80	1.50	3.00	4.50	6.00	9.00	12.00
A_e(mg)	0.179	0.680	1.635	4.991	15.288	27.461	40.298	66.524	92.903

1. Fraction of dose excreted unchanged

The regression equation of the last four data points is

$$A_e^{\infty} = 8.73t - 11.97$$

$$f_e = \frac{8.73}{15} = 0.582$$

2. Overall elimination rate constant

$$K = \frac{8.73}{11.97} = 0.72 \text{ h}^{-1}$$

3. Excretion and metabolic rate constants

$$k_e = 0.582 \times 0.72 = 0.42 \text{ h}^{-1}$$

$$k_m = 0.72 - 0.42 = 0.3 \text{ h}^{-1}$$

9.6 A single dose (500 mg) of a drug was administered orally to a 70-kg volunteer. A set of plasma concentrations were obtained and analyzed according to a one-compartment model. The analysis yielded the equation

$$C_p = 40(e^{-0.1155t} - e^{-1.386t})$$

The total amount of drug excreted unchanged in the urine during a period that exceeded $7T_{1/2}$ was also measured and reported as 350 mg. The drug is known to have an apparent volume of distribution of 10 L. Calculate the following:

1. Excretion rate constant

$$F = \frac{40 \text{ mg/L} \times 10 \text{ L} \times (1.386 - 0.1155) \text{ h}^{-1}}{500 \text{ mg} \times 1.386} = 0.734$$

$$f_e = \frac{350}{0.734 \times 500} = 0.95$$

$$k_e = 0.95 \times 0.1155 = 0.109 \text{ h}^{-1}$$

2. ARE equation for this drug

$$ARE = 275.48(1.386e^{-0.1155t} - 0.1155e^{-1.386t})$$

or

$$ARE = 381.81e^{-0.1155t} - 31.81e^{-1.386t}$$

3. Rate equation for this drug

$$\frac{\Delta A_e}{\Delta t} = 43.6(e^{-0.1155t_{midpoint}} - e^{-1.386t_{midpoint}})$$

ASSIGNMENT

9.1 The cumulative amounts of unchanged drug appearing in the urine following an IV injection of 500 mg of an antibiotic are reported in Table 9.10. Determine the following:
   9.1.1 Linear regression equation of log ARE versus time
   9.1.2 Overall elimination rate constant
   9.1.3 Half-life
   9.1.4 Fraction of dose excreted unchanged
   9.1.5 Metabolic rate constant
   9.1.6 Linear regression equation of log rate versus time

9.2 Four grams of an antibiotic was administered intravenously to a patient with normal renal function. The total amount of unchanged drug recovered in urine within 24 hours of the injection was 2083 mg. The half-life of the drug is 1.25 h and the initial plasma concentration is 285 mg/L. Calculate the following:
   9.2.1 Renal and metabolic clearances
   9.2.2 Fraction of dose excreted unchanged
   9.2.3 Fraction of dose eliminated as metabolite(s)

9.3 Use the data presented in Application 9.3 (Table 9.7) and determine the linear regression equation of log ARE versus time.

9.4 A 65-kg hospitalized urology patient with renal failure was given 4 g of an antibiotic intravenously. The total amount of drug excreted unchanged in urine 10 hours after the injection was 3 g. The apparent volume of distribution is 0.4 L/kg and $T_{1/2}$ = 300 minutes. Determine the following:
   9.4.1 Rate constant of excretion
   9.4.2 Renal clearance

TABLE 9.10 Data Related to Assignment 9.1

t (h)	0.5	1	2	3	4	5	6	8	11	14	20	∞
A_e (mg)	27	52	98	137	171	200	226	268	314	343	375	400

9.4.3 Fraction of dose in the body at $t = 10$ h
9.4.4 Rate and ARE equations

9.5 The effect of rest compared with intermittent exercise was investigated in male volunteers after intravenous bolus injection of 750 mg of a cephalosporin. Urine was collected and assayed, and the following two linear regression equations were reported based on the amount of free drug in urine:

$$\log \text{ARE} = 1.778 - 0.1t$$

$$\log \frac{\Delta A_e}{\Delta t} = 1.29 - 0.2t_{\text{midpoint}}$$

(The units of amount and time are "mg" and "h", respectively.) Fill in the blanks of Table 9.11.

9.6 The following are the rate and ARE equations of two structurally similar investigational drugs (A and B). Both drugs were given in a crossover design to a 60-kg patient by IV bolus injection of 500 mg. The apparent volume of distribution for both drugs, estimated from plasma data, was approximately 10% body weight.

Drug A: $\text{ARE} = 50e^{-0.5t}$

Drug B: $\log \text{rate} = 1.398 - 0.175t_{\text{midpoint}}$

(The units of amount and time are "mg" and "h", respectively.) Fill in the blanks of Table 9.12.

9.7 A male patient (60 years old, 80 kg) with normal renal function receives a new drug by intravenous infusion at the rate of 60 mg/h. The urine was collected during the infusion and the cumulative amounts of drug were determined as reported in Table 9.13. Calculate the following:
    9.7.1 Overall elimination rate constant
    9.7.2 Fraction of dose excreted unchanged
    9.7.3 Fraction of dose eliminated as metabolite(s)
    9.7.4 Half-life of drug

TABLE 9.11 Assignment 9.5

Condition	A_e^{∞} (mg)	k_e (h^{-1})	k_m (h^{-1})	A_m^{∞} (mg)	$(f_{el})_{3\,h}$
Rest					
Exercise					

TABLE 9.12 Assignment 9.6

Parameter/Constant	Drug A	Drug B
Metabolic rate constant (h^{-1})		
Total amount excreted unchanged (mg)		
Total amount eliminated as metabolite(s) (mg)		
Metabolic clearance (mL/min)		
AUC (mg h/L)		

9.8 Simulate the ARE and rate curves based on the equations of Applications 9.6.2 and 9.6.3.

$$\text{ARE} = 381.81e^{-0.1155t} - 31.81e^{-1.386t} \quad \text{and} \quad \frac{\Delta A_e}{\Delta t} = 43.6\ (e^{-0.1155t_{midpoint}} - e^{-1.386t_{midpoint}})$$

9.9 The following is the ARE equation of a drug given by IV bolus:

$$\log \text{ARE} = 2 - 0.1t$$

The amount was measured in milligrams and time in hours. By using the parameter and constant of this equation answer the following questions:

9.9.1 If the dose were 200 mg what would be the total amount eliminated as metabolites?

9.9.2 If the dose were 1000 mg what would be the fraction of dose excreted unchanged?

9.9.3 If the dose were 250 mg what would be the excretion rate constant?

9.9.4 If 40% of the dose were excreted unchanged what would be the dose?

9.9.5 If 30% of the dose were eliminated as metabolite(s) and the volume of distribution is 10 L what would be the renal clearance?

9.10 After an IV bolus injection of an antibiotic to a 70-kg, 55-year-old male patient, the cumulative amounts of unchanged drug excreted in urine were measured as reported in Table 9.14. Ultimately a total of 1 g was excreted unchanged. The plasma concentration of the drug 4 hours after injection was determined as 6.25 mg/L. The total amount of drug eliminated as metabolites was approximated as 40% of the dose. By using the rate plot determine the following:

9.10.1 Overall elimination rate constant

9.10.2 Dose

9.10.3 First-order excretion rate constant

TABLE 9.13 Data Related to Assignment 9.7

Time (h)	0.25	0.50	0.80	1.50	3.00	4.50	6.00	9.00	12.00
A_e (mg)	0.719	2.724	6.540	19.964	61.153	109.847	161.194	266.099	371.612

TABLE 9.14 Data Related to Assignment 9.10

Amount (mg)	0	160	300	500	750	938	984
Time (h)	0	0.25	0.50	1.00	2.00	4.00	6.00

9.10.4 Renal and metabolic clearance

9.10.5 ARE equation

ASSIGNMENT (EXTRA CREDIT)

EC-9.1 On the basis of data presented in the following article, answer the questions of this assignment:

Carchman SH, Crowe Jr, JT, Wright GJ. The bioavailability and pharmacokinetics of guanfacine after oral and intravenous administration to healthy volunteers. *J Clin Pharmacol* 1987;27:762–7.

■ Because the time of intravenous infusion is less than 2% of the half-life of the drug you can assume that the drug was given as an IV bolus injection. Based on the reported data calculate the estimated A_e^∞ and excretion rate constant.

■ Explain why the investigators have reported the ratio of renal guanfacine clearance to creatinine clearance.

■ Does the difference between the A_e^∞ values for oral administration and IV injection correspond to the differences between the AUC values for oral administration and IV injection?

■ To what does the ratio $(A_e^\infty)_{po}/(A_e^\infty)_{iv}$ correspond?

EC-9.2 The major metabolites of 5-fluorouracil in the urine according to Heggie et al are α-fluoro-β-alanine (FBAL) and α-fluoro-ureidopropionic acid (FUPA). Read the article and answer the questions for this assignment.

Heggie GD, Sommadossi JP, Cross DS, Huster WJ, Diasio RB. Clinical pharmacokinetics of 5-fluorouracil and its metabolites in plasma, urine, and bile. *Cancer Res* 1987;47:2203–6.

■ Approximate the fraction of dose excreted unchanged from Figure 2 of the article.

■ Estimate the fraction of each major metabolite in the urine.

■ Calculate the clearance of each metabolite and compare with the reported data.

■ From Table 3 of the article calculate the metabolic rate constants of the following metabolites of 5-fluorouracil: dihydrofluorouracil, α-fluoro-ureidopropionic acid, α-fluoro-β-alanine.

EC-9.3 According to the data reported in the following article, the total amounts of ciprofloxacin excreted unchanged in the urine 48 hours after IV and oral administration of 200 mg were 119 ± 17.67 and 83.77 ± 18.46 mg, respectively. Assume the data follow a one-compartment model and the average amounts excreted unchanged are 120 and 84 mg. Use the relevant data from Table 1 of the article and develop the ARE and rate equations. Simulate the related ARE and rate curves as a linear plot and the related lines as a semilogarithmic plot over a period of 48 hours.

Drusano GL, Standiford HC, Plaisance K, Forrest A, Leslie J, Caldwell J. Absolute bioavailability of ciprofloxacin. *Antimicrob Agents Chemother* 1986;30:444–6.

BIBLIOGRAPHY

1. Cummings AJ, Martin BK, Park GS. Kinetic considerations relating to the accrual and elimination of drug metabolites. *Br J Pharmacol Chemother* 1967;29:150.
2. Galloway JA, McMahon RE, Culp HW, Marshal FJ, Young EC. Metabolism, blood levels and rate of excretion of acetohexamide in human subjects. *Diabetes* 1967;16:118.
3. Gibaldi M, Perrier D. *Pharmacokinetics.* New York: Marcel Dekker, 1975:6.
4. Houston JB. Drug metabolite kinetics. In: Rowland M, Tucker G, editors. *Pharmacokinetics: theory and methodology.* Oxford: Pergamon Press, 1986:131.
5. Pang KS, Gillette JR. Metabolite pharmacokinetics: methods for simultaneous estimates of elimination rate constants of a drug and its metabolite. *Drug Metab Dispos* 1980;8:39.
6. Wagner JG. Some possible errors in the plotting and interpretation of semilogarithmic plots of blood level and urinary excretion data. *J Pharm Sci* 1958;52:1097.
7. Wagner JG. Fundamentals of clinical pharmacokinetics. Hamilton, IL: *Drug Intelligence,* 1975:38.

CHAPTER 10

MULTIPLE DOSING KINETICS: ONE-COMPARTMENT MODEL

Right thinking is the greatest excellence, and wisdom is to speak the truth
and act in accordance with nature, while paying attention to it.
STOBAEUS (SELECTIONS)

OBJECTIVES

- To discuss multiple dosing kinetics of intravenous bolus injection, short-term infusion, and oral administration.

- To discuss the concept of steady-state levels in multiple dosing.

- To interpret the plasma concentration–time fluctuation before and after achieving steady-state levels.

- To estimate important parameters of multiple dosing before, during, and after achieving steady-state levels.

- To discuss various methods of designing a dosing regimen.

10.1 INTRODUCTION

The purpose of a multiple-dosing regimen is to achieve a consistent pharmacologic response for a period longer than the duration of action of a single dose administration. Similar to intravenous infusion (Chapter 7), this type of continuous therapy is achieved by accumulating drug in the body following uninterrupted administration of drug based on a fixed dose and dosing interval and achievement of a steady-state level within the therapeutic range of the drug. Unlike continuous infusion, however, the plasma concentration of drug fluctuates in multiple dosing. After each dose it reaches a maximum level (peak) and then declines to a minimum concentration (trough). The dose is usually kept constant and dosing interval, τ, is selected as a fixed interval approximately equal to the half-life of the drug. This means that during each dosing interval approximately 50% of the total amount of drug in the body is eliminated and 50% remains in the body. Thus, peak and trough levels of each dose are higher than those of previous doses. As dose and dosing interval are kept constant, after a finite time the administered dose is equal to the amount eliminated from the body. This is when the steady-state levels (ie, peak and trough) are achieved and the amount accumulated in the body is at its anticipated maximum level of the dosing regimen. A well-designed dosing regimen would maintain the fluctuation at steady state within the therapeutic range. The concept is similar to intravenous infusion; that is, we maintain the steady state if and only if the rate of input is equal to the rate of output, or the administered dose is equal to the amount eliminated from the body during a dosing interval. The fixed dose that is given on a regular basis is also known as the maintenance dose.

10.2 KINETICS OF MULTIPLE IV BOLUS INJECTIONS

The kinetics of multiple-dosing regimens are based on geometric series that was discussed in Chapter 1, Section 1.15. Assume a course of therapy starts with a fixed dose and dosing interval. The dose is either injected rapidly through the tubing of an IV set, close to the vein, or injected directly by syringe intravenously. The injection takes place at a fixed interval of τ. The summary of this regimen in terms of peak and trough levels is presented in Table 10.1. A^0 is the initial amount in the body, and A_{max} and A_{min} are the maximum and minimum amounts, respectively. The parentheses of the table, as we discussed in Chapter 1, Section 1.15, are the geometric series of the multiple-dosing function after each dose. As the number of doses increases, the number of exponential terms increases. Thus, after administration of too many doses, the equation becomes longer and using these terms for the purpose of calculating the concentration of drug in plasma becomes awkward (Table 10.1). To make the calculation more manageable we solve for the solution of the geometric series of the nth dose as follows:

Step 1: The difference between peak and trough levels of the nth dose (Table 10.1) is

$$(A_{max})_n - (A_{min})_n = A^0(S_n) - A^0(S_n)e^{-K\tau} = A^0(S_n)(1 - e^{-K\tau}) \qquad (10.1)$$

where S_n, as is identified in the table, corresponds to the geometric series of the nth dose.

Step 2: The difference between peak and trough levels can also be obtained by subtracting $(A_{min})_n = A^0(e^{-K\tau} + e^{-K\tau} + e^{-2K\tau} + e^{-3K\tau} + e^{-4K\tau} + \cdots + e^{-(n-1)\tau} + e^{-n\tau})$ from $(A_{max})_n = A^0(1 + e^{-K\tau} + e^{-2K\tau} + e^{-3K\tau} + e^{-4K\tau} + \cdots + e^{-(n-1)\tau})$, which yields the relationship

$$(A_{max})_n - (A_{min})_n = A^0(1 - e^{-n\tau}) \qquad (10.2)$$

Setting Equation 10.1 equal to Equation 10.2 and solving for S_n provides the relationships

$$S_n = \frac{1 - e^{-nK\tau}}{1 - e^{-K\tau}} \qquad (10.3)$$

We could also use Equation 1.48 (Chapter 1) to generate the above equation.

TABLE 10.1 Summary of Peaks and Trough Levels in Multiple Intravenous Injections and the Related Geometric Series

τ	Dose	A_{max}	A_{min}
τ_1	D_1	$(A_{max})_1 = A^0$	$(A_{min})_1 = A^0 e^{-K\tau}$
τ_2	D_2	$(A_{max})_2 = A^0(1 + e^{-K\tau})$	$(A_{min})_2 = A^0(e^{-K\tau} + e^{-2K\tau})$
τ_3	D_3	$(A_{max})_3 = A^0(1 + e^{-K\tau} + e^{-2K\tau})$	$(A_{min})_3 = A^0(e^{-K\tau} + e^{-2K\tau} + e^{-3K\tau})$
τ_4	D_4	$(A_{max})_4 = A^0(1 + e^{-K\tau} + e^{-2K\tau} + e^{-3K\tau})$	$(A_{min})_4 = A^0(e^{-K\tau} + e^{-2K\tau} + e^{-3K\tau} + e^{-4K\tau})$
⋮	⋮	⋮	⋮
τ_n	D_n	$(A_{max})_n = A^0 \underbrace{(1 + e^{-K\tau} + e^{-2K\tau} + e^{-3K\tau} + e^{-4K\tau} + \cdots + e^{-(n-1)\tau})}_{S_n}$	$(A_{min})_n = A^0 \underbrace{(e^{-K\tau} + e^{-K\tau} + e^{-2K\tau} + e^{-3K\tau} + e^{-4K\tau} + \cdots + e^{-(n-1)\tau} + e^{-n\tau})}_{S_n e^{-K\tau}}$

Equation 10.3 summarizes all the exponential terms of $(A_{max})_n$ in Table 10.1 and represents the solution of geometric series of multiple dosing after the nth dose. As $n \to \infty$, that is, when the accumulation reaches the expected maximum level and steady state is achieved, $e^{-nK\tau} \to 0$, and Equation 10.3 converts to the following form that represents the solution of the geometric series of multiple dosing at steady state:

$$(S_n)_{ss} = \frac{1}{1 - e^{-K\tau}} \tag{10.4}$$

10.2.1 Equations of Peak and Trough Levels

The usefulness of Equations 10.3 and 10.4 is that they enable us to develop equations of multiple-dosing kinetics for any concentration after any dose. For example, by multiplying equations of first dose by S_n or $(S_n)_{ss}$ several relationships are developed that can be used to calculate plasma concentration at any time during therapy. Equations of first dose are:

$$(C_{p_{max}})_1 = C_p^0 \tag{10.5}$$

$$(C_{p_{min}})_1 = (C_{p_{max}})_1 e^{-K\tau} = C_p^0 e^{-K\tau} \tag{10.6}$$

$$(C_{p_t})_1 = (C_{p_{max}})_1 e^{-Kt} = C_p^0 e^{-Kt} \tag{10.7}$$

Equation 10.7 represents plasma concentration at any time between peak and trough levels of the first dose.

By multiplying Equations 10.5 to 10.7 by Equation 10.3, the following relationships are obtained that are used to predict plasma concentrations ($C_{p_{max}}$, $C_{p_{min}}$, and C_{p_t}) after the nth dose before achieving the steady-state level (Figure 10.1):

$$(C_{p_{max}})_n = C_p^0 \left(\frac{1 - e^{-nK\tau}}{1 - e^{-K\tau}} \right) \tag{10.8}$$

$$(C_{p_{min}})_n = C_p^0 \left(\frac{1 - e^{-nK\tau}}{1 - e^{-K\tau}} \right) e^{-K\tau} = (C_{p_{max}})_n e^{-K\tau} \tag{10.9}$$

$$(C_{pt})_n = C_p^0 \left(\frac{1 - e^{-nK\tau}}{1 - e^{-K\tau}} \right) e^{-Kt} = (C_{p_{max}})_n e^{-Kt} \tag{10.10}$$

Multiplying Equations 10.5 to 10.7 by Equation 10.4 gives equations of steady-state levels:

$$(C_{p_{max}})_{ss} = C_p^0 \left(\frac{1}{1 - e^{-K\tau}} \right) \tag{10.11}$$

$$(C_{p_{min}})_{ss} = C_p^0 \left(\frac{e^{-K\tau}}{1 - e^{-K\tau}} \right) = (C_{p_{max}})_{ss} e^{-K\tau} \tag{10.12}$$

$$(C_{p_t})_{ss} = C_p^0 \left(\frac{e^{-K\tau}}{1 - e^{-K\tau}} \right) = (C_{p_{max}})_{ss} e^{-K\tau} \tag{10.13}$$

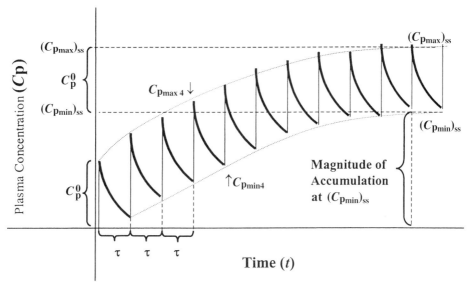

FIGURE 10.1 Plasma concentration–time profile of multiple intravenous bolus injections of the same dose given every fixed dosing interval of τ. The fluctuation between peak and trough levels is equal to the initial plasma concentration of the maintenance dose, and the magnitude of accumulation depends on the dose and dosing interval.

C_p^0 in the above equations represents the initial plasma concentration of the maintenance dose, that is, D_M/V_d. The difference between peak and trough levels of the steady-state level is also equal to C_p^0 (Figure 10.1).

10.2.2 Time Required to Achieve Steady-state Plasma Levels

Similar to intravenous infusion (Chapter 7), if the therapy starts with the maintenance dose, it would take some time to attain the steady-state level. Contrary to intravenous infusion, in which the amount and time of input are continuous, however, in multiple-dosing kinetics, this time consists of several dosing intervals and, hence, cannot be expressed as continuous t, but rather as $n\tau$. The equation of $n\tau$, or the time needed to achieve any fraction of steady-state level, is determined by comparing the numerators of Equations 10.3 and 10.4. In both equations "1" corresponds to 100% of steady-state level, e^{-nK^τ} is the fraction left to reach the steady-state level, and $1 - e^{-nK^\tau}$ of Equation 10.3 represents the fraction of steady-state level:

$$f_{ss} = 1 - e^{-nK^\tau} \tag{10.14}$$

Solving for $n\tau$ by taking the natural logarithm of Equation 10.14, we obtain

$$n\tau = -\frac{\ln(1 - f_{ss})}{K} \tag{10.15}$$

or

$$n\tau = -3.3T_{1/2} \log(1 - f_{ss}) \tag{10.16}$$

According to Equation 10.16 and similar to intravenous infusion, the time required to achieve any fraction of steady state is directly proportional to half-life, or indirectly proportional to the overall elimination rate constant. For example, to achieve 50% of the steady-state level, that is, for $f_{ss} = 0.5$, $n\tau = 1T_{1/2}$; for 75%, $f_{ss} = 0.75$, $n\tau = 2T_{1/2}$; for 90%, $f_{ss} = 0.9$, $n\tau = 3.3T_{1/2}$; for 95%, $f_{ss} = 0.95$, $n\tau = 4.3T_{1/2}$; for 99%, $f_{ss} = 0.99$, $n\tau = 6.6T_{1/2}$. Clinically the time required to reach a steady-state fluctuation is between four and five half-lives. For the assignments of this chapter it is assumed to be approximately seven half-lives.

10.2.3 Average Steady-state Plasma Concentration

The average plasma concentration at steady state is another concentration parameter that is developed based on the definition of steady state. At steady state the rate of input is equal to the rate of output. In the case of intravenous infusion the rate of input is zero-order and continuous, whereas in multiple dosing it is sequential and the rate is defined as maintenance dose given every dosing interval. The rate of output during infusion at steady state, although first-order, remains constant because of the constant steady-state plasma level. In multiple dosing the rate of output changes during a dosing interval and declines from a maximum to a minimum because of the change in plasma level. Therefore, to define a single rate of output during a dosing interval, similar to intravenous infusion, we have to relay on the average rate of elimination, which corresponds to the average steady-state plasma level:

$$\text{rate of Input} = \text{maintenance dose/dosing interval} = D_M/\tau$$

$$\text{rate of output} = Cl_t \times (C_{p_{ave}})_{ss} = K \times (A_{ave})_{ss}$$

where $(C_{p_{ave}})_{ss}$ and $(A_{ave})_{ss}$ are average concentration and average amount at steady state, respectively.

Setting the rate of input equal to the rate of output and solving for $(C_{p_{ave}})_{ss}$ lead to the equation of average steady-state plasma concentration, which can be presented in various forms:

$$(C_{p_{ave}})_{ss} = \frac{D}{Cl_t\tau} = \frac{D}{KV_d\tau} = \frac{1.44T_{1/2}D}{V_d\tau} = \frac{C_p^0}{K\tau} = \frac{(AUC)_\tau}{\tau} \tag{10.17}$$

The definition of the average steady-state plasma concentration based on Equation 10.17 can be either the average rate of input divided by clearance or the area under the plasma concentration–time curve of a maintenance dose at steady state divided by the dosing interval. Equation 10.17 is used in designing and adjusting dosing regimens for patients. The shortcoming of the equation is that it provides no information about the peak or trough level, fluctuation, within the therapeutic range. The magnitude of the fluctuation, however, can be estimated from D/V_d, where $D = D_M$.

10.2.4 Loading Dose and Maintenance Dose

To avoid waiting four to five half-lives to achieve quasi-steady-state levels, a loading dose (D_L) can be administered at the start of therapy. This one-time dose should provide an initial concentration equal to the maximum plasma concentration at steady state. Thus, the loading dose is equal to the maximum amount of drug in the body at steady state:

$$D_L = (C_{p_{max}})_{ss}V_d = (A_{max})_{ss} \tag{10.18}$$

The maintenance dose (D_M) is that portion of the loading dose that is eliminated from the body by all routes of elimination during steady state in the first dosing interval:

$$(f_{el})_\tau = 1 - e^{-K\tau} \tag{10.19}$$

$$D_M = D_L(1 - e^{-K\tau}) \tag{10.20}$$

The maintenance dose can also be defined as the fluctuation at steady state multiplied by the volume of distribution. The fluctuation is the difference between the peak and trough levels:

$$D_M = V_d(C_{p_{max}} - C_{p_{min}}) \tag{10.21}$$

It can also be calculated from Equation 10.17:

$$D_M = (C_{p_{ave}})_{ss}Cl_t\tau \tag{10.22}$$

Equation 10.22 also indicates that the maintenance dose is the average rate of elimination at steady state $(C_{p_{ave}})_{ss}Cl_t$ in one dosing interval multiplied by the dosing interval.

Thus in a multiple-dosing regimen if a loading dose is followed by a maintenance dose at every fixed dosing interval, the steady-state fluctuation can be achieved immediately and maintained as long as therapy is continued (Figure 10.2).

Equation 10.20 represents the relationship between loading dose and maintenance dose:

$$D_L = \frac{D_M}{1 - e^{-K\tau}} = \frac{D_M}{1 - (1/2)^{T_{1/2}/\tau}} = \frac{D_M}{(f_{el})_\tau} \tag{10.23}$$

Based on the relationship between the $T_{1/2}$ of a drug and dosing interval, three scenarios can be perceived:

1. If $\tau \gg T_{1/2}$, the ratio $T_{1/2}/\tau$ would be very small and the denominator would approach one. Under this assumption $D_L = D_M$. An example is administering a drug with wide therapeutic range and very short half-life, say less than 30 minutes given every 4 hours. Under this condition no loading dose would be necessary.

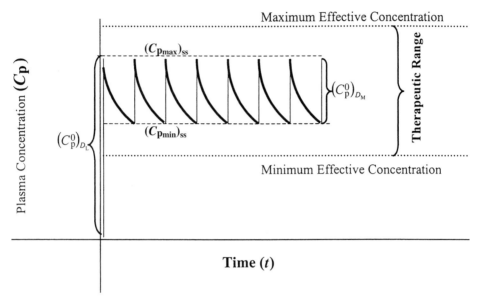

FIGURE 10.2 Profile of fluctuation of plasma concentration following administration of loading dose and six maintenance doses. Note that the fluctuation is shown within the therapeutic range. Thus, the steady state peak and trough levels may or may not be equal to the maximum and minimum effective concentrations, respectively.

2. If $\tau = T_{1/2}$, the denominator would be equal to 0.5 and the loading dose would be twice the maintenance dose. An example is giving a drug with a half-life of 6 hours four times a day.
3. If $\tau << T_{1/2}$, the denominator approaches zero and the relationship would become undefined. An example is giving a drug with a half-life of 7 days once a day. Needless to say, having a very long half-life may not be a good characteristic for a therapeutic agent. In this type of situation we can set the loading dose equal to the average amount at steady state and define the relationship according to the equation

$$D_L = (A_{ave})_{ss} = \frac{D_M}{K\tau} \tag{10.24}$$

10.2.5 Extent of Accumulation

We may estimate the degree of accumulation of a drug in the body at steady state by a number known as the accumulation ratio, which is determined by dividing the peak or trough level of steady state by the peak or trough level of the first dose. The first dose here refers to the maintenance dose according to the profile of Figure 10.1. The ratio, as presented in Equation 10.25, is the same as Equation 10.4, which we identified as the solution of geometric series of multiple dosing at steady state. The ratio indicates how many -fold of a drug is accumulated in the body at the peak or trough level of steady state with respect to first dose for a given dosing regimen. It also corresponds to the ratio D_L/D_M, which is the reciprocal of the fraction of dose eliminated from the body by all routes of elimination during a dosing interval at steady state. For example, if the ratio $1/(1 - e^{-K^\tau}) = 1/(f_{el})_\tau = 5$, this means that the amount of drug accumulated is five times more than what was accumulated after the first dose and $(C_{p_{max}})_{ss} = 5(C_{p_{max}})_1$ or $(C_{p_{min}})_{ss} = 5(C_{p_{min}})_1$:

$$R = \frac{(C_{p_{max}})_{ss}}{(C_{p_{max}})_1} = \frac{(C_{p_{max}})_{ss}}{(C_p^0)_{D_M}} = \frac{(C_{p_{min}})_{ss}}{(C_{p_{min}})_1} = \frac{D_L}{D_M} = \frac{1}{1 - e^{-K\tau}} = \frac{1}{(f_{el})_\tau} \qquad (10.25)$$

10.2.6 Decline of Plasma Concentration after Last Dose

We may need to know how much of a drug is left in the body after the last dose of a dosing regimen, whether or not steady state is achieved. This type of information may be called for when the course of therapy for a patient is revised, a different drug is recommended, and there a drug–drug interaction is probable. Knowledge of the plasma concentration after the last dose of the first drug may help to determine when the second drug should be initiated. The following equations, which are modified versions of Equation 6.10, can be used to estimate the plasma concentration after the last dose:

$$C_{p_{t'}} = C_{p_{max}} e^{-Kt'} \quad \text{or} \quad C_{p_{t'}} = C_{p_{min}} e^{-K(t'-\tau)} \qquad (10.26)$$

See Figure 10.3.

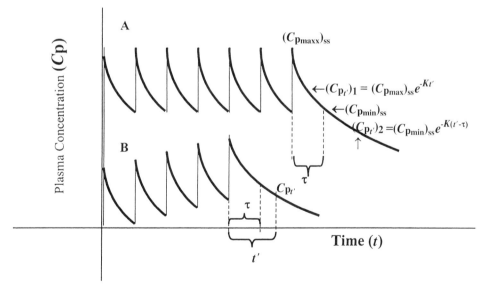

FIGURE 10.3 Decline of plasma concentration after the last dose of a multiple dosing regimen before (B) and after (A) achieving steady-state level. For drugs that follow a one-compartment model and are given by intravenous injection, the plasma concentration after the last dose can be estimated with respect to peak level, $(C_{p_{t'}})_1$, or trough level, $(C_{p_{t'}})_2$.

10.2.7 Design of a Dosing Regimen

The purpose of designing a dosing regimen is to determine the loading dose, maintenance dose, and dosing interval for a given drug based on the pharmacokinetics of the drug in a population of patients. A few practical methods for designing a dosing regimen are discussed here.

10.2.7.1 Calculation of Dosing Regimen Based on a Target Concentration within the Therapeutic Range:

　Step 1: Select a target concentration within the therapeutic range of the drug and set it equal to the average steady-state plasma concentration.

　Step 2: Based on the half-life of the drug, select a dosing interval. For example, if the half-life is 3–4, 4–6, 6–8, 8–12, or 24 hours, we can set $\tau = T_{1/2}$ and give the dose every 4 hours, four times daily, three times daily, twice daily, and daily.

　Step 3: Determine the maintenance dose according to the equation

$$D_M = (C_{p_{ave}})_{ss}V_d\tau K \tag{10.27}$$

Because dosing interval is set equal to half-life, $D_L = 2D_M$. If the dosing interval is different from the half-life, for example $T_{1/2} = 6h$ and you set $\tau = 4h$, the loading dose is determined according to equation 10.23. For drugs with very short half-life the dosing interval is usually set equal to four hours for convenience of administration and $D_L = D_M$.

　It would be advisable to verify whether the peak and trough levels of dosing regimen are within the therapeutic range. This is particularly important for drugs with low therapeutic range. A quick approach would be:

$$(C_{p_{max}})_{ss} = \frac{D_L}{V_d} \tag{10.28}$$

$$(C_{p_{min}})_{ss} = (C_{p_{max}})_{ss} - \frac{D_M}{V_d} \tag{10.29}$$

10.2.7.2 Calculation of Dosing Regimen Based on Steady-state Peak and Trough Levels (Fluctuation) within the Therapeutic Range:

　Step 1: Select the desired peak and trough levels within the therapeutic range.

　Step 2: Determine the fluctuation of plasma concentrations, which is equal to the initial plasma concentration of the maintenance dose

$$\text{fluctuation} = (C_{p_{max}})_{ss} - (C_{p_{min}})_{ss} = (C_p^0)_{D_M}$$

　Step 3: Calculate the maintenance dose as

$$D_M = V_d \times (C_{p_{max}} - C_{p_{min}})_{ss} \tag{10.30}$$

Step 4: Select the dosing interval. A trough level equal to half of the peak level would indicate that the dosing interval is equal to the half-life of drug. The loading dose would then be equal to twice the maintenance dose. If the trough level is not half of the peak level, the dosing interval can be estimated as

$$\tau = \frac{2.303}{K} \log \frac{(C_{p_{max}})_{ss}}{(C_{p_{min}})_{ss}} \tag{10.31}$$

10.2.7.3 Calculation of Dosing Regimen Based on Minimum Steady-state Plasma Concentration within the Therapeutic Range: We can also determine the dosing regimen based on the minimum steady-state plasma concentration. First we select a dosing interval, preferentially equal to the half-life of the drug. Then, by using the equation of plasma concentration at steady state, we calculate the maintenance dose:

$$D_M = \frac{(C_{p_{min}})_{ss} V_d \left(1 - e^{-K\tau}\right)}{e^{-K\tau}} \tag{10.32}$$

Depending on the dosing interval, the loading dose is calculated as described previously.

10.3 KINETICS OF MULTIPLE ORAL ADMINISTRATION

The basic premise of the kinetics of multiple oral administration is the same as that for multiple intravenous injections. The only difference is that we must be mindful of the effect of the absorption process on the plasma concentration of drug. Similar to the elimination process, multiple absorption can also be defined in terms of a geometric series. Therefore, for multiple oral administration there are two geometric series: one for absorption and one for elimination. The solutions of the geometric series are:

1. Before achieving the steady state,

$$(S_n)_K = \frac{1 - e^{-nK\tau}}{1 - e^{-K\tau}} \quad \text{and} \quad (S_n)_{k_a} = \frac{1 - e^{-nk_a\tau}}{1 - e^{-k_a\tau}} \tag{10.33}$$

2. During the steady state,

$$(S_n)_K = \frac{1}{1 - e^{-K\tau}} \quad \text{and} \quad (S_n)_{k_a} = \frac{1}{1 - e^{-k_a\tau}} \tag{10.34}$$

The profile of plasma concentration following multiple oral administration is presented in Figure 10.4. The only striking difference from the profile for multiple intravenous bolus injections is the bell-shaped characteristic of the oral dose.

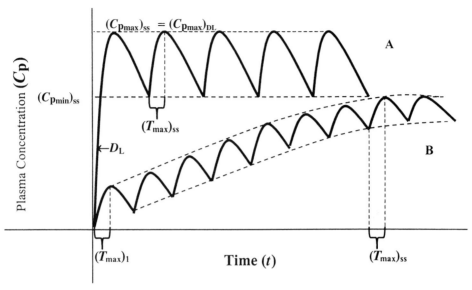

FIGURE 10.4 Plasma concentration–time profile of multiple oral administration. (A) Immediate attainment of peak and trough levels of steady state following administration of a loading dose and four maintenance doses. (B) Gradual accumulation of drug attained in the body by giving a smaller maintenance dose in shorter dosing interval.

10.3.1 Peak, Trough, and Average Plasma Concentrations of Multiple Oral Dosing before and after Achieving Steady State

As was discussed for multiple intravenous injections, one way of developing the equations of plasma concentration during multiple dosing is to multiply the equations of the first dose by the solutions of the geometric series. For example, for equations of trough levels we multiply the trough level of the first dose by Equations 10.33 and 10.34. The equation of the trough level of the first dose is

$$(C_{p_{min}})_1 = \overleftarrow{C}_p^0 (e^{-K\tau} - e^{-k_a\tau}) \tag{10.35}$$

The equation of the trough level after the nth dose before achieving steady state is

$$(C_{p_{min}})_n = \overleftarrow{C}_p^0 \left[\left(\frac{1 - e^{-nK\tau}}{1 - e^{-K\tau}} \right) e^{-K\tau} - \left(\frac{1 - e^{-nk_a\tau}}{1 - e^{-k_a\tau}} \right) e^{-k_a\tau} \right] \tag{10.36}$$

The equation of the trough level during steady state is

$$(C_{p_{min}})_{ss} = \overleftarrow{C}_p^0 \left[\frac{e^{-K\tau}}{1 - e^{-K\tau}} - \frac{e^{-k_a\tau}}{1 - e^{-k_a\tau}} \right] \tag{10.37}$$

If, however, the absorption process is fast and the dosing interval is set to be equal to or greater than $7(T_{1/2})_{k_a}$, the absorption exponential approaches zero $(e^{-k_a\tau} \to 0)$ and the trough level is only a function of the elimination process:

$$(C_{p_{min}})_n = \overleftarrow{C}_p^0 \left(\frac{1 - e^{-nk\tau}}{1 - e^{-K\tau}} \right) e^{-K\tau} \tag{10.38}$$

$$(C_{p_{min}})_{ss} = \overleftarrow{C}_p^0 \left(\frac{e^{-K\tau}}{1 - e^{-K\tau}} \right) \tag{10.39}$$

In other words, the maintenance dose is given when the absorption process is complete. In clinical practice it can be assumed that the amount of drug left at the site of absorption would be insignificant after four or five half-lives of absorption. In this chapter, we follow the rule that $7T_{1/2}$ is the time for completion of a first-order process.

Estimation of the peak levels depends on the value of T_{max}. As the T_{max} of steady-state levels remains constant and reproducible, it is considered a more reliable value than the T_{max} of doses before achieving steady state. By taking the first derivative of the following function that describes the plasma concentration at any time during the steady state, we can develop the equation of T_{max} for multiple oral dosing at steady state:

$$(C_{p_t})_{ss} = \overleftarrow{C}_p^0 \left[\frac{e^{-K\tau}}{1 - e^{-K\tau}} - \frac{e^{-k_a t}}{1 - e^{-k_a \tau}} \right] \tag{10.40}$$

The first derivative of Equation 10.40 is

$$\frac{d(C_{p_t})_{ss}}{dt} = \overleftarrow{C}_p^0 \left[\frac{-Ke^{-Kt}}{1 - e^{-K\tau}} + \frac{k_a e^{-k_a t}}{1 - e^{-k_a \tau}} \right] \tag{10.41}$$

Setting equation 10.41 equal to zero and solving for T_{max} lead to

$$\frac{e^{-KT_{max}}}{e^{-k_a T_{max}}} = \frac{k_a(1 - e^{-K\tau})}{K(1 - e^{-k_a\tau})} \tag{10.42}$$

$$(T_{max})_{ss} = \frac{2.303}{k_a - K} \log \left(\frac{k_a(1 - e^{-K\tau})}{K(1 - e^{-k_a\tau})} \right) \tag{10.43}$$

Therefore, by multiplying the equation of maximum plasma concentration after the first dose (Equation 8.28) by Equation 10.34 and substituting $(T_{max})_{ss}$ for t, we obtain the following equation for maximum plasma concentration at steady state:

$$(C_{p_{max}})_{ss} = \frac{FD}{V_d} \left(\frac{e^{-K(T_{max})ss}}{1 - e^{-K\tau}} \right) \tag{10.44}$$

The average plasma concentration at steady state for multiple oral dosing is similar to Equation 10.17:

$$(C_{p_{ave}})_{ss} = \frac{FD}{Cl_t \tau} = \frac{FD}{KV_d \tau} = \frac{1.44T_{1/2}FD}{V_d \tau} = \frac{(AUC)_\tau}{\tau} \qquad (10.45)$$

10.3.2 Extent of Accumulation

The extent of accumulation at steady state is also determined as described earlier for Equation 10.25:

$$R = \frac{(C_{p_{min}})_{ss}}{(C_{p_{min}})_1} = \frac{1}{(1 - e^{-K\tau})(1 - e^{-k_a \tau})} \quad \text{when } \tau < 7(T_{1/2})_{k_a} \qquad (10.46)$$

or

$$R = \frac{1}{(1 - e^{-K\tau})} \quad \text{when } \tau > 7(T_{1/2})_{k_a} \qquad (10.47)$$

10.3.3 Loading Dose, Maintenance Dose, and Designing a Dosing Regimen

The procedure for designing a regimen for multiple oral dosing is the same as described for multiple intravenous injections; however, we should be mindful of the bioavailability factor, F, in calculating D_M or D_L. For example, Equation 10.27 changes to

$$D_M = \frac{(C_{p_{ave}})_{ss} V_d \tau K}{F} \qquad (10.48)$$

The relationship between loading dose and maintenance dose, assuming F values are equal, can be described as

$$D_L = \frac{D_M}{(1 - e^{-K\tau})(1 - e^{-k_a \tau})} \quad \text{when } \tau < 7(T_{1/2})_{k_a} \qquad (10.49)$$

or

$$D_L = \frac{D_M}{1 - e^{-K\tau}} \quad \text{when } \tau > 7(T_{1/2})_{k_a} \qquad (10.50)$$

The time required to reach any fraction of steady state during multiple oral dosing is calculated with Equation 10.16.

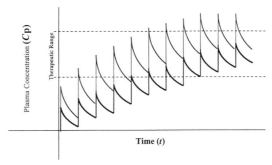

FIGURE 10.5 Keeping the dosing interval the same and increasing the dose would raise the fluctuation, accumulation, and steady-state level. For drugs with a narrow therapeutic range, increasing the dose may elevate the plasma concentration beyond the maximum effective level.

10.4 EFFECT OF CHANGING DOSE, DOSING INTERVAL, AND HALF-LIFE ON ACCUMULATION OF DRUG IN THE BODY AND FLUCTUATION OF PLASMA CONCENTRATION

In the following discussion we consider (i) the difference between the peak and trough levels, which is equal to the initial plasma concentration of a single maintenance dose, as a measure of fluctuation; and (ii) the average amount or concentration of drug in the body as a measure of accumulation. For a given dosing regimen, if the dosing interval is kept constant and dose is increased, the following parameters increase: peak and trough levels before and after achieving steady state; average plasma concentration at steady state; fluctuation of plasma concentration; accumulation of drug in the body.

Decreasing the dose would reduce the steady-state level, plasma fluctuation, and drug accumulation in the body (Figure 10.5).

If the dose is kept constant and dosing interval is altered, increasing the dosing interval would increase the fluctuation; lower the steady-state level; and reduce the accumulation in the body.

If the dosing interval is shortened, a reduced dosing interval would increase the accumulation, reduce the fluctuation, and increase the steady-state level (Figure 10.6).

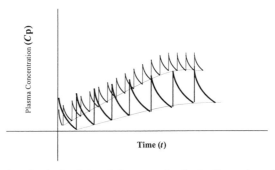

FIGURE 10.6 Reducing the dosing interval decreases the fluctuation, raises steady-state level, and increases accumulation.

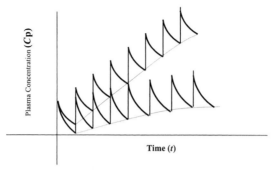

FIGURE 10.7 If the regular dosing regimen of a drug is used for patients with moderate to severe renal impairment or hepatic failure, because of the increase in half-life of elimination in these patients, steady-state level and accumulation would be significantly higher than in patients with normal renal function.

Patients with renal failure usually have a longer half-life for a given drug. Recommending the dose and dosing interval that are designed for patients with normal renal function would increase the steady-state level and accumulation in patients with renal failure. The fluctuation changes but not noticeably (Figure 10.7).

10.5 EFFECT OF IRREGULAR DOSING INTERVAL ON THE PLASMA CONCENTRATION OF DRUGS

It is obvious that designing a dosing regimen with a fixed dosing interval is intended for around-the-clock administration. If the dosing interval is changed irregularly and arbitrarily by the patient, the fluctuation, accumulation, and steady-state level would be affected. This issue may not be crucial for drugs with a very wide therapeutic range; however, it should be considered extremely important for drugs with a low therapeutic index and narrow therapeutic range. Consider Figure 10.8 for a hypothetical plasma concentration of a drug with a narrow therapeutic range that is taken on a regular dosing interval of 6–12–6–12 (four times daily or every 6 hours) versus the plasma concentration of the irregular dosing interval 8–12–4–8 (so-called 4 tablets a day). Clearly, taking the drug according to the latter schedule would create inconsistency in accumulation of drug in the body and reduce the plasma level below the minimum effective concentration. If the therapeutic range of the drug were wide, as shown in Figure 10.8, The inconsistency may not be of concern because the lowest concentration would remain within the range, and both schedules may be considered reasonable.

APPLICATION

10.1 Three patients are prescribed a drug 300-mg every six hours by IV bolus injection. The initial plasma concentrations of the first dose and the half-lives are reported in Table 10.2. Determine the following:

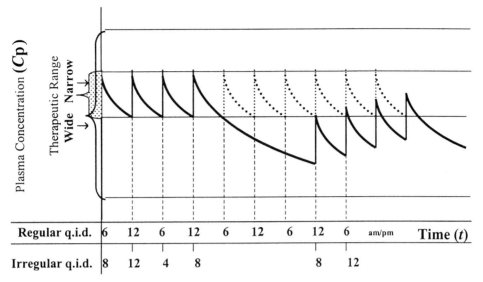

FIGURE 10.8 Comparison of fluctuation of plasma levels between regular and irregular dosing regimens. The regular q.i.d is given every 6 hours around the clock. The irregular q.i.d. is when "four tablets a day" is understood as four tablets between 7 AM and 10 PM, between 8 AM and 8 PM, and so on. The latter schedule may become problematic for some drugs with a narrow therapeutic range, as the plasma concentration may fall below the minimum effective concentration during sleep (eg, during the interval 8 PM to 8 AM in the preceding schedule).

1. Steady-state peak and trough levels for all three patients

$$K_A = 0.1155 \ h^{-1}, \quad K_B = 0.0866 \ h^{-1}, \quad K_C = 0.1155 \ h^{-1}$$

Patient A

$$(C_{p_{max}})_{ss} = 6/(1 - e^{-0.1155 \times 6}) = 12 \ \mu g/mL$$

$$\tau = T_{1/2}; \text{ therefore, } (C_{p_{min}})_{ss} = 12/2 = 6 \ \mu g/mL$$

TABLE 10.2 Data Related to Application 10.1

Patient	$T_{1/2}$ (h)	Initial Plasma Level ($\mu g/mL$)
A	6	6
B	8	8
C	6	10

Patient B

$$(C_{p_{max}})_{ss} = 8/(1 - e^{-0.0866 \times 6}) = 19.73 \ \mu g/mL$$

$$(C_{p_{min}})_{ss} = 19.73 \ e^{-0.0866 \times 6} = 11.73 \ \mu g/mL$$

Patient C

$$(C_{p_{max}})_{ss} = 10/(1 - e^{-0.1155 \times 6}) = 20 \ \mu g/mL$$

$$\tau = T_{1/2}; \text{ therefore, } (C_{p_{min}})_{ss} = 20/2 = 10 \ \mu g/mL$$

NOTE
- Dosing at intervals less than the $T_{1/2}$ of a drug (eg, Patient B) results in a higher steady-state level and a greater degree of accumulation.
- The smaller volume of distribution or the larger initial plasma concentration results in a greater fluctuation between the peak and trough levels (eg, Patients A and C).

2. Trough level of the second dose for Patient A

$$(C_{p_{min}})_2 = 6(1 - e^{-2 \times 0.1155 \times 6}) \ e^{-0.1155 \times 6}/(1 - e^{-0.1155 \times 6}) = 4.5 \ \mu g/mL$$

NOTE
- For Patient A, $\tau = 6$ hours, after second dose $n = 2$ (ie, $n\tau = 12$ hours $< 7T_{1/2}$). Also, $2\tau = 2(T_{1/2})_A$; therefore, the minimum concentration after the second dose is 75% of $(C_{p_{min}})_{ss}$.

$$(C_{p_{min}})_2 = 0.75(C_{p_{min}})_{ss} = 0.75(6) = 4.5 \ \mu g/mL$$

- In practice, "quasi-steady-state levels," that is, the levels achieved after four to five half-lives, are considered steady-state levels.
- The time required to reach any fraction of steady-state level is dependent solely on the half-life of a drug. The same concept was discussed in Chapter 7.

3. Design a reasonable dosing regimen for Patient A if it is desired to maintain the fluctuation between 10 and 20 mg/L:

Method 1: Set $(C_{p_{ave}})_{ss} = 15$ mg/L and $\tau = T_{1/2}$.

$$D_M = (15 \text{ mg/L})(0.1155 \text{ h}^{-1})(50 \text{ L})(6 \text{ h}) = 519 \text{ mg} \cong 0.5 \text{ g}$$

Because $\tau = T_{1/2}$, $D_L = 2D_M = 1.038$ g. The dosing regimen would then be $D_L \cong 1$ g followed by $D_M \cong 0.5$ g four times daily.

Method 2

$$V_d = 300 \text{ mg}/6 \text{ (mg/L)} = 50 \text{ L}$$

$$D_M = (20 \text{ mg/L} - 10 \text{ mg/L})50 \text{ L} = 0.5 \text{ g}$$

$$\tau = T_{1/2}, \quad \text{ie}, \quad D_L = 2D_M, \quad \text{ie}, \quad D_L = 1 \text{ g}$$

Therefore, the dosing regimen according to the criteria set in this problem would be $D_L = 1$ g and $D_M = 0.5$ g four times daily.

The following calculations are for a dosing interval less than the half-life eg $\tau = 4$ h.

$$D_M = (15 \text{ mg/L})(0.1155)(50)(4 \text{ h})$$

$$D_M = 346.5 \text{ mg}$$

$$D_L = 346.5/1 - e^{-0.1155 \times 4} = 936.5 \text{ mg}$$

To check whether the fluctuation remains within the therapeutic range 10–20 mg/L

$$(C_{p_{max}})_{ss} = 936.5/50 = 18.73 \text{ mg/L}$$

$$(C_{p_{min}})_{ss} = 18.73e^{-0.115 \times 4} = 11.8 \text{ mg/L}$$

Therefore, the dosing regimen is a 1-g loading dose (ie. 936.5 mg $\cong$ 1 g), followed by 350-mg maintenance dose every 4 hours.

4. Plasma concentration 2 hours after giving the second dose to Patient A

$$(C_{p_{t=2 \text{ h}}})_n = \frac{6(1 - e^{-2 \times 0.1155 \times 6})e^{-0.1155 \times 2}}{1 - e^{-0.1155 \times 6}} = 7.15 \text{ mg/L}$$

5. Plasma levels 6 and 12 hours after the last dose for Patient A assuming the steady-state fluctuation is achieved

$$C_{p_{6 \text{ h after last dose}}} = (C_{p_{min}})_{ss} = 6 \text{ mg/L}$$

$C_{p_{12 \text{ h}}}$ occurs one half-life after the $(C_{p_{min}})_{ss}$ and two half-lives after $(C_{p_{max}})_{ss}$; therefore,

$$C_{p_{12 \text{ h}}} = 6 \text{ (mg/L)}/2 = 3 \text{ mg/L}$$

or

$$C_{p_{12 \text{ h}}} = (C_{p_{max}})_{ss} \, e^{-0.1155 \times 12 \text{ h}} = 3 \text{ mg/L}$$

6. Loading dose to attain steady-state level immediately: For Patients A and C, $\tau = T_{1/2}$; therefore,

$$D_L = 2D_M = 2(300) = 600 \text{ mg}$$

For Patient B

$$D_L = 300/(1 - e^{-0.0866 \times 6}) = 740 \text{ mg}$$

7. Average amount of drug in the body at plateau for Patient A

$$(A_{ave})_{ss} = D_M/K\tau = 300/((0.693/T_{1/2})(T_{1/2})) = 300/0.693 = 432 \text{ mg}$$

8. Average rates of input and output during steady state for Patient A

$$\text{average rate of input} = 300 \text{ mg four times daily}$$

$$\text{average rate of output} = 300 \text{ mg every 6 hours}$$

10.2 The following equations represent the decline of plasma concentration of drug X in patients with normal renal function (Group A) and patients with renal insufficiency (Group B) following a 4-g IV injection:

$$\log C_p = 2.5 - 0.25t \quad \text{(Group A)}$$

$$C_p = 320e^{-0.16t} \quad \text{(Group B)}$$

(Plasma concentrations were measured in $\mu g/mL$ and t in h.) Assume the drug was administered intravenously (bolus) every 4 h to both groups for 3 days. Calculate the following:

1. Maximum plasma concentration after first dose

$$(C_{p_{max}})_{1A} = C_p^0 = \text{antilog } 2.5 = 316.23 \ \mu g/mL$$

$$(C_{p_{max}})_{1B} = 320 \ \mu g/mL$$

2. Minimum plasma concentration just before 4th and 12th doses

$$K_A = (0.25)(2.303) = 0.576 \text{ h}^{-1} \quad K_B = 0.16 \text{ h}^{-1}$$

$$(T_{1/2})_A = 1.2 \text{ h} \quad (T_{1/2})_B = 4.33 \text{ h}$$

Patient A

$$(C_{p_{min}})_{3A} = (C_{p_{min}})_{11A} = (C_{p_{min}})_{ss} = \frac{316e^{-0.576 \times 4}}{1 - e^{-0.576 \times 4}} = 35 \text{ mg/L}$$

Patient B

$$(C_{p_{min}})_{3B} = \frac{320(1 - e^{-3\times0.16\times4})e^{-0.16\times4}}{1 - e^{-0.16\times4}} = 303.72 \text{ mg/L}$$

$$(C_{p_{min}})_{11B} = (C_{p_{min}})_{ss} = 357.71 \text{ mg/L}$$

3. Average plateau concentration

$$Cl_{tA} = (4 \text{ g}/0.316)(0.576) = 7.29 \text{ L/h}$$

$$(C_{p_{ave}})_{ssA} = 4g/(7.29 \times 4) = 0.137 \text{ g/L} = 137 \text{ mg/L}$$

$$Cl_{tB} = (0.16)(4 \text{ g}/0.320) = 2 \text{ L/h}$$

$$(C_{p_{ave}})_{ssB} = 4 \text{ g}/(2 \times 4) = 0.5 \text{ g/L} = 500 \text{ mg/L}$$

4. Plasma concentration 4 and 8 hours after last dose

$$C_{p_{4h} A} = (C_{p_{min}})_{ss} = 35 \text{ mg/L} \quad C_{p_{4h} B} = 357.71 \text{ mg/L}$$

$$C_{p_{8h} A} = 35e^{-0.576\times4} = 3.5 \text{ mg/L} \quad C_{p_{8h} B} = 357.71e^{-0.16\times4} = 188.61 \text{ mg/L}$$

5. Total amount eliminated in one dosing interval at steady state

$$\text{total amount eliminated} = D_M = 4 \text{ g}$$

10.3 A solid dosage form of a β-adrenergic receptor agonist drug with an elimination half-life of 8 hours and an apparent volume of distribution equal to 50% of body weight is given to a male patient (age 29, weight 80 kg) to relieve bronchospasm. The plasma level of the drug that provides adequate airway ventilation is approximately 10 μg/mL. The patient is advised to take the medication four times daily.

1. What maintenance dose would you recommend? Assume the drug is 90% available.

$$D_M = \frac{(C_{p_{ave}})_{ss}V_d\tau}{1.44 \times T_{1/2} \times F} = \frac{(10 \text{ mg/L}) \times 40 \text{ L} \times 6 \text{ h}}{1.44 \times 8 \text{ h} \times 0.9} = 231.5 \text{ mg}$$

Note. A limitation that may be encountered in multiple oral dosing is the type of solid dosage form (capsule, caplet, soft gelatin, etc) and the amount of active ingredient in each dose. For example, if the commercially available form of this drug is a 250-mg capsule, you may recommend one capsule as the maintenance dose. The challenge of designing a regimen for oral multiple dosing is when, for a very narrow therapeutic index drug, you wish to avoid significant fluctuation within the therapeutic range, the calculated maintenance dose is 250 mg but the commercially available capsule is 375 mg. Having a lower-strength capsule may help in designing a better regimen that provides smaller fluctuation.

10.4 A solid dosage form of an antibiotic with an absorption half-life of 30 minutes and elimination half-life of 10 hours is given to a female patient (45 years old, 85 kg) three times daily. The bioavailability of the drug is 0.9 and the apparent volume of distribution is 10 L. Calculate the following:

1. T_{max} of first dose

$$k_a = 0.693/30 \text{ min} = 0.0231 \text{ min}^{-1} = 1.386 \text{ h}^{-1}$$

$$T_{max} = \frac{2.303}{1.386 - 0.0693} \log \frac{1.386}{0.0693} = 2.275 \text{ h}$$

$$K = 0.693/10 \text{ h} = 0.0698 \text{ h}^{-1}$$

2. T_{max} at steady state

$$(T_{max})_{ss} = \frac{2.303}{1.386 - 0.0693} \log \left(\frac{1.386}{0.0693} \left(\frac{1 - e^{-0.0693 \times 8}}{1 - e^{-1.386 \times 8}} \right) \right) = 1.626 \text{ h}$$

3. Average steady-state plasma concentration

$$(C_{p_{ave}})_{ss} = \frac{0.9 \times 250}{0.0693 \times 10 \times 8} = 40.58 \text{ mg/L} \cong 41 \text{ mg/L}$$

4. Peak and trough levels at steady state

$$\tilde{C}_p^0 = \frac{0.9 \times 250 \times 1.386}{10(1.386 - 0.0693)} = 23.68 \text{ mg/L} \cong 24 \text{ mg/L}$$

$$(C_{p_{min}})_{ss} = 24 \left(\frac{e^{-0.0693 \times 8}}{1 - e^{-0.0693 \times 8}} \right) = 32.40 \text{ mg/L}$$

$$(C_{p_{max}})_{ss} = 24 \left(\frac{e^{-0.0693 \times 1.626}}{1 - e^{-0.0693 \times 8}} \right) = 50.40 \text{ mg/L}$$

5. Loading dose

$$D_L = \frac{250}{1 - e^{-0.0693 \times 8}} = 587.43 \text{ mg} \cong 2D_M$$

6. Time it takes to achieve 90% of average steady-state plasma level

$$n\tau = 3.3 T_{1/2} = 33 \text{ h}$$

ASSIGNMENT

10.1 Two grams of a drug was given twice a day to a 65-kg patient. We know the following information about the drug:

$$\text{apparent } V_d = 26.2 \text{ L/100 kg}$$

$$Cl_t = 116.4 \text{ mL/min per 70 kg}$$

$$Cl_r = 82.2 \text{ mL/min per 70 kg}$$

Calculate the following:

10.1.1 Trough level after the first dose.

10.1.2 Maximum steady-steady plasma concentration.

10.1.3 Plasma levels 6 and 12 hours after the last dose, assuming steady-state levels are achieved.

10.1.4 Average amount in the body during and after achieving the steady-state levels.

10.1.5 Total amount eliminated per dosing interval at steady state.

10.1.6 Total amount eliminated as metabolite(s) per dosing interval at plateau.

10.1.7 Time it takes to reach to 60% of the average steady-state plasma concentration.

10.1.8 Time it takes to reach to 75% of the average plateau level.

10.2 Three patients receive a 500-mg IV bolus injection of an antibiotic every 6 hours. The half-life and initial plasma concentrations of the first dose for each patient are reported in Table 10.3. Determine the following for all three patients:

10.2.1 Trough level of the third dose.

10.2.2 Steady-state peak and trough levels.

10.2.3 Plasma levels 4 and 8 hours after the last dose, assuming the steady-state levels are achieved.

10.2.4 Average steady-state plasma concentration.

10.2.5 A reasonable dosing regimen (D_L, D_M, and τ) to achieve a fluctuation within a therapeutic range of 50 to 150 mg/L.

10.3 The following equations represent the decline of plasma concentration of an antibiotic in a patient with normal renal function (Patient A) and a patient with renal impairment (Patient B) following a 0.5-g IV injection.

TABLE 10.3 Data Related to Assignment 10.2

Patient	$T_{1/2}$ (h)	Initial Plasma Level (mg/L)
A	4	40
B	6	50
C	8	70

$$Y = 0.6 - 0.1t \quad \text{(Patient A)}$$

$$C_p = 5 \, e^{-0.0693t} \quad \text{(Patient B)}$$

(Plasma concentrations were measured in mg/L and time in h.) Assume the drug was given to both patients every 4 hours for 3 days. Calculate the following:

10.3.1 Plasma levels (peak and trough) after the last dose.
10.3.2 Plasma levels after the last dose of the first day.
10.3.3 Average steady-state plasma concentration.
10.3.4 Accumulation index.

10.4 Recommend a reasonable regimen for multiple oral dosing of a drug with an elimination half-life of 4 hours and absorption half-life of 0.5 hours. The dosage forms of the drug available are 150- and 300-mg capsules. The minimum and maximum effective therapeutic concentrations of this drug are 15 and 55 mg/L. The apparent volume of distribution is 10 L and its absolute bioavailability is 0.9. Design the regimen based on a target concentration of 41 mg/L. Determine whether the fluctuaion remains within the therapeutic range.

ASSIGNMENT (EXTRA CREDIT)

EC-10.1 Prepare a short description of the article by Demibas et al. Include in your report the objectives and significance of the article, a brief description of methodology, and a summary of the results and conclusions.

Demibas, S, Reyderman, L, Stavchansky, S. Bioavailability of dextromethorphan (as dextrophan) from sustained release formulations in the presence of guaifenesin in human volunteers. *Biopharm Drug Disp* 1998;19:541–5.

Complete your assignment by answering the following questions:

- Discuss the significance of calculating the fluctuation index in this study.
- On day 6 according to Figure 2 of the article, the mean minimum plasma concentration is approximately 200 μg/L. Is this value consistent with the reported accumulation index?
- Determine the percentage accumulation of the drug based on the AUCs of the first and sixth days:

$$\% = (\text{AUC}_{6th\ day} - \text{AUC}_{1st\ day}) / \text{AUC}_{1st\ day}$$

EC-10.2 Review the article by Cheng et al and answer the questions for this assignment:

Cheng CL, Smith DE, Carver PL, Cox SR, Watkins PB, Blake DS, Kauffman CA, Meyer KM, Amidon GL and Stetson PL. Steady-state pharmacokinetics of delavirdine in HIV-positive patients: effect on erythromycin breath test. *Clin Pharmacol Ther* 1997;61:531–43.

- Summarize the experimental design of the project as a flow chart.
- Discuss the significance of the erythromycin breath test.
- What was the rationale for administration of Heidelberg capsules.

TABLE 10.4 Data Related to Assignment EC-10.3

Drug	Trade Name	$T_{1/2}$ (h)	F	Initial Dose[a] (mg)	Maintenance Dose[a] (mg)	Maximum Dose[a] (mg/d)
Benazepril/benazeprilat	Lotensin	21–22	0.37	10 q.i.d.	20–40/d	80
Captopril	Capoten	2	0.70	25 b.i.d./t.i.d.	50 b.i.d./t.i.d.	450
Enalapril/enalaprilat	Vasotec	11	0.7	5 q.i.d.	10–40 q.i.d./b.i.d.	40
Fosinopril/fosinoprilat	Monopril	12–15	0.36	10 q.i.d.	20–40 q.i.d./b.i.d.	80
Lisinopril	Prinivil/Zestril	12	0.25	10 q.i.d.	20–40 q.i.d.	80
Ramipril/ramiprilat	Altace	>50	0.6	2.5 q.i.d.	2.5–20 q.i.d./b.i.d.	—
Quinapril/quinaprilat	Accupril	25	0.8	10 q.i.d.	20–80 q.i.d./b.i.d.	80

[a]For controlling hypertension (*Source:* maufacturer's publication).

- Explain whether the increase in T_{max} is expected in this type of escalating dosing regimen.
- Determine the accumulation index for all three dosing regimens.
- Based on what information in this investigation would you consider delavirdine or its metabolites a potent inhibitor of CYP3A4?
- What are the ramifications of inhibition of CYP3A4 for HIV-positive patients?

EC-10.3 This assignment requires a literature search (library/internet). The commercially available angiotensin-converting enzyme (ACE) inhibitors are equally effective in controlling hypertension and some of them are also effective in controlling congestive heart failure. There are, however, significant differences between these drugs with respect to their pharmacokinetic properties. Some of these differences are given in Table 10.4.

- Search the literature and report the apparent volume(s) of distribution and minimum and maximum effective concentrations for each drug. Cite the reference.
- Explain the reason(s) for variation of bioavailability among these compounds.
- Determine the average steady-state plasma concentration for the maintenance dosing regimen and the related fluctuation of plasma concentration.
- Identify the major route(s) of elimination for each drug.
- Calculated the total amount excreted unchanged in each dosing interval at steady state.
- Simulate the fluctuations of plasma concentration following initial and maintenance doses at steady state.
- Report the percentage protein binding of each drug.

EC-10.4 de Repentigny et al evaluated the multiple dosing kinetics of an orally active antifungal agent in small children at different ages from 6 months to 12 years. Based on the mean values presented in Table 2 of the article complete the following:

de Repentigny L, Ratelle J, Leclerc JM, Cornu G, Sokal EM, Jacqmin P, de Beule K. Repeated-dose pharmacokinetics of an oral solution of itraconazole in infant and children. *Antimicrob Agents Chemother* 1998;42:404–8.

- Calculate $C_{p_{min}}$ for ages 0.5–2, 2–5, and 5–12.
- Calculate the accumulation index based on $C_{p_{max}}$, $C_{p_{min}}$ and AUC for ages 0.5–2, 2–5, and 5–12.
- Calculate the average plasma concentration for all three age groups.
- How long would it take to reach steady-state levels in children 0.5–2 and 5–12 years old?
- What is the purpose of adding 400 mg hydroxypropyl-β-cyclodextrin per milliliter of dose?
- Does the addition of hydroxy-β-cyclodextrin influence the pharmacokinetics of itraconazole? How?

BIBLIOGRAPHY

1. Buell J, Jelliffe R, Kalaba R, Sridhar R. Modern control theory and optimal drug regimens. I. The plateau effect. *Math Biosci* 1969;5:285.

2. Colburn WA. Estimating the accumulation of drugs. *J Pharm Sci* 1983;72:833.

3. Gibaldi M, Perrier D. *Pharmacokinetics,* 2nd ed. New York: Marcel Dekker, 1982:113.

4. Krüger-Thiemer E. Formal theory of drug dosage regimens, I. *J Theor Biol* 1966;13:212.

5. Krüger-Thiemer E. Formal theory of drug dosage regimens. II. The exact plateau effect. *J Theor Biol* 1969;23:169.

6. Krüger-Thiemer E, Bünger P. The role of the therapeutic regimen. Part I. *Chemotherapia* 1965/1966;10:61.

7. Levy G. Pharmacokinetic control and clinical interpretation of steady-state blood levels of drugs. *Clin Pharmacol Ther* 1976;16(1, pt 2):130.

8. Perrier D, Gibaldi M. Relationship between plasma or serum drug concentration and amount of drug in the body at steady state upon multiple dosing. *J Pharmacokinet Biopharm* 1973;1:17.

9. Slattery JT, Gibaldi M, Koup JR. Prediction of maintenance dose required to attain a desired drug concentration at steady state from a single determination of concentration after an initial dose. *Clin Pharmacokinet* 1980;5:377.

10. Van Rossum JM, Tomey AHM. Rate of accumulation and plateau plasma concentration of drugs after chronic medication. *J Pharm Pharmacol* 1968;20:390.

11. Wagner JG, Northam JI, Always CD, Carpenter OS. Blood levels of drug at equilibrium state after multiple dosing. *Nature* 1965;207:1301.

12. Wagner JG. Clinical pharmacokinetics. Hamilton, IL: *Drug Intelligence,* 1975:133.

MULTICOMPARTMENT MODELS: LINEAR TWO-COMPARTMENT MODEL WITH INSTANTANEOUS INPUT AND FIRST-ORDER DISPOSITION

Let these things be believed as resembling the truth.
PLUTARCH (TABLE TALK)

OBJECTIVES

- To discuss the pharmacokinetics of drugs that follow a two-compartment model.

- To compare the plasma concentration–time profiles of drugs that follow a two-compartment model with those of drugs that follow a one-compartment model.

- To discuss the meaning of various hybrid rate constants of the model.

- To discuss methods of determining initial estimates of rate constants of distribution and elimination.

- To estimate important pharmacokinetic parameters and constants such as initial plasma concentration, total body clearance, and apparent volume of distribution.

11.1 INTRODUCTION

For most drugs the two-compartment model is considered a more realistic model for interpretation of their behavior in the body. The model assumes that a drug distributes between two compartments, moves between the first and second in proportion to the concentration difference between the compartments, and is eliminated from the first compartment in proportion to its concentration there. The first compartment, also known as the central compartment, may represent blood, extracellular fluid, and highly perfused tissues such as liver, kidneys, and lungs etc. As was discussed in Chapter 2, highly perfused tissues achieve rapid equilibrium with the systemic circulation and these tissues are kinetically impossible to tell apart from the systemic circulation. Thus, the central compartment is assumed kinetically a homogeneous compartment. The second compartment, known as the peripheral compartment, represents tissues and regions of the body with less blood perfusion. The equilibration of free drug between these tissues and the systemic circulation occurs more slowly. Kinetically, the less accessible tissues, because of their lower rate of uptake, behave as a compartment. Examples of tissues that may be included in the second compartment are adipose tissue, muscle, and skin etc.

On bolus injection of a drug that follows a two-compartment model, the drug distributes very quickly. The mixing of drug in the central compartment is extremely rapid in relation to its removal by distribution to the peripheral compartment and elimination via the liver and kidneys. Simultaneously with its dilution in the central compartment, which is a physical process, the drug also distributes to the second compartment and is eliminated from the first compartment. Obviously, as the model is linear and assuming the organs of elimination are part of the central compartment, the rate of elimination is proportional to the concentration in the central compartment and the rate of distribution is proportional to the difference in concentrations between the two compartments.

11.2 EQUATIONS OF THE MODEL

Figure 11.1 is a diagram of the model. To develop the equations of the model we start with the rate equation of each compartment. The rate of change in amount of drug in the central compartment (compartment 1) depends on the rates of distribution and elimination. The input is instantaneous and has no rate. The related differential equation is

$$\frac{dA_1}{dt} = k_{21}A_2 - k_{12}A_1 - k_{10}A_1 \tag{11.1}$$

The rate of change in amount of drug in the peripheral compartment (compartment 2) is a function of rates of distribution in and out of the compartment and the assumption here is that no elimination occurs from the peripheral compartment:

$$\frac{dA_2}{dt} = k_{12}A_1 - k_{21}A_2 \tag{11.2}$$

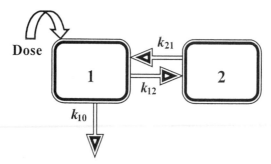

FIGURE 11.1 Diagram of two-compartment model with instantaneous input and first-order distribution and elimination.

A_1 and A_2 are the amounts of drug at any time in the central and peripheral compartments, respectively. The rate constants of distribution are k_{12} and k_{21}. The first subscript number represents the departure compartment and the second number represents the arrival compartment.

By using the Laplace method of integration (Chapter 1, Sections 1.11 and 1.12) or the method of input-disposition functions (Chapter 1, Section 1.13), we can integrate Equations 11.1 and 11.2 simultaneously to obtain the following relationships for the amounts of drug in the central and peripheral compartments:

$$A_1 = \frac{D(\alpha - k_{21})}{\alpha - \beta} e^{-\alpha t} + \frac{D(k_{21} - \beta)}{\alpha - \beta} e^{-\beta t} \qquad (11.3)$$

$$A_2 = \frac{k_{12}D}{\alpha - \beta} (e^{-\beta t} - e^{-\alpha t}) \qquad (11.4)$$

Here A_1 and A_2 are the amounts of drug at any time in the central and peripheral compartments, respectively. The rate constants α and β are first-order hybrid rate constants that are considered the roots of the quadratic equations generated during the integration. These rate constants can be estimated from the slopes of the logarithm of plasma concentration versus time plot.

By dividing Equation 11.3 by the apparent volume of distribution of the central compartment we obtain the equation of the model in terms of plasma concentration:

$$C_p = \underbrace{\frac{D(\alpha - k_{21})}{V_1(\alpha - \beta)}}_{a} e^{-\alpha t} + \underbrace{\frac{D(k_{21} - \beta)}{V_1(\alpha - \beta)}}_{b} e^{-\beta t} \qquad (11.5)$$

By substituting a and b for the coefficients of each exponential term the equation of the model can be simplified to

$$C_p = ae^{-\alpha t} + be^{-\beta t} \qquad (11.6)$$

The plot of log of plasma concentration versus time for a drug that follows a two compartment model has two distinct phases (Figure 11.2). The early phase, called the distributive phase, is formed by the rapid decline in the plasma concentration of the drug in the central compartment. This rapid decline is the result of a number of physical and physiologic processes that occur simultaneously with and immediately after the injection. Among these processes are the rapid distribution and dilution of the drug into those fluids and tissues that make up the central compartment, transfer of drug to the peripheral compartment, and elimination of drug from the central compartment. After a certain period, which varies from drug to drug, this initial phase comes to an end and the drug concentration in various tissues and fluids declines steadily. This slower, gradual decline appears as a second phase of the curve of logarithm of plasma concentration–time curve. The second phase is also called the postdistributive phase or disposition phase. During this phase all physiologic processes (excretion, metabolism, and distribution) contribute

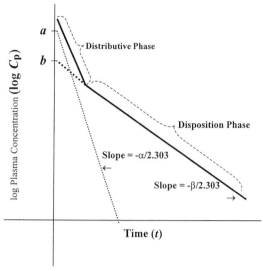

FIGURE 11.2 Diagram of plasma concentration–time profile of a drug that follows a two-compartment (biexponential) model.

to the consistent decline of drug concentration in the central compartment, which is also a function of physicochemical characteristics of the drug and its interaction with biologic molecules (Figure 11.2). Therefore, the rate constant calculated from the slope of the second phase of the curve, β, can only be identified as the disposition (ie, distribution and elimination (metabolism and excretion)) rate constant and the related half-life as physiologic or biologic or disposition half-life. This is one of the important differences between one- and two-compartment models.

Extrapolation of the terminal portion of the curve to the y axis gives the y intercept, which is equal to the coefficient b. This extrapolated line represents the biologic processes that are involved in the disposition of a drug. Therefore, subtracting the data points of the extrapolated line that correspond to the early time points from the observed plasma concentrations of the distributive phase leads to a number of residual values that represent all other processes that with disposition influence the early sharp decline of plasma concentration. Plotting the residuals against the early time points forms a straight line with slope of $-\alpha/2.303$ and y intercept of a. Both α and β are first-order hybrid rate constants; α represents the rate constant of all physical and physiologic processes other than the distribution and elimination that occur simultaneously with and immediately after injection of a drug into the body during the distributive phase. The rate constant β represents the physiologic process of disposition.

11.3 PARAMETERS AND CONSTANTS OF TWO-COMPARTMENT MODEL

The initial estimates of a, b, α, and β can be obtained by linear regression analysis of the extrapolated and residual lines as will be described below; however, the best approach would be to use specialized pharmacokinetic software developed for the purpose of selecting the correct model and estimating the related parameters and constants. The appropriate software would be that which would analyze the entire plasma level/time data, that is both the distributive and postdistributive phases of the curve together, by nonlinear regression analysis.

11.3.1 Estimation of a, b, α, and β

When the data set is ideal and free of systemic and random errors, we use the last two data points to estimate the slope and y intercept of the extrapolated line:

$$\text{slope} = \frac{\log C_{p_n} - \log C_{p_{n-1}}}{t_n - t_{n-1}} = -\frac{\beta}{2.303} \tag{11.7}$$

$$b = y \text{ intercept} = \frac{C_{p_n}}{e^{-\beta t}} \tag{11.8}$$

Therefore, the equation of the extrapolated line is

$$\tilde{C}_p = be^{-\beta t} \tag{11.9}$$

When the data are real and scatter, first, by plotting the logarithm of plasma concentration versus time, we identify those data points that form the disposition phase. Then, by using linear regression analysis, we determine the equation of the extrapolated line:

$$\log \tilde{C}_p = \log b - \frac{\beta}{2.303} t \tag{11.10}$$

By knowing the equation of the extrapolated line (ie, the disposition phase) one can estimate the data points on the extrapolated portion of the disposition line and subtract them from the data points of the distributive phase to determine the residual values. The procedure is similar to the calculation of the residual line in oral absorption (Chapter 8) except that here the extrapolated values are less than the observed plasma concentrations.

TABLE 11.1 Stepwise Calculations of Residual Line with Slope = $-\alpha/2.303$

Time Points of Distributive Phase	Plasma Concentrations of Distributive Phase	Extrapolated Values	Residual Values
t_1	C_{p_1}	$be^{-\beta t_1}$	$C_{p_1} - be^{-\beta t_1}$
t_2	C_{p_2}	$be^{-\beta t_2}$	$C_{p_2} - be^{-\beta t_2}$
t_3	C_{p_3}	$be^{-\beta t_3}$	$C_{p_3} - be^{-\beta t_3}$
t_4	C_{p_4}	$be^{-\beta t_4}$	$C_{p_4} - be^{-\beta t_4}$
$\vdots$	$\vdots$	$\vdots$	$\vdots$

The stepwise calculations of the residual values are presented in Table 11.1. Regression analysis of the logarithm of residuals versus time according to the equation

$$\log(C_p - \tilde{C}_p) = \log a - \frac{\alpha}{2.303} t \qquad (11.11)$$

provides the initial values of a and α.

$$(C_p - \tilde{C}_p) = ae^{-\alpha t} \qquad (11.12)$$

11.3.2 Estimation of Initial Plasma Concentration and Apparent Volume of Distribution of the Central Compartment

Setting t equal to zero in Equation 11.6 gives us an estimate of the plasma concentration at time zero:

$$C_p^0 = a + b \qquad (11.13)$$

Replacing the coefficients a and b with their formulas according to Equation 11.5 leads to a different version of Equation 11.13:

$$C_p^0 = \frac{D(\alpha + k_{21})}{V_1(\alpha - \beta)} + \frac{D(k_{21} - \beta)}{V_1(\alpha - \beta)} = \frac{D}{V_1} \qquad (11.13a)$$

Therefore,

$$V_1 = \frac{D}{C_p^0} = \frac{D}{a + b} \qquad (11.14)$$

Similar to a one-compartment model, the apparent volume of distribution of the central compartment is only a proportionality constant that is used to determine the amount in the central compartment:

$$(A_1)_t = C_{p_t} V_1 \qquad (11.15)$$

Equations 11.13 and 11.14 emphasize the importance of taking early plasma samples after the injection of a drug that follows a two compartment model for the purpose of identifying the distributive phase. If the first blood sample is taken sometime after the end of the distributive phase, the profile of log C_p versus time constitutes only the disposition phase. This profile would be similar to that discussed for a one-compartment model in Chapter 6. Therefore, one mistakenly would analyze the data according to a one-compartment model, in which case some parameters such as initial plasma concentration would be underestimated.

11.3.3 Estimation of the Rate Constants of Distribution and Elimination

The first-order distribution rate constants are k_{12} and k_{21}. The miniature rate constant k_{21}, representing the rate constant for transfer from the peripheral compartment to the central compartment, is determined from the formula of a or b:

$$b = \frac{(a + b)(k_{21} - \beta)}{(\alpha - \beta)} \qquad (11.16)$$

Therefore, $\qquad k_{21} = \frac{a\beta + b\alpha}{a + b} \qquad (11.17)$

Because the denominator of Equation 11.17 is the initial plasma concentration, a and b in the numerator can be normalized with respect to the initial plasma concentration:

$$a_N = a/(a + b) \quad \text{and} \quad b_N = b/(a + b)$$

Therefore, $\qquad k_{21} = a_N\beta + b_N\alpha \qquad (11.18)$

where a_N and b_N are the normalized values of a and b.

To determine the equations of other miniature rate constants we need to review the disposition function of the model. According to the criteria set forth in Chapter 1 (Section 1.13), the disposition function of the model, $(\text{Disp})_s$, is

$$(\text{Disp})_s = \frac{s + k_{21}}{s^2 + (k_{12} + k_{21} + k_{10}) + k_{21}k_{10}} = \frac{s + E_2}{(s + \alpha)(s + \beta)} \qquad (11.19)$$

The denominator of Equation 11.19, $(s + \alpha)(s + \beta)$, can be written as $s^2 + s(\alpha + \beta) + \alpha\beta$, which corresponds to $s^2 + s(k_{12} + k_{21} + k_{10}) + k_{21}k_{10}$. The comparison yields two relationships:

$$\alpha + \beta = k_{12} + k_{21} + k_{10} \qquad (11.20)$$

$$\alpha\beta = k_{21}k_{10} \qquad (11.21)$$

Therefore, the overall elimination rate constant, k_{10}, and the rate constant for transfer from the central to the peripheral compartment can be determined by the equations

$$k_{10} = \frac{\alpha\beta}{k_{21}} \qquad (11.22)$$

$$k_{12} = \alpha + \beta - k_{10} - k_{21} \qquad (11.23)$$

There are other relationships for calculating the miniature rate constants that are beyond the scope of this textbook.

11.3.4 Half-lives of Two-compartment Model

Contrary to the one-compartment model with intravenous bolus injection, which offers only one rate constant and one half-life of elimination, the two-compartment model enables us to estimate various half-lives. Some are useful in practice and some are used only for the calculation of the rate constants.

1. The half-life of β, known as the physiologic half-life or biologic half-life or half-life of disposition, represents the combined effects of distribution and elimination. This half-life should not be mistaken for the half-life of elimination; it would take seven biologic half-lives for a drug to be completely eliminated from the body. This means that after $2(T_{1/2})_{biol}$, $f_{el} = 0.75$ and $f_b = 0.25$; after $3.3(T_{1/2})_{biol}$, $f_{el} = 0.9$ and $f_b = 0.1$; after $4.3(T_{1/2})_{biol}$, $f_{el} = 0.95$ and $f_b = 0.95$; and so on.

$$(T_{1/2})_{biol} = 0.693/\beta \tag{11.24}$$

2. The half-life of k_{10}, known as the half-life of elimination, represents the collective effects of metabolism and excretion:

$$(T_{1/2})_{elim} = 0.693/k_{10} \tag{11.25}$$

3. The half-life of α represents all physical and physiologic processes other than distribution and elimination that occur immediately after the injection during the distributive phase. This half-life is neither the biologic nor elimination half-life and is used only to calculate α:

$$(T_{1/2})_\alpha = 0.693/\alpha \tag{11.26}$$

4. The half-life of k_{12} is the half-life of drug transfer from the central to the peripheral compartment:

$$(T_{1/2})_{k_{12}} = 0.693/k_{12} \tag{11.27}$$

5. The half-life of k_{21} is the half-life of drug transfer from the peripheral to the central compartment:

$$(T_{1/2})_{k_{21}} = 0.693/k_{21} \tag{11.28}$$

11.3.5 Area under the Curve, Volume of Distribution, and Clearance

The area under the plasma concentration–time curve of a drug that follows a two-compartment model can be estimated by the trapezoidal rule (Chapter 1, Section 1.9) or by integration of the equation of the model (Equation 11.6). The integration can be carried out from zero to infinity or from zero to any time t:

$$\text{AUC}_0^\infty = \int_0^\infty ae^{-\alpha t} + be^{-\beta t} = \frac{a}{\alpha} + \frac{b}{\beta} \tag{11.29}$$

$$\text{AUC}_0^t = \int_0^t ae^{-\alpha t} + be^{-\beta t} = \frac{ae^{-\alpha t}}{-\alpha} + \frac{be^{-\beta t}}{-\beta} \tag{11.30}$$

By substituting the formulas for a and b in Equation 11.29 we can obtain a different version of the parameter between zero and infinity:

$$\text{AUC}_0^\infty = \frac{D(\alpha - k_{21})}{V_1(\alpha - \beta)\alpha} + \frac{D(k_{21} - \beta)}{V_1(\alpha - \beta)\beta} = \frac{\beta C_p^0(\alpha - k_{21}) + \alpha C_p^0(k_{21} - \beta)}{\alpha\beta(\alpha - \beta)} = \frac{(\alpha - \beta)k_{21}C_p^0}{(\alpha - \beta)\alpha\beta}$$

Therefore, $$\text{AUC}_0^\infty = \frac{C_p^0}{k_{10}} \tag{11.31}$$

Note: Equation 11.31 also enables us to calculate k_{10} as

$$k_{10} = \frac{C_p^0}{\text{AUC}_0^\infty} = \frac{a + b}{a/\alpha + b/\beta} = \frac{1}{a_N/\alpha + b_N/\beta} \tag{11.32}$$

The volume of distribution, as was discussed in Chapters 4 and 6 (Section 6.3.3), is only a conversion factor that is used to change concentration of a drug in plasma to total amount of drug in the body or vice versa. It has very limited or no physiologic significance and its magnitude depends on what particular model is used and what kinetic pool is considered. For a two-compartment model we can estimate the volumes of distribution of the central compartment and of the peripheral compartment and the overall volume of distribution that encompasses both compartments.

The volume of distribution of the central compartment, V_1, was discussed earlier and can be estimated with Equation 11.14.

To estimate the overall volume of distribution of a drug that follows a two-compartment model various formulas have been recommended. Among them the following relationship known as $(V_d)_{\text{area}}$ or $(V_d)_\beta$ has been accepted as a more practical formula. The formula is derived from the model independent relationship of clearance = dose/AUC. Therefore,

$$(V_d)_{\text{area}} = \frac{D}{\beta \times \text{AUC}_0^\infty} = \frac{D}{\beta(a/\alpha + b/\beta)} \tag{11.33}$$

The apparent volume of distribution of the peripheral compartment cannot be determined directly, mainly because it is not a sampling compartment and it is not as homogeneous as the central compartment. The indirect determination of this volume term by subtracting the volume of the central compartment from the overall volume of distribution yields a value that is somewhat fictitious. As a result any "concentration" term for the peripheral compartment would also be considered a fictitious parameter. Therefore, it is preferable to use the "amount," rather than "concentration," to characterize the time course of a drug in the peripheral compartment.

The definition of total body clearance here is the same as described in Chapter 5 (Section 5.4). Some useful equations in determining the total body clearance of a drug that follows a two-compartment model are:

$$Cl_t = \frac{D}{AUC_0^\infty} \tag{11.34}$$

$$Cl_t = V_1 k_{10} \tag{11.35}$$

$$Cl_t = (V_d)_{area}\, \beta \tag{11.36}$$

Equations 11.35 and 11.36 also indicate that the rate of elimination from the body is equal to the rate of elimination from the central compartment as long as no elimination occurs from the peripheral compartment. To prove this point we set the total amount of drug in the body to be equal to the combined amount of drug in compartments 1 and 2: i.e. $A = A_1 + A_2$. Thus, the fraction of drug in the central compartment at any time would be $f_c = A_1/A$ and the amount of drug in the body would be $A = A_1/f_c$. Based on this fractional relationship we can define the amount of drug in the central compartment as a fraction of the total amount in the body: $A_1 = f_c \times A$. Therefore, the overall rate of elimination from the body can be defined as

$$\frac{dA}{dt} = -\beta A = -k_{10}A_1 = -k_{10}f_c A \tag{11.37}$$

Therefore,

$$\beta = k_{10}f_c = k_{10}\frac{A_1}{A} = k_{10}\frac{C_p V_1}{A} \tag{11.38}$$

$$\frac{\beta A}{C_p} = (V_d)_{area}\,\beta = k_{10}V_1 \tag{11.39}$$

Other clearance terms such as renal and metabolic clearances are estimated as discussed in Chapter 9; that is,

$$Cl_r = f_e Cl_t = \frac{A_e^\infty}{D}\, Cl_t = \frac{D - A_m^\infty}{D}\, Cl_t \tag{11.40}$$

$$Cl_m = f_m Cl_t = \frac{A_m^\infty}{D}\, Cl_t = \frac{D - A_e^\infty}{D}\, Cl_t \tag{11.41}$$

11.3.6 Time Course of Amount of Drug in the Peripheral Compartment

The equation of the change in amount of drug with respect to time in the peripheral compartment (Equation 11.4) is developed by integration of differential Equation 11.2 and by using the method of input-disposition function or method of substitution as described in Chapter 1. The magnitude of uptake by the peripheral compartment for a given drug depends on a number of factors such as lipid solubility of the drug, extent of elimination from the central compartment, degree of protein binding, and type of interaction and accumulation in the tissues (Figure 11.3). The AUC of Figure 11.3 that represents the extent of accumulation of drug in the second compartment can be estimated as

$$(\text{AUC}_0^\infty)_{\text{peripheral}} = \frac{k_{12}D}{\alpha - \beta} \left(\frac{1}{\beta} - \frac{1}{\alpha} \right) \tag{11.42}$$

The curve also has a maximum amount that corresponds to $T_{\max}$ of the curve:

$$(T_{\max})_{\text{peripheral}} = \frac{2.303}{\alpha - \beta} \log \frac{\alpha}{\beta} \tag{11.43}$$

$$(A_{\max})_{\text{peripheral}} = \frac{k_{12}D}{\alpha - \beta} (e^{-\beta T_{\max}} - e^{-\alpha T_{\max}}) \tag{11.44}$$

At $T_{\max}$ the rate of input into the peripheral compartment is equal to the rate of output from the compartment. Thus at that instant we achieve a steady-state level:

$$\frac{dA_2}{dt} = 0; \quad \text{therefore, } k_{12}A_1 = k_{21}A_2 \tag{11.45}$$

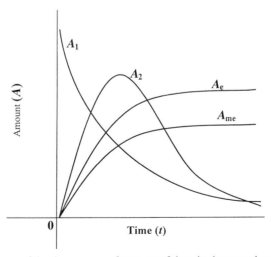

FIGURE 11.3 Diagram of the time course of amount of drug in the central compartment (A_1), and peripheral compartment (A_2), and cumulative amount eliminated unchanged (A_e) and as metabolites (A_{me}). The mass balance of drug at any time t is equal to dose (ie, dose $= A_1 + A_2 - A_e + A_{\text{me}}$).

Based on this concept a different overall volume of distribution is proposed, $(V_d)_{ss}$. It is assumed that at T_{max}

$$A_1 = C_p(V_1)_{ss}$$

$$A_2 = C_2(V_2)_{ss}$$

$$(V_d)_{ss} = (V_1)_{ss} + (V_2)_{ss}$$

$$C_2 = C_p$$

Therefore, $k_{12}C_p(V_1)_{ss} = k_{21}C_2(V_2)_{ss}$ and

$$(V_2)_{ss} = \left(\frac{k_{12}}{k_{21}}\right)V_1 \tag{11.46}$$

and in terms of $(V_d)_{ss}$, we obtain

$$(V_d)_{ss} = \left(\frac{k_{12}}{k_{21}}\right)V_1 + V_1 = \left(\frac{k_{12} + k_{21}}{k_{21}}\right)V_1 \tag{11.47}$$

It is important to note that $(V_d)_{ss}$ calculated with Equation 11.47 is different from V_{ss} of the noncompartmental analysis that will be discussed in Chapter 17 and is based on statistical moments. Equation 11.47 may represent the volume of distribution of a drug only at the point where the amount of drug in the peripheral compartment reaches its maximum.

By comparing the equations of the central compartment, 11.3, with the peripheral compartment, 11.4, we can conclude that the terminal portion of log A_2 versus time has the same slope as the disposition phase of log A, versus time and thus they are parallel (Figure 11.4).

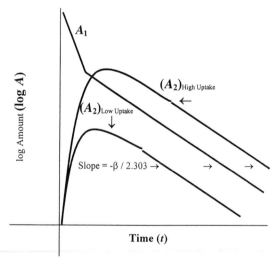

FIGURE 11.4 In linear pharmacokinetics, irrespective of the magnitude of uptake by the peripheral compartment, the terminal portion of the log amount of free drug versus time curve of the peripheral compartment would be parallel to the disposition phase of the central compartment with slope of $-\beta/2.303$.

11.4 OTHER MULTICOMPARTMENT MODELS

In addition to the two-compartment model discussed in this chapter there are other multicompartment models. Selection of any of these models for any compound is not predetermined. Mathematical and statistical criteria must be considered and satisfied in fitting an equation to a set of data in order to identify the most appropriate model. Obviously, finding the most appropriate model enables us to estimate the pharmacokinetic parameters and constants more accurately. Commercially available specialized software for pharmacokinetic analysis do include these criteria in their curve fitting process and analysis of data. It is necessary that we define the purpose and the reason for selection of a model as clearly as possible. There are times we may encounter the following situations:

■ A compound undergoes metabolism in the peripheral compartment and we need to know the peripheral rate constant of metabolism.
■ The drug is preferentially taken up by one organ and we are interested in the rate of uptake of that organ and the relationship between the amount of uptake and the pharmacologic response.
■ The drug undergoes enterohepatic recirculation and we need to know what fraction of dose returns to the systemic circulation.
■ The compound is administered as a prodrug and we are interested in determining how quickly conversion to the therapeutically active form takes place and what is the bioavailability of the drug.

The selection of biologic samples and related mathematical models should be such that the pharmacokinetic parameters and constants of interest, similar to the aforementioned situations, can be calculated. We should also keep the following points in mind:

■ In compartmental analysis, the compartments refer only to the amount of drug in a distinct kinetic pool. They do not correspond to physiologic or physical identifiable processes or compartments.
■ A set of data may be defined by more than one mathematical relationship. Thus, the uniqueness of the solution should also be confirmed.
■ It is necessary to consider the established and well-defined criteria of curve fitting for the selection of a compartment model.

A discussion of the selection criteria for the most appropriate model for one or more sets of biological data is beyond the scope of this textbook. The preceding short discussion was presented only to highlight a few dilemmas in selecting a pharmacokinetic model and inform students that we cannot arbitrarily select a model.

Two other examples of two-compartment model are presented in Figure 11.5. The main difference between these models is where elimination of the compound occurs. The general equation of these models, based on the free concentration of drug in plasma, is the same as Equation 11.6; however, their disposition functions are different and the calculation of the miniature rate constants is based on different formulas for $\alpha\beta$ or $\alpha + \beta$. Diagrams of more complex models are presented in Figure 11.6. Using Laplace transform or input-disposition functions as described in Chapter 1, we can easily develop the equations of these models (Figures 11.5 and 11.6).

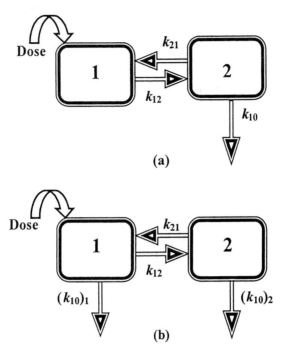

FIGURE 11.5 Diagram of two-compartment model with elimination from the peripheral compartment (a) or from the peripheral and central compartments (b).

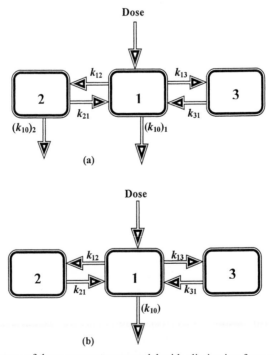

FIGURE 11.6 Diagram of three-compartment model with elimination from central and peripheral compartments (a) or elimination from only the central compartment (b). There might be cases where the elimination occurs from all three compartments.

TABLE 11.2 Data Related to Application 11.1

Time (h)	Serum Concentration (μg/mL)
0.1	520
0.3	310
0.4	250
0.5	190
0.7	120
1.5	72
2.5	36
4.0	18
5.0	7.2
6.0	6.0

APPLICATION

11.1 A clinically stable hospitalized urology adult patient receives 4 g of an antibiotic intravenously every 4h. Serial blood samples are obtained after the first dose and serum concentration is determined as presented in Table 11.2. The drug is known to follow a two-compartment model. Determine the following:

1. Disposition rate constant: The regression equation of the last six data points (ie, the postdistributive phase or β phase) is

$$\log \tilde{C}_p = 2.28 - 0.278t$$

$$\tilde{C}_p = 190.54(\text{mg/L})e^{-0.64 \text{ h}^{-1}t}$$

Therefore, $$\beta = 0.64 \text{ h}^{-1}$$

2. Biologic half-life

$$(T_{1/2})_\beta = 0.693/0.64 = 1.08 \text{ h}$$

3. Equation of the model: The residual concentrations are listed in Table 11.3. The regression equation of the residual concentrations is

$$\log(C_p - \tilde{C}_p) = 2.76 - 1.99t$$

Therefore, $$(C_p - \tilde{C}_p) = 575.44(\text{mg/L})e^{-4.55 \text{ h}^{-1}t}$$

The biexponential equation of the model is

$$C_p = 575.44(\text{mg/L})e^{-4.55 \text{ h}^{-1}t} + 190.54(\text{mg/L})e^{-0.64 \text{ h}^{-1}t}$$

TABLE 11.3 Calculation of Residual Line of Application 11.1

t	$\bar{C}_p$ (mg/L)	C_p (mg/L)	$\bar{C}_p - C_p$ (mg/L)
0.1	178.73	520	341.27
0.3	157.25	310	152.75
0.4	147.50	250	102.50
0.5	138.35	190	51.65

4. Half-life of elimination

$$k_{21} = \frac{(190.54 \times 4.55) + (575.44 \times 0.64)}{574.44 + 190.54} = 1.61 \text{ h}^{-1}$$

$$k_{10} = \frac{4.55 \times 0.64}{1.61} = 1.81 \text{ h}^{-1}$$

Therefore

$$(T_{1/2})_{\text{elimination}} = \frac{0.693}{1.81} = 0.383 \text{ h}$$

5. Total body clearance

$$\text{Cl}_t = V_1 k_{10}$$

$$V_1 = 4000 \text{ mg}/(575.44 + 190.54) \text{ mg/L} = 5.22 \text{ L}$$

$$\text{Cl}_t = (5.22)(1.81 \text{ h}^{-1}) = 9.45 \text{ L/h} = 157.47 \text{ mL/min}$$

or

$$\text{Cl}_t = (V_d)_{\text{area}} (\beta)$$

$$\text{AUC} = (575.44/4.55) + (190.54/0.64) = 424.2 \text{ mg h/L}$$

$$(V_d)_{\text{area}} = 4000 \text{ mg}/(424.2)(0.64) \text{ mg/L} = 14.77 \text{ L}$$

$$\text{Cl}_t = (14.77 \text{ L})(0.64 \text{ h}^{-1}) = 9.43 \text{ L/h}$$

or

$$\text{Cl}_t = \text{dose/AUC}$$

$$\text{Cl}_t = 4000 \text{ (mg)}/424.2 \text{ (mg h/L)} = 9.43 \text{ L/h}$$

6. Total amount of drug in central compartment 1 hour after injection

$$A_1 = A(V_1)e^{-\alpha_t} + B(V_1)e^{-\beta_t}$$

$$A_1 = 575.44(5.22)e^{-4.55(1)} + 190.54(5.22)e^{-0.64(1)} = 556.2 \text{ mg}$$

7. Plasma concentrations at $t = 6$ min and $t = 7$ hours

$$C_{p_{6 \text{ min}}} = 575.44e^{-4.55(0.1)} + 190.54e^{-0.64(0.1)} = 543.81 \text{ mg/L}$$

$$(T_{1/2})_\alpha = 0.693/4.55 = 0.152 \text{ h}; \text{ therefore, } 7 \text{ h} > 7 \ (T_{1/2})_\alpha$$

$$C_{p_{7 \text{ h}}} = 190.54e^{-0.64 \ (7 \text{ h})} = 2.61 \text{ mg/L}$$

8. Distribution rate constants

$$k_{21} = 1.61 \text{ h}^{-1}$$

$$k_{12} = 4.55 + 0.64 - 1.61 - 1.81 = 1.77 \text{ h}^{-1}$$

9. Renal and metabolic clearances if the drug is cleared 75% as unchanged via the kidneys, and the balance by hepatic metabolism:

$$f_e = 0.75$$

$$Cl_r = (9.4 \text{ L/h})(0.75) = 7.05 \text{ L/h}$$

$$Cl_m = (9.4 \text{ L/h}) \ (0.25) = 2.35 \text{ L/h}$$

11.2 After an IV bolus injection of a single dose of 250 mg of an antibiotic to a 70-kg patient, blood samples were collected and plasma concentration of the drug was determined at different intervals and reported as milligrams per liter versus hours. Analysis of the data following curve fitting and consideration of related criteria revealed the following two-compartment model:

$$C_p = 35(\text{mg/L})e^{-3.465(\text{h}^{-1})t} + 15(\text{mg/L})e^{-0.1155(\text{h}^{-1})t}$$

Determine the following:

1. Apparent volume of distribution of central compartment

$$V_1 = \frac{250 \text{ mg}}{(35 + 15) \text{ mg/L}} = 5 \text{ L}$$

2. Biologic half-life of drug

$$(T_{1/2})_\beta = \frac{0.693}{0.1155} = 6 \text{ h}$$

3. Distribution rate constants

$$k_{21} = \frac{(35 \times 0.1155) + (15 \times 3.465)}{35 + 15} = 1.12 \text{ h}^{-1}$$

$$k_{12} = 0.1155 + 3.465 - 1.12 - \left(\frac{0.1155 \times 3.465}{1.12} \right) = 2.10 \text{ h}^{-1}$$

4. Amount of drug in central compartment 12 hours after injection

$$(T_{1/2})_\beta = 6 \text{ h} \quad (T_{1/2})_\alpha = 0.2 \text{ h} \quad t = 12 \text{ h}$$

$$12 \text{ h} = 2(T_{1/2})_\beta = 60(T_{1/2})_\alpha$$

$$C_{p_{12 \text{ h}}} = 15 \text{ mg/L} \times 0.25 = 3.75 \text{ mg/L}$$

$$A_1 = 3.75 \text{ mg/L} \times 5 \text{ L} = 18.75 \text{ mg}$$

5. Amount of drug in peripheral compartment 12 hours after injection

$$A_2 = \frac{2.1 \times 250}{3.465 - 0.1155} (0.25) = 39.18 \text{ mg}$$

ASSIGNMENT

11.1 One gram of a semisynthetic parenteral cephalosporin was administered intravenously to two male patients (A and B) on a multiple-dosing basis. Patient A is a 45-year-old, 75-kg male with normal renal function. Patient B is a 49-year-old, 58-kg male with chronic renal failure secondary to diabetic nephropathy. Serum concentrations of the drug were determined and are reported in Table 11.4. Calculate the following:

    11.1.1 Disposition rate constant
    11.1.2 Biologic half-life
    11.1.3 Equation of the residual line
    11.1.4 Biexponential equation of the model
    11.1.5 Apparent volume of distribution of the central compartment
    11.1.6 Area under plasma concentration–time curve
    11.1.7 Distribution and elimination rate constants
    11.1.8 Elimination half-life
    11.1.9 Total body clearance
    11.1.10 Area under the curve of amount of drug in peripheral compartment versus time

11.2 The decline in serum concentration of an antibiotic is known to follow a two-compartment model, and the fraction excreted unchanged in urine on average is about 60% of the dose. An IV injection of 10 mg/kg of this drug was recommended four times daily to the patients in Table 11.5. Serum concentration after the first dose was measured at different intervals and is reported in Table 11.6. Patient B undergoes hemodialysis and

TABLE 11.4 Data Related to Assignment 11.1

	Serum Concentration (mg%)	
Time (h)	Patient A (Normal Renal Function)	Patient B (Renal Failure)
0.05	1.050	1.100
0.10	0.920	1.050
0.20	0.820	0.960
0.30	0.720	0.900
0.40	0.620	0.820
0.50	0.500	0.740
1.00	0.420	0.530
2.00	0.295	0.455
4.00	0.145	0.330
6.00	0.071	0.240
8.00	0.035	0.175
10.00	0.017	0.125

the serum samples in Table 11.6 were measured in the interdialysis period. Calculate the following for both patients:

11.2.1 Biologic half-life
11.2.2 Distribution rate constants
11.2.3 Elimination half-life

TABLE 11.5 Data Related to Assignment 11.2

	Patient A	Patient B
Age	29	46
Weight (kg)	67	75
Renal function	Normal	Severe impairment
Dose (mg/kg)	10	10
Time (h)	Serum Conc. (mg/L)	Serum Conc. (mg/L)
0.05	80.00	88.00
0.10	70.00	82.00
0.20	56.00	72.00
0.30	40.00	64.00
0.40	30.00	56.00
0.60	18.00	43.00
1.00	14.00	25.00
2.00	7.80	21.00
3.00	4.50	18.50
4.00	2.30	14.50
5.00	1.25	12.20
7.00	0.37	8.27

TABLE 11.6 Assignment 11.4

Parameter/Constant	Answer	Units
Plasma concentration 6 hours after injection		μg/mL
Half-life of disposition		h
Rate constant of distribution		min^{-1}
Apparent volume of distribution of central compartment		L
Amount of drug in peripheral compartment at $t = 6$ hours		mg
Area under plasma concentration-time curve		mg h/L
Total body clearance		mL/min

11.2.4 Amount of drug in first and second compartments at $t = 0$

11.2.5 Biexponential equation of the model

11.2.6 Apparent volume of distribution of central compartment

11.2.7 Total body clearance

11.2.8 Metabolic clearance

11.2.9 Total amount in peripheral compartment 4 hours after injection

11.2.10 Total amount in central compartment 4 hours after first dose

11.2.11 Total amount in body 4 hours after first dose

11.2.12 Plasma concentration 6 hours after injection of first dose and just before giving second dose

11.2.13 Plasma concentration just after giving second dose

11.2.14 $(V_d)_{area}$

11.2.15 T_{max} and A_{max} of amount in peripheral compartment

11.3 Hemodialysis was initiated immediately after the injection of second dose for patient B from Assignment 11.2 and continued for 6 hours. Six serum samples were collected during last 2 hours of hemodialysis. The related regression equation of the six data points is

$$C_p = 32e^{-0.533t}$$

Calculate the biologic half-life during dialysis. Comment on the effect of hemodialysis on the calculated parameters and constants in comparison with patient A and B (interdialysis period).

11.4 After an IV bolus injection of 1 g of a drug to a 60-kg patient, blood samples were collected and plasma concentration of the drug was determined at different intervals and reported as micrograms per liter versus hours. Analysis of the data following curve fitting and consideration of related criteria revealed the following two-compartment model.

$$C_p = 70e^{-1.7325t} + 30e^{-0.1155t}$$

Fill in the blanks in Table 11.6.

11.5 If after injection of 3 g of a drug that follows a two-compartment model, the area under the plasma concentration−time curve is estimated as 750 mg h/L, what is the biologic half-life if $(V_d)_{area}$ is 20 L?

11.6 If the overall elimination rate constant of a drug following injection of 500 mg is 0.5 h^{-1}, what is the area under the plasma concentration–time curve if the initial plasma concentration is 100 μg/mL? (Assume the drug follows a two-compartment model.)

BIBLIOGRAPHY

1. Benet LZ. *General treatment of linear mammillary models with elimination from any compartment as used in pharmacokinetics.* 1972;61:536.
2. Braunberg H. Mathematical models in the study of steroid dynamics. In: Raspé G, editor. *Advances in biosciences.* Vieweg: Pergamon Press, 1969:145.
3. Dost FH. An explicit function for rate constant of entrance concerning a two-compartment model. In: Raspé G, editor. *Advances in biosciences.* Vieweg: Pergamon Press, 1969:137.
4. Gibaldi M, Perrier D. *Pharmacokinetics,* 2nd ed. New York: Marcel Dekker, 1982:45.
5. Locker A. The formulation of models to explain blood and tissue data on distribution of drugs and tracers (with special reference to multicompartment model). In: Raspé G, editor. *Advances in biosciences.* Vieweg: Pergamon Press, 1969:115.
6. Rescigno A, Segre G. *Drug and tracer kinetics.* Waltham, MA: Blaisdell, 1966:44.
7. Schneider B. Mathematical and statistical problems in pharmacokinetics. In: Raspé G, editor. *Advances in biosciences.* Vieweg: Pergamon Press, 1969:103.
8. Wagner JG. Clinical pharmacokinetics. Hamilton, IL: *Drug Intelligence,* 1975:57.

CHAPTER 12

MULTIPLE-DOSING KINETICS: TWO-COMPARTMENT MODEL

Our discussion will be adequate if its degree of clarity fits the subject-matter;
for we should not seek the same degree of exactness in all sorts of arguments alike,
any more than in the products of different crafts.
ARISTOTLE (NICOMACHEAN ETHICS)

OBJECTIVES

■ To discuss the multiple-dosing kinetics of a drug that follows a two-compartment model.

■ To define the differences between one- and two-compartment models related to multiple dosing.

■ To discuss methods of determining peak, trough, and average plasma concentrations.

■ To estimate the time required to achieve any fraction of steady state and accumulation index.

■ To design a dosing regimen.

12.1 INTRODUCTION

The theory and principles of multiple-dosing kinetics for drugs that follow a two-compartment model are very much the same as those for a one-compartment model. The equations of the model are based on solving the related geometric series and transforming the single-dose equations into multiple-dosing relationships. The noticeable difference in the plasma concentration–time profile is the decline in plasma concentration after each dose according to the two-compartment model. This means that a fast distributive phase and slow disposition phase occur after each dose (Figure 12.1). The hybrid rate constants α and β remain the same as for the first dose; however, the parameters a and b may change for concentration curves of doses given before or after steady state is reached. An important factor that may simplify some of the relationships of peak or trough levels is the length of dosing interval in relation to $7(T_{1/2})_{\alpha}$, as will be discussed in the following sections.

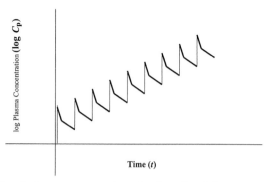

FIGURE 12.1 Profile of plasma concentration of a drug that follows a two-compartment model and is given on a multiple-dosing basis. The biphasic characteristic of the disposition is usually apparent after each dose.

12.2 EQUATIONS OF THE MODEL

Solutions of the geometric series of α and β for concentrations of drug before and during steady state are similar to those discussed for a one-compartment model in Chapter 10. Before steady state is reached,

$$S_n(e^{-\alpha\tau})_n = \frac{1 - e^{-n\alpha\tau}}{1 - e^{-\alpha\tau}} \quad S_n(e^{-\beta\tau})_n = \frac{1 - e^{-n\beta\tau}}{1 - e^{-\beta\tau}} \tag{12.1}$$

For steady state to be reached without a loading dose, a number of maintenance doses should be given. This means that n increases and the numerators of Equations 12.1 approach one:

$$S_n(e^{-\alpha\tau})_{ss} = \frac{1}{1 - e^{-\alpha\tau}} \quad S_n(e^{-\beta\tau})_{ss} = \frac{1}{1 - e^{-\beta\tau}} \tag{12.2}$$

12.2.1 Equations of Plasma Concentration before Steady State: Peak and Trough Levels

The peak and trough levels of the first dose are:

$$(C_{p_{max}})_1 = a + b \tag{12.3}$$

$$(C_{p_{min}})_1 = ae^{-\alpha\tau} + be^{-\beta\tau} \tag{12.4}$$

By multiplying Equations 12.3 and 12.4 by Equation 12.1 we can develop relationships for peak and trough levels before steady state:

$$(C_{p_{max}})_n = a\left(\frac{1 - e^{-n\alpha\tau}}{1 - e^{-n\alpha\tau}}\right) + b\left(\frac{1 - e^{-n\beta\tau}}{1 - e^{\beta\tau}}\right) \tag{12.5}$$

$$(C_{p_{min}})_n = a\left(\frac{1 - e^{-n\alpha\tau}}{1 - e^{\alpha\tau}}\right)e^{-\alpha\tau} + b\left(\frac{1 - e^{-n\beta\tau}}{1 - e^{-\beta\tau}}\right)e^{-\beta\tau} \tag{12.6}$$

It is important to recognize that when the dosing interval is equal to or greater than seven half-lives of α (ie, $\tau \geq 7(T_{1/2})_\alpha$), $e^{-\alpha\tau}$ and $e^{-n\alpha\tau}$ approach zero and Equations 12.5 and 12.6 convert to

$$(C_{p_{max}})_n = a + b\left(\frac{1 - e^{-n\beta\tau}}{1 - e^{-\beta\tau}}\right) \tag{12.7}$$

$$(C_{p_{min}})_n = b\left(\frac{1 - e^{-n\beta\tau}}{1 - e^{-\beta\tau}}\right)e^{-\beta\tau} \tag{12.8}$$

To calculate plasma concentration at any time between the peak and trough levels of any dose before steady state, we can apply the following relationship, which is the product of Equation 12.4 at time t and Equation 12.1:

$$(C_{p_t})_n = a\left(\frac{1 - e^{-n\alpha\tau}}{1 - e^{\alpha\tau}}\right)e^{-\alpha t} + b\left(\frac{1 - e^{-n\beta\tau}}{1 - e^{-\beta\tau}}\right)e^{-\beta t} \tag{12.9}$$

Obviously, if $t \geq 7(T_{1/2})_\alpha$, Equation 12.9 will be modified:

$$(C_{p_t})_n = b\left(\frac{1 - e^{-n\beta\tau}}{1 - e^{-\beta\tau}}\right)e^{-\beta t} \tag{12.10}$$

12.2.2 Equations of Plasma Concentration after Achieving Steady State

A similar approach is used to develop equations of peak and trough levels after achieving the steady-state fluctuation:

$$(C_{p_{max}})_{ss} = \frac{a}{1 - e^{-\alpha\tau}} + \frac{b}{1 - e^{\beta\tau}} \tag{12.11}$$

$$(C_{p_{min}})_{ss} = \frac{ae^{-\alpha\tau}}{1 - e^{-\alpha\tau}} + \frac{be^{-\beta\tau}}{1 - e^{-\beta\tau}} \tag{12.12}$$

When $\tau \geq 7(T_{1/2})_\alpha$, Equations 12.11 and 12.12 convert to

$$(C_{p_{max}})_{ss} = a + \frac{b}{1 - e^{\beta\tau}} \tag{12.13}$$

$$(C_{p_{min}})_{ss} = \frac{be^{-\beta\tau}}{1 - e^{-\beta\tau}} \tag{12.14}$$

Plasma concentrations between the peak and trough levels of any dose during steady state can be estimated by

$$(C_{p_t})_{ss} = \frac{ae^{-\alpha t}}{1 - e^{-\alpha\tau}} + \frac{be^{-\beta t}}{1 - e^{-\beta\tau}} \tag{12.15}$$

When $t \geq 7(T_{1/2})_\alpha$,

$$(C_{p_t})_{ss} = \frac{be^{-\beta t}}{1 - e^{-\beta \tau}} \qquad (12.16)$$

The average steady-state plasma concentration is also calculated similarly to that for a one-compartment model. The definition is the same as described in Chapter 10:

$$(C_{p_{ave}})_{ss} = \frac{D}{Cl_t \tau} = \frac{AUC}{\tau} = \frac{D}{k_{10} V_1 \tau} = \frac{D}{\beta V_{d\,area} \tau} = \frac{C_p^0}{k_{10} \tau} = \frac{1.44 (T_{1/2})_{biol} D}{V_{d\,area} \tau} \qquad (12.17)$$

It is important to note that for nearly every therapeutic agent in practice the dosing interval is equal to or greater than the $7(T_{1/2})_\alpha$. Under this condition the time required to achieve any fraction of steady state can be estimated with

$$n\tau = -3.3(T_{1/2})_\beta \log(1 - f_{ss}) \qquad (12.18)$$

According to Equation 12.18, the time required to achieve any fraction of steady state is dependent solely on the biologic half-life:

$$\text{To achieve} \quad f_{ss} = 0.5 \quad n\tau = 1(T_{1/2})_{biol}$$

$$\text{To achieve} \quad f_{ss} = 0.75 \quad n\tau = 2(T_{1/2})_{biol}$$

$$\text{To achieve} \quad f_{ss} = 0.90 \quad n\tau = 3.3(T_{1/2})_{biol}$$

$$\text{To achieve} \quad f_{ss} = 0.95 \quad n\tau = 4.3(T_{1/2})_{biol}$$

$$\text{To achieve} \quad f_{ss} = 0.99 \quad n\tau = 6.6(T_{1/2})_{biol}$$

12.2.3 Fraction of Steady State, Accumulation Index, and Relationship between Loading Dose and Maintenance Dose

Equation 12.18 is derived from the numerator of multiple dosing function of Equation 12.8, which represents the fraction of steady state (see Chapter 10):

$$f_{ss} = 1 - e^{-n\beta \tau} \qquad (12.19)$$

This is a useful equation for estimating maximum and minimum plasma concentrations before steady state without knowing the values of a and α and based on the steady-state peak and trough levels (see Application 12.1).

The accumulation index and the relationship between the loading dose and maintenance dose are similar to those for equations of a one-compartment model as described in Chapter 10. The only difference is the rate constant of the equations; in a one-compartment model it is based on the overall elimination rate constant, K, whereas in a two-compartment model it is based on the disposition rate constant β:

$$R = \frac{(C_{p_{min}})_{ss}}{(C_{p_{min}})_1} = \frac{1}{1 - e^{-\beta\tau}} \tag{12.20}$$

$$D_L = \frac{D_M}{1 - e^{-\beta\tau}} = \frac{D_M}{1 - (1/2)^{(T_{1/2})_{biol}/\tau}} \tag{12.21}$$

Combination of loading dose and maintenance dose provides immediate steady-state levels (Figure 12.2). Equation 12.21 indicates that for drugs with a very short biologic half-life no loading dose is necessary. Setting the dosing interval equal to the biologic half-life in the equation indicates that the loading dose is twice the maintenance dose. For drugs with a very long half-life, because the denominator of the equation approaches zero, the loading dose is set equal to the average amount in the body at steady state:

$$D_L = \frac{D_M}{\beta\tau} \tag{12.22}$$

12.2.4 Decline of Plasma Concentration after Last Dose

After the last dose is given, regardless of whether the steady state is achieved, the plasma concentration declines biexponentially according to the two-compartment model. To estimate plasma concentration at $t' < \tau$ we may need to use Equations 12.9 and 12.10 or 12.15 and 12.16. However, if $t' > \tau$, the simple approach to calculating the plasma concentration of less than $C_{p_{min}}$ is:

$$\log C_{p_{t'}} = \log C_{p_{min}} - \frac{\beta(t' - \tau)}{2.303} \quad \text{or} \quad C_{p_{t'}} = C_{p_{min}} e^{-\beta(t' - \tau)} \tag{12.23}$$

Using $C_{p_{max}}$ as the initial plasma concentration of the monoexponential decline after the last dose would add some error to the estimation of $C_{p_{t'}}$ (ie, $C_{p_{t'}} \neq C_{p_{max}} e^{-\beta t'}$, Figure 12.3).

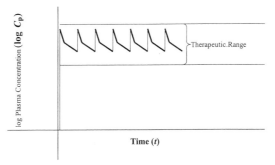

FIGURE 12.2 Profile of logarithm of plasma concentration versus time after multiple intravenous dosing of a drug that follows a two-compartment model with the first dose given as a loading dose.

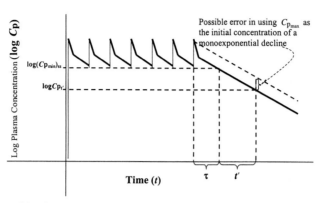

FIGURE 12.3 Profile of plasma concentration of multiple-dosing kinetics of a drug that follows a two-compartment model with loading dose and biexponential decline of plasma concentration after the last dose.

12.2.5 Designing a Dosing Regimen

Among the approaches discussed in Chapter 10 (Section 10.2.7) for a one-compartment model, the most practical approach for a two-compartment model would be the method based on a selected average plasma concentration within the therapeutic range. After selecting a target concentration, we set the dosing interval equal to the biologic half-life and estimate the maintenance dose according to the relationships

$$D_M = (C_{p_{ave}})_{ss} \times (V_d)_{area} \tau \beta \tag{12.24}$$

or

$$D_M = (C_{p_{ave}})_{ss} V_1 \tau k_{10} \tag{12.25}$$

If the dosing interval is equal to the biologic half-life of the drug, $D_L = 2D_M$. If it is less or greater than the half-life, then Equation 12.21 can be used to determine the loading dose.

APPLICATION

12.1 The following equation represents the two-compartment model of the first maintenance dose of an antibiotic after IV bolus injection of 4 g to a hospitalized patient.

$$C_p = 575.44e^{-4.55t} + 190.54e^{-0.64t}$$

(Plasma concentration of the drug was measured in mg/L and time in h.) It is recommended that the patient receive this medication every 4 hours for 4 days. Calculate the following:

1. Minimum steady-state amount of drug in the body

$$\tau = 4 \text{ h} > (T_{1/2})_\alpha$$

$$(C_{p_{min}})_{ss} = 190.54 e^{-0.64 \times 4}/(1 - e^{-0.64 \times 4}) = 15.96 \text{ mg/L}$$

$$V_1 = 4 \text{ g}/(0.575 + 0.190) = 5.23 \text{ L}$$

$$(A_{min})_{ss} = (15.96)(5.23) = 83.47 \text{ mg} = 0.083 \text{ g}$$

2. Accumulation index

$$R = (C_{p_{min}})_{ss}/(C_{p_{min}})_1$$

$$R = (15.96)/(190.54 e^{-0.64(4)}) = 1.08 \quad \text{when } \tau > 7(T_{1/2})_\alpha$$

NOTE

■ Dosing at intervals greater than the $(T_{1/2})_{biol}$ of a drug may result in low or no accumulation, as is apparent in this case from the value of the accumulation index.
■ The ratio of loading dose to maintenance dose is equal to the accumulation index.
■ Because $R \cong 1$, $D_L = D_M$.

3. Average steady-state plasma concentration

$$(C_{p_{ave}})_{ss} = D/(Cl_t \times \tau)$$

$$Cl_t = (V_d)_{area}\beta$$

$$(V_d)_{area} = D/AUC$$

$$AUC = (575.4/4.55) + (190.54/0.64) = 424.18 \text{ mg h/L}$$

$$(V_d)_{area} = 4000/(424.18 \times 0.64) = 14.73 \text{ L}$$

$$Cl_t = 14.73 \times 0.64 = 9.427 \text{ L/h} = 157.12 \text{ mL/min}$$

$$(C_{p_{ave}})_{ss} = 4000/9.427 \times 4 = 106.08 \text{ mg/L}$$

or

$$(C_{p_{ave}})_{ss} = AUC/\tau = (424.18 \text{ mg h/L})/4 \text{ h} = 106.04 \text{ mg/L}$$

4. Time required to achieve 50 and 65% of plateau levels

$$(n\tau)_{50\%} = 1(T_{1/2})_{biol} = 1.08 \text{ h}$$

$$(n\tau)_{65\%} = -3.3(1.08)\log(1 - 0.65) = 1.625 \text{ h}$$

5. Plasma concentration 8 hours after last dose

$$C_{p_{8\,h}} = (C_{p_{min}})_{ss}\, e^{-\beta(4)} = 15.96 e^{-0.64 \times 4} = 1.234 \text{ mg/L}$$

12.2 A dose of 0.25 mg of a drug that follows a two-compartment model was given to a 70-kg patient intravenously every 24 hours for 20 consecutive days. The following data are known: $(T_{1/2})_{biol} = 48$ h, $(V_d)_{area} = 7.38$ L/kg, $(C_{p_{min}})_{ss} = 1$ μg/L, $(C_{p_{max}})_{ss} = 2$ μg/L, $f_e = 0.8$, $V_1 = 1$ L/kg. Calculate the following:

1. Half-life of elimination

$$\beta = 0.0144 h^{-1}$$

$$V_1 = 70L$$

$$(V_d)_{area} = 7.38 \times 70 = 516.60 \text{ L}$$

$$Cl_t = \beta(V_d)_{area} = k_{10}V_1$$

$$k_{10} = (0.0144 \times 516.6)/70 = 0.106 \text{ h}^{-1}$$

Therefore,

$$(T_{1/2}) = 0.693/0.106 = 6.54 \text{ h}$$

2. Average steady-state plasma concentration

$$(C_{p_{ave}})_{ss} = 0.25/(0.0144 \times 516.60 \times 24) = 0.0014 \text{ mg/L} = 1.4 \text{ ng/ml}$$

3. Metabolic clearance

$$Cl_m = (1 - 0.8) \times 0.0144 \times 516.67 = 1.488 \text{ L/h}$$

4. Maximum amount of drug in central compartment 1 week after first dose (ie, amount in body immediately after 7th dose)

$$(f_{ss})_{week} = 1 - e^{-7 \times 0.0144 \times 24} = 0.911$$

$$(A_1)_{week} = 0.911 \times 2 \text{ mg/L} \times 70 \text{ L} = 127.54 \text{ mg}$$

5. Loading dose

$$D_L = 0.25/(1 - e^{-0.0144 \times 24}) = 0.855 \text{ mg}$$

6. Plasma concentration 48 hours after last dose (ie, 20th dose)

$$C_{p_{t'}} = 48 \text{ h} = (1 \text{ mg/L})\, e^{-0.0144 \times (48-24)} = 0.707 \text{ }\mu\text{g/L}$$

7. Total amount of drug excreted unchanged per dosing interval at steady state

$$(A_e)_\tau = 0.25 \times 0.8 = 0.2 \text{ mg}$$

8. Time it would take to achieve average plasma concentration of 0.7 ng/mL

$$0.7 \text{ ng/mL} = 50\% \ (C_{p_{ave}})_{ss}$$

$$n\tau = (T_{1/2})_{biol} = 48 \text{ h}$$

ASSIGNMENT

12.1 A 60-kg hospitalized male patient with atrial fibrillation was given a cardiac glycoside by IV bolus injection every 24 hours for 10 consecutive days. Based on the analysis of plasma concentration the following data are known about the patient: $(V_d)_{area} = 7.38 \text{L/kg}$, $V_1 = 1 \text{ L/kg}$, $(C_{p_{min}})_{ss} = 1 \ \mu g/L$, $Cl_t = 0.213 \text{L h}^{-1}/\text{kg}$, $(C_{p_{max}})_{ss} = 2 \ \mu g/L$. Calculate the following:

12.1.1 Plasma concentration 72 hours after last dose
12.1.2 Peak level after third dose
12.1.3 Time it would take to achieve 65% of average steady-state plasma concentration
12.1.4 Time it would take to achieve maximum plasma concentration of 1 $\mu g/L$

12.2 A 25-year-old female receives 50 mg of an antibiotic intravenously four times daily. The drug follows a two-compartment model and the related data for the first dose are: $a = 11.25 \text{ mg/L}$, $b = 3.75 \text{ mg/L}$, $\alpha = 1.8 \text{ h}^{-1}$, $\beta = 0.2 \text{ h}^{-1}$.

12.2.1 Calculate the average steady-state plasma concentration.
12.2.2 Determine the loading dose necessary to attain steady state immediately.
12.2.3 Calculate the trough level at steady state.
12.2.4 What is the plasma concentration 12 hours after the last dose? Assume the steady state is achieved.
12.2.5 How long would it take to reach 80% of steady-state levels?
12.2.6 Calculate the accumulation index.
12.2.7 If the fraction of dose eliminated as metabolites is 0.46, what is the total amount excreted and metabolized in a dosing interval at steady state.

ASSIGNMENT (EXTRA CREDIT)

EC-12.1 Ben Korman et al describe the theory of determining an infusion regimen with controlled fluctuation for drugs of low therapeutic index. The regimen involves combination of an IV bolus and several IV infusions. Read the article and answer the questions for this assignment.

Korman B, Jennings LS, Rigg RA. Rapid attainment of steady-state plasma concentration within precise limits. *J Pharmacokinet Biopharm* 1998;26:319–28.

■ Discuss the clinical application of the proposed methodology.
■ How would you simplify the equation to fit drugs that follow a one-compartment model?
■ How can the method facilitate the induction of anesthesia?

BIBLIOGRAPHY

1. Colburn WA. Estimating the accumulation of drugs. *J Pharm Sci* 1983;72:833.
2. Gibaldi M, Perrier D. *Pharmacokinetics,* 2nd ed. New York: Marcel Dekker, 1982:113.
3. Krüger-Thiemer E. Formal theory of drug dosage regimens, I. *J Theor Biol* 1966;13:212.
4. Krüger-Thiemer E. Formal theory of drug dosage regimens. II. The exact plateau effect. *J Theor Biol* 1969;23:169.
5. Krüger-Thiemer E, Bünger P. The role of the therapeutic regimen, Part I. *Chemotherapia* 1965/1966;10:61.
6. Levy G. Pharmacokinetic control and clinical interpretation of steady state blood levels of drugs. *Clin Pharmacol Ther* 1976;16(1, pt 2):130.
7. Perrier D, Gibaldi M. Relationship between plasma or serum drug concentration and amount of drug in the body at steady state upon multiple dosing. *J Pharmacokinet Biopharm* 1973;1:17.
8. Slattery JT, Gibaldi M, Koup JR. Prediction of maintenance dose required to attain a desired drug concentration at steady state from a single determination of concentration after an initial dose. *Clin Pharmacokinet* 1980;5:377.
9. Van Rossum JM, Tomey AHM. Rate of accumulation and plateau plasma concentration of drugs after chronic medication. *J Pharm Pharmacol* 1968;20:390.
10. Wagner JG, Northam JI, Always CD, Carpenter OS. Blood levels of drug at equilibrium state after multiple dosing. *Nature* 1965;207:1301.
11. Wagner JG. Clinical pharmacokinetics. Hamilton, IL: *Drug Intelligence,* 1975:133.

MULTICOMPARTMENT MODELS: LINEAR TWO-COMPARTMENT MODEL WITH FIRST-ORDER INPUT AND FIRST-ORDER DISPOSITION

Time is a thought or a measure, not a reality.
AETIUS

OBJECTIVES

■ To discuss the pharmacokinetics of orally administered drugs that follow a two-compartment model.

■ To interpret the influence of the hybrid rate constants α, β, and k_a on the profile of the plasma concentration–time curve.

■ To develop the equations of the model.

■ To discuss the method of determination of the absorption rate constant.

■ To estimate parameters and constants such as initial plasma concentration, total body clearance, and apparent volume of distribution.

13.1 INTRODUCTION

As was discussed in Chapter 3, first-order input refers to when the drug is administered orally, intramuscularly, rectally, sublingually, and so on and absorption from the site of administration is governed by passive diffusion and first-order kinetics. In this chapter, similar to Chapter 8, we focus on oral absorption as the first-order input. The profile of the plasma concentration–time curve of drugs that are given orally and are known to follow a two-compartment model is somewhat different from the skewed bell-shaped curve of a one-compartment model. The difference is due mainly to the combined effect and contribution of the three biologic processes of absorption, distribution, and elimination in handling a drug in the body. In the chapter related to one-compartment models with first-order input (Chapter 8) we observed the influence of absorption and elimination processes on the C_p-versus-time curve without the distribution process. In this chapter we explore the joint influence of all three biologic processes on the profile of the curve. Obviously, the overall representation of the equations of the model will be more complex than that for the one-compartment model. Having a more complex model would necessitate the use of a specialized computer program for calculation of the parameters and constants of the model. Additionally, because visual determination of two-compartmental characteristics of an orally administered drug is not always possible, the curve fitting criteria of specialized pharmacokinetic software are needed to select the appropriate model. Frequently, when it is possible, the drug is also given intravenously to establish with certainty whether the drug follows a two- or more-compartment model. However, from time to time the two-compartmental characteristics of a drug can be obvious after plotting plasma data of an orally administered dose of a drug. For example, when absorption is rapid and the plasma concentration reaches a maximum within the interval of the distributive phase, a distinctive distributional nose appears that identifies the two-compartment characteristic of the drug. As was discussed earlier, however, depending on the influence of the combined rates of absorption, distribution, and elimination, the shape of the curve may not be so noticeably that of a two-compartment model.

13.2 EQUATIONS OF THE MODEL

The diagram of the model is presented in Figure 13.1. It represents the site of absorption, central compartment or compartment 1, and peripheral compartment or compartment 2. Compartment 1 represents the systemic circulation and highly perfused tissues. Compartment 2 represents the less accessible or slow-equilibrating tissues and organs. The site of absorption is the GI tract and the barrier between the systemic circulation and this compartment is the GI tract wall. The amount of drug declines in the GI tract by diffusion through the wall into the systemic circulation. Other parallel processes, such as GI metabolism by enzymes like CYP3A4 (Chapter 3, Section 3.2.1.7), or degradation at low or

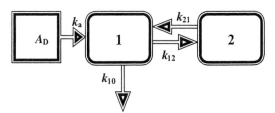

FIGURE 13.1 Diagram of a two-compartment model with first-order absorption and first-order elimination. A_D represents the amount of drug at the site of absorption; compartment 1 is the central compartment; compartment 2 is the peripheral compartment; k_a is the first-order absorption rate constant; k_{12} and k_{21} are the distribution rate constants; and k_{10} is the overall elimination rate constant.

high pH of the GI tract, or adsorption to food particles, may also remove the drug concurrently from this compartment. The amount of drug that permeates the membrane of the wall may be pumped back into the GI tract by P-glycoprotein or, after permeation, can be subjected to hepatic first-pass metabolism. The equations of the model represent the overall outcome and combined effect of all processes involved. The rate equations are:

$$\frac{dA_D}{dt} = -k_a A_D \tag{13.1}$$

$$\frac{dA_1}{dt} = k_a A_D + k_{21} A_2 - k_{12} A_1 - k_{10} A_1 \tag{13.2}$$

$$\frac{dA_2}{dt} = k_{12} A_1 - k_{21} A_2 \tag{13.3}$$

The input function of the model is Equation 1.42 (Chapter 1):

$$\text{input} = \frac{k_a FD}{s + k_a}$$

The disposition function of the central compartment using Equation 1.43 (Chapter 1) yields the general form of the disposition function of a two-compartment model:

$$(\text{Disp})_{s1} = \frac{s + E_2}{(s + E_1)(s + E_2) - k_{12}k_{21}} = \frac{s + k_{21}}{s^2 + s(k_{21} + k_{10} + k_{12}) + k_{21}k_{10}} = \frac{s + E_2}{(s + \alpha)(s + \beta)}$$

where E_1 is the sum of the exit rate constants of the central compartment, E_2 is the sum of the exit rate constants of the peripheral compartment, and the quadratic form of the denominator is expressed as $(s + \alpha)(s + \beta)$. Multiplying the input by the disposition function yields the Laplace transform of the central compartment:

$$\mathcal{L}(A_1) = \frac{k_a FD(s + k_{21})}{(s + k_a)(s + \alpha)(s + \beta)} \tag{13.4}$$

By use of the method of partial fractions (Chapter 1, Section 1.13.3) or the table of Laplace transforms (Chapter 1, Table 1.9 Equation 21), Equation 13.4 can be integrated to define the amount in the central compartment as a function of time:

$$A_1 = \frac{k_a FD(k_{21} - k_a)}{(\alpha - k_a)(\beta - k_a)} e^{-k_a t} + \frac{k_a FD(k_{21} - \alpha)}{(k_a - \alpha)(\beta - \alpha)} e^{-\alpha t} + \frac{k_a FD(k_{21} - \beta)}{(k_a - \beta)(\alpha - \beta)} e^{-\beta t} \tag{13.5}$$

where F is the absolute bioavailability, D is the administered dose, k_a is the first-order absorption rate constant, k_{21} is the first-order distribution rate constant from the peripheral compartment to the central compartment, and α and β are the first-order hybrid rate constants estimated from the slopes of the distributive and postdistributive phases. Dividing Equation 13.5 by the apparent volume of distribution of the central compartment yields

$$C_p = \underbrace{\frac{k_a FD(k_{21} - k_a)}{V_1(\alpha - k_a)(\beta - k_a)}}_{c^*} e^{-k_a t} + \underbrace{\frac{k_a FD(k_{21} - \alpha)}{V_1(k_a - \alpha)(\beta - \alpha)}}_{a^*} e^{-\alpha t} + \underbrace{\frac{k_a FD(k_{21} - \beta)}{V_1(k_a - \beta)(\alpha - \beta)}}_{b^*} e^{-\beta t} \qquad (13.6)$$

which, by denoting the coefficients of exponential terms as a^*, b^*, and c^*, is further simplified to

$$C_p = a^* e^{-\alpha t} + b^* e^{-\beta t} + c^* e^{-k_a t} \qquad (13.7)$$

13.3 INFLUENCE OF THE RATE CONSTANTS OF THE MODEL ON THE PLASMA CONCENTRATION–TIME CURVE

Depending on the frequency of plasma sampling and the relationship between α and k_a, the plot of log plasma concentration versus time of an orally administered drug that follows a two-compartment model may exhibit a typical maximum peak or distributional nose (Figure 13.2). Therefore, a preliminary plot of log C_p against time may help to identify the two-compartmental characteristics of a drug and differentiate it from a one-compartment model.

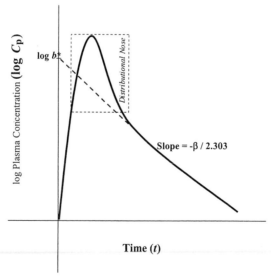

FIGURE 13.2 Typical plasma concentration–time profile of an orally administered drug that exhibits two-compartment model characteristics.

Analysis of the C_p–t curve is not as simple and straightforward as for the one-compartment model. For example, the only definite assumption that can be made about Figure 13.2 or Equation 13.7 is that β, the slower first-order rate constant of disposition, is smaller than α and k_a. Thus, it can be estimated from the slope of the linear terminal portion of the curve. Extrapolation of the linear segment then provides the y intercept b^*. Theoretically we should be able to estimate the other two rate constants, α (the fast disposition rate constant) and k_a (the absorption rate constant), from the residuals of the curve and the extrapolated line. The problem, however, is that without knowing the magnitude of α it would be impossible to determine which of the two rate constants is the fastest. The equation of the first residual curve is determined by subtraction of the equation of the β phase from Equation 13.7:

$$(C_p - \overleftarrow{C}_p) = (a^*e^{-\alpha t} + b^*e^{-\beta t} + c^*e^{-k_a t}) - (b^*e^{-\beta t})$$

$$(C_p - \overleftarrow{C}_p) = a^*e^{-\alpha t} + c^*e^{-k_a t} \qquad (13.8)$$

Hence, the first residual concentrations are the positive values of $C_p - \overleftarrow{C}_p$, which when plotted as $\log(C_p - \overleftarrow{C}_p)$ versus time exhibit a profile similar to that in Figure 13.3. The positive values of $C_p - \overleftarrow{C}_p$ are the residuals of the distributional nose.

This first bell-shaped residual curve will have a linear terminal portion with a slope equal to $-\alpha/2.303$ (if $\alpha < k_a$) or $-k_a/2.303$ (if $\alpha > k_a$). The y intercept of the line is either a^* or c^*, depending on which rate constant is smaller. Having this first residual curve

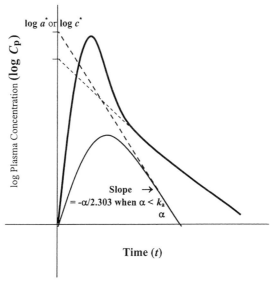

FIGURE 13.3 A plot of positive residuals of Equation 13.8 versus time may produce a residual curve with a linear terminal portion that has a slope of one of the remaining rate constants divided by 2.303 and a y intercept equal to one of the remaining coefficients a^* or c^*.

with the linear terminal portion will allow us to determine a second set of residual concentrations that can be calculated by subtracting the equation of the linear extrapolated segment of the first residual curve from Equation 13.8.

That is, when $\alpha < k_a$,

$$[(C_p - \tilde{C}_p) - \bar{\bar{C}}_p] = (a^*e^{-\alpha t} + c^*e^{k_a t}) - a^*e^{-\alpha t} = c^*e^{-k_a t} \qquad (13.9)$$

When $\alpha > k_a$,

$$[(C_p - \tilde{C}_p) - \bar{\bar{C}}_p] = (a^*e^{-\alpha t} + c^*e^{k_a t}) - c^*e^{-k_a t} = a^*e^{-\alpha t} \qquad (13.10)$$

Therefore, the slope of the line of the second residual would be either $-\alpha/2.303$ or $-k_a/2.303$ depending on which rate constant is the largest. The y intercept of the line is the coefficient associated with the largest rate constant (Figure 13.4).

When α and k_a have very similar values ($\alpha \cong k_a$) the plasma concentration–time curve behaves as if the drug follows a one-compartment model with first-order input. As the compartmental analysis in general is based on the principles of curve fitting, the selection of the appropriate model, one- versus two-compartment, should be determined based on the criteria of curve fitting such as Akaike and/or Schwartz criteria.

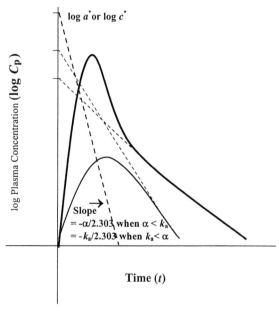

FIGURE 13.4 A plot of the second residual concentrations versus time is a straight line with a slope equal to $-\alpha/2.303$ and y intercept of a^* when $\alpha < k_a$, or slope of $-k_a/2.303$ and y intercept of c^* when $\alpha > k_a$.

13.4 PARAMETERS AND CONSTANTS OF THE MODEL

13.4.1 Initial Plasma Concentration

By setting $t = 0$ in Equation 13.7 the exponential terms $e^{-\alpha t}$, $e^{-\beta t}$, and $e^{-k_a t}$ become equal to one and the initial plasma concentration can be defined as

$$C_p^0 = a^* + b^* + c^* \tag{13.11}$$

13.4.2 Area under Plasma Concentration–Time Curve

Integration of Equation 13.7 yields the following relationship for the area under the plasma concentration–time curve:

$$\mathrm{AUC}_0^\infty = \frac{a^*}{\alpha} + \frac{b^*}{\beta} + \frac{c^*}{k_a} \tag{13.12}$$

Equation 13.12 can be expanded by substituting the equations of a^*, b^*, and c^* from Equation 13.6:

$$\mathrm{AUC}_0^\infty = \frac{k_a FD(k_{21} - \alpha)}{\alpha V_1(k_a - \alpha)(\beta - \alpha)} + \frac{k_a FD(k_{21} - \beta)}{\beta V_1(k_a - \beta)(\alpha - \beta)} + \frac{k_a FD(k_{21} - k_a)}{k_a V_1(\alpha - k_a)(\beta - k_a)}$$

Therefore,

$$\mathrm{AUC}_0^\infty = \frac{k_a FD}{k_a V_1 \alpha \beta} \left[\frac{\alpha\beta(k_{21} - k_a)(\alpha - \beta) + k_a\beta(k_{21} - \alpha)(\beta - k_a) - k_a\alpha(k_{21} - \beta)(\alpha - k_a)}{(\alpha - k_a)(\beta - k_a)(\alpha - \beta)} \right]$$

$$\mathrm{AUC}_0^\infty = \frac{FD}{V_1 \alpha \beta} \left[\frac{k_{21}(k_a^2\alpha - \alpha^2 k_a - \alpha\beta^2 + \alpha^2\beta + k_a\beta^2 - k_a^2\beta)}{(k_a^2\alpha - \alpha^2 k_a - \alpha\beta^2 + \alpha^2\beta + k_a\beta^2 - k_a^2\beta)} \right] = \frac{FDk_{21}}{V_1 \alpha \beta}$$

Because for the two-compartment model $\alpha \times \beta = k_{21}k_{10}$,

$$\mathrm{AUC}_0^\infty = \frac{FD}{V_1 k_{10}} = \frac{FD}{\mathrm{Cl_t}} = \frac{FD}{V_{d_\beta}\beta} \tag{13.13}$$

The trapezoidal rule is also the method of choice in determining the area under the curve from 0 to ∞ and from 0 to t. In estimation of AUC_0^∞ by the trapezoidal rule the terminal area is determined by dividing the last plasma concentration by β.

13.4.3 Apparent Volumes of Distribution

The overall volume of distribution, $V_{d\beta}$, and the volume of the central compartment are determined from Equation 13.13:

$$V_{d\beta} = \frac{FD}{\beta \times \text{AUC}_0^\infty} \tag{13.14}$$

$$V_1 = \frac{FD}{k_{10} \times \text{AUC}_0^\infty} \tag{13.15}$$

13.4.4 Total Amount Eliminated between Times 0 and t and between Times 0 and ∞

The differential equation defining the total amount of drug eliminated from the body is

$$\frac{dA_{el}}{dt} = k_{10}A_1 \tag{13.16}$$

Integration of Equation 13.16 between 0 and t gives

$$A_{el} = \int_0^t k_{10}A_1 dt = k_{10}V_1 \int_0^t C_p dt \tag{13.17}$$

Therefore, the total amount eliminated between 0 and t is

$$A_{el} = k_{10}V_1 \text{AUC}_0^t = \text{Cl}_t \text{AUC}_0^t \tag{13.18}$$

When t approaches infinity, $A_{el} = FD$, which is the same as Equation 13.15; that is, the total amount eliminated between 0 and ∞ is equal to the total amount absorbed:

$$FD = k_{10}V_1 \text{AUC}_0^\infty = \text{Cl}_t \text{AUC}_0^\infty \tag{13.19}$$

Therefore, the total amount excreted unchanged between 0 and t and between 0 and ∞ can be estimated according to the equations

$$A_e = f_e(k_{10}V_1 \text{AUC}_0^t) = \text{Cl}_r \times \text{AUC}_0^t \tag{13.20}$$

$$A_e^\infty = f_e(k_{10}V_1 \text{AUC}_0^\infty) = \text{Cl}_r \times \text{AUC}_0^\infty = f_e FD \tag{13.21}$$

The fractions of dose excreted unchanged and eliminated as metabolites are given

$$f_e = \frac{A_e^\infty}{FD} \tag{13.22}$$

$$f_m = \frac{FD - A_e^\infty}{FD} \tag{13.23}$$

The total amount of drug eliminated as metabolites can be estimated as

$$A_m = f_m(k_{10}V_1 \text{AUC}_0^t) = \text{Cl}_m \times \text{AUC}_0^t \qquad (13.24)$$

$$A_m^\infty = f_m(k_{10}V_1 \text{AUC}_0^\infty) = \text{Cl}_m \times \text{AUC}_0^\infty = f_m FD \qquad (13.25)$$

13.4.5 Estimation of Distribution and Elimination Rate Constants

The elimination rate constant, k_{10}, is determined according to Equations 11.22, and the rate constants of distribution, k_{12} and k_{21}, are determined according to Equations 11.17, 11.18, and 11.23 (Chapter 11).

13.4.6 Estimation of First-order Absorption Rate Constant: Loo–Riegelman Method

This method is based on the mass balance equation of the amount or concentration of a drug between the site of absorption, the central and peripheral compartments, and the total amount eliminated from the body. The method requires a prior knowledge of the distribution rate constants, k_{12} and k_{21}, and also the overall elimination rate constant, k_{10}. These rate constants are usually determined following intravenous injection of the drug. Application of the method requires a good understanding of the principles and assumptions of the equations. There are some similarities between this method and the Wagner–Nelson method (Chapter 8, Section 8.5.2.4). Both methods are popular in determining the first-order absorption rate constant and are included in various commercially available pharmacokinetic software. The Wagner–Nelson method is favored for one-compartment models, whereas the Loo–Riegelman method is preferred for two-compartment models.

To develop the equations of the Loo–Riegelman method we start with the mass balance equation at time t:

$$A_{\text{total}} = A_1 + A_2 + A_{\text{el}} \qquad (13.26)$$

where A_{total} is the total amount of drug absorbed; A_1 is the amount in the central compartment; A_2 is the amount in the peripheral compartment; and A_{el} is the amount eliminated.

The total amounts of drug eliminated at times t and ∞ according to Equations 13.18 and 13.19 are

$$A_{\text{el}} = k_{10}V_1 \text{AUC}_0^t$$

$$A_{\text{el}}^\infty = k_{10}V_1 \text{AUC}_0^\infty = FD$$

Therefore, the percentage of the total amount of drug absorbed is

$$\left(\frac{A_{\text{total}}}{FD} \right) \times 100 = \%A_1 + \%A_2 + \left[\frac{k_{10}V_1 \text{AUC}_0^t}{k_{10}V_1 \text{AUC}_0^{\infty t}} \right] \times 100 \qquad (13.27)$$

In Equation 13.27 the amount eliminated from the body, A_{el}, is expressed in terms of the volume of the central compartment and the area under the plasma concentration–time curve from 0 to t and from 0 to ∞. As was mentioned earlier, prior knowledge of k_{10} is also required.

The second term of the equation is the amount of drug in the peripheral compartment, which for the orally administered dose is unknown. By using the following equations and methodology we can express the amount in the peripheral compartment in terms of the amount of drug in the central compartment, which is the sampling compartment. Assume we are considering only the change in the amount of drug between two adjacent time points, t_n and t_{n-1} (ie, $t_n - t_{n-1} = \Delta t$). Therefore, the amount in the body at t_n is

$$(A_1)_n = (A_1)_{n-1} + \left(\frac{\Delta A_1}{\Delta t}\right)(\Delta t) \tag{13.28}$$

The rate of change in the amount of drug in the peripheral compartment is the same as described in Chapter 11, Equation 11.2:

$$\frac{dA_2}{dt} = k_{12}A_1 - k_{21}A_2$$

Substituting Equation 13.28 for A_1 in the above equation yields

$$\frac{(dA_2)_{t_n}}{dt} = k_{12}\left[(A_1)_{t_{n-1}} + \frac{\Delta A_1}{\Delta t}(\Delta t)\right] - k_{21}A_2 \tag{13.29}$$

$$\frac{(dA_2)_{t_n}}{dt} = k_{12}(A_1)_{t_{n-1}} + k_{12}\left[\frac{\Delta A_1}{\Delta t}\right]\Delta t - k_{21}A_2 \tag{13.30}$$

By using the Laplace transform and recalling the following relationships from Chapter 1, Table 1.9, we integrate Equation 13.30:

$$\mathscr{L}(1) = 1/s$$

$$\mathscr{L}(t) = 1/s^2$$

$$\mathscr{L}(A_1) = \overline{A}_1$$

$$\mathscr{L}(A_2) = \overline{A}_2$$

$$\mathscr{L}\left(\frac{dA_2}{dt}\right) = s(\overline{A}_2) - (\overline{A}_2)_{t_{n-1}}$$

$(\overline{A})_{t_{n-1}}$ is considered the initial condition of the interval Δt. Therefore, the Laplace transform of Equation 13.30 is

$$s(\overline{A}_2)_{t_n} - (\overline{A}_2)_{t_{n-1}} = \frac{k_{12}(\overline{A}_1)_{t_{n-1}}}{s} + \frac{k_{12}(\Delta A_1/\Delta t)\Delta t}{s^2} - k_{21}(\overline{A}_2)_{t_n} \tag{13.31}$$

Rearranging Equation 13.31 to solve for $(\overline{A_2})_{t_n}$ yields

$$(\overline{A_2})_{t_n} = \frac{(\overline{A_2})_{t_{n-1}}}{s + k_{21}} + \frac{k_{12}(\overline{A_1})_{t_{n-1}}}{s(s + k_{21})} + \frac{k_{12}(\Delta A_1/\Delta t)\Delta t}{s^2(s + k_{21})} \tag{13.32}$$

The inverse Laplace transform of Equation 13.32 is

$$(A_2)_{t_n} = \underbrace{(A_2)_{t_{n-1}}e^{-k_{21}\Delta t}}_{\text{1st term}} + \underbrace{\frac{k_{12}}{k_{21}}(A_1)_{t_{n-1}}[1 - e^{-k_{21}\Delta t}]}_{\text{2nd term}} + \underbrace{\frac{k_{12}}{k_{21}}\Delta A_1 - \frac{k_{12}}{k_{21}^2} \times \frac{\Delta A_1}{\Delta t}[1 - e^{-k_{21}\Delta t}]}_{\text{3rd term}}$$

$$\tag{13.33}$$

To simplify Equation 13.33 Taylor series expansion is applied to the exponential function of the third term:

$$e^{-k_{21}\Delta t} \cong 1 - k_{21}\Delta t + \frac{k_{21}^2(\Delta t)^2}{2} \tag{13.34}$$

Substituting Equation 13.34 for the third term of Equation 13.33 yields

$$(A_2)_{t_n} = \underbrace{(A_2)_{t_{n-1}}e^{-k_{21}\Delta t}}_{\text{1st term}} + \underbrace{\frac{k_{12}}{k_{21}}(A_1)_{t_{n-1}}[1 - e^{-k_{21}\Delta t}]}_{\text{2nd term}} + \underbrace{\frac{k_{12}}{k_{21}}\Delta A_1 - \frac{k_{12}}{k_{21}} \times \frac{\Delta A_1}{\Delta t}\left[1 - k_{21}\Delta t + \frac{k_{21}^2(\Delta t)^2}{2}\right]}_{\text{3rd term}}$$

$$\tag{13.35}$$

Further simplification of the third term of Equation 13.35 yields the following relationship which represents the $(A_2)_{t_n}$ term in Equations 13.26 and 13.27:

$$(A_2)_{t_n} = (A_2)_{t_{n-1}}e^{-k_{21}\Delta t} + \frac{k_{12}}{k_{21}}(A_1)_{t_{n-1}}[1 - e^{-k_{21}\Delta t}] + \frac{k_{12}}{2}\Delta A_1\Delta t \tag{13.36}$$

Therefore,

$$A_{\text{total}} = \underbrace{(A_1)_{t_n}}_{A_1} + \underbrace{(A_2)_{t_{n-1}} + \frac{k_{12}}{k_{21}}(A_1)_{t_{n-1}}[1 - e^{-k_{21}\Delta t}] + \frac{k_{12}}{2}\Delta A_1\Delta t}_{A_2} + \underbrace{k_{10}V_1\text{AUC}_0^t}_{A_{\text{el}}} \tag{13.37}$$

By dividing Equation 13.37 by the volume of the central compartment we obtain the following equation in terms of the concentration of free drug:

$$C_{\text{total}} = (C_p)_{t_n} + (C_2)_{t_{n-1}} + \frac{k_{12}}{k_{21}}(C_p)_{t_{n-1}}[1 - e^{-k_{21}\Delta t}] + \frac{k_{12}}{2}\Delta C_{p_1}\Delta t + k_{10}\text{AUC}_0^t \tag{13.38}$$

The advantage of Equation 13.38 is that the terms on the right-hand side of the equal sign, except $(C_2)_{t_{n-1}}$, are expressed in terms of the concentration of drug in plasma. The term $(C_2)_{t_{n-1}}$ can be estimated by the following equation which is the same as equation 13.36 except that it is expressed in terms of concentration of the second compartment. The starting point for calculation of the concentration of the second compartment is $(C_2)_{t_{n-1}} = 0$:

$$(C_2)_{t_n} = (C_2)_{t_{n-1}} e^{-k_{21}\Delta t} + \frac{k_{12}}{k_{21}} (C_p)_{t_{n-1}}[1 - e^{-k_{21}\Delta t}] + \frac{k_{12}}{2} \Delta C_p \Delta t \qquad (13.39)$$

Now with the help of Equations 13.37 and 13.38, we can expand Equation 13.27 to express "% absorbed" (ie, $(A_{total}/FD) \times 100$):

$$\frac{A_{total}}{FD} \times 100 = \%(A_1)_{t_n} + \%\left[(A_2)_{t_{n-1}} + \frac{k_{12}}{k_{21}} (A_1)_{t_{n-1}}[1 - e^{-k_{21}\Delta t}] + \frac{k_{12}}{2} \Delta A_1 \Delta t \right]$$

$$+ \frac{k_{10}V_1 AUC_0^t}{k_{10}V_1 AUC_0^\infty} \times 100 \quad (13.40)$$

The last step of this method is to plot the logarithm of percentage remaining to be absorbed, which is $\log[100 - ((A_{total}/FD) \times 100)]$, against time. This plot should be linear with a slope of $-k_a/2.303$.

APPLICATION

13.1 A new drug was administered intravenously and orally in a crossover design to a group of volunteers. Blood samples were collected at different intervals; the plasma portion was separated, extracted with ethyl acetate, evaporated under nitrogen, reconstituted in methanol, and analyzed by HPLC to determine the concentration of the drug. Pharmacokinetic analysis of the intravenous data provided the following values for α and β: ($\alpha = 3.04$ h^{-1} and $\beta = 0.70$ h^{-1}). The oral data were also analyzed according to a two-compartment model. The predicted plasma concentrations for oral absorption are reported in Table 13.1.

Estimate the first and second residual concentrations of the oral dose and determine α, β, and k_a.

1. First residual concentrations: Regression analysis of the last four data points of log plasma concentration versus time gives the slope of the first extrapolated line, 0.0056 min^{-1}; therefore,

$$\beta = 2.303 \times 0.0056 = 0.0129 \ min^{-1} = 0.774 \ h^{-1}$$

The calculations of the first residual curve are presented in Table 13.2.

Regression analysis of the second extrapolated line estimated from the last four data points gives a slope of 0.0235 min^{-1}; therefore,

$$\alpha = 2.303 \times 0.0235 = 0.0541 \ min^{-1} = 3.247 \ h^{-1}$$

The calculations of the second residual curve are presented in Table 13.3.

TABLE 13.1 Data Related to Application 13.1

Time (h)	Predicted Concentration of Drug in Plasma, C_p (mg/L)	Logarithm of C_p
10	6.0	0.77815
25	40.5	1.60746
40	110.0	2.04139
55	220.0	2.34242
70	300.0	2.47712
100	350.0	2.54407
125	300.0	2.47712
140	250.0	2.39794
155	160.0	2.20412
175	70.0	1.84510
200	30.0	1.47712
225	19.0	1.27875
270	10.0	1.00000
300	6.8	0.83251
350	3.8	0.57978

The slope of the regression line of the second residual concentrations is 0.0276 min^{-1}; therefore,

$$k_a = 0.0276 \times 2.303 = 0.0635 \text{ min}^{-1} = 3.814 \text{ h}^{-1}$$

13.2 Plasma concentration of a drug at different time points was measured in a group of volunteers following oral and IV administration of 1 g in a crossover design. The data are

TABLE 13.2 Calculations of the First Residual Curve: Application 13.1

Time (min)	$\tilde{C}_p$	$C_p - \tilde{C}_p$	Time (min)	First Residual Concentration	Log First Residual Concentration
10	291.743	−285.743	70	56.695	1.75354
25	240.436	−199.936	100	165.414	2.21857
40	198.153	−88.153	125	258.589	2.41261
55	163.305	56.695	140	233.778	2.36880
70	134.586	165.414	155	195.424	2.29098
100	91.411	258.589	175	115.022	2.06078
125	66.222	233.778	200	35.246	1.54711
140	54.576	195.424	225	4.823	0.68334
155	44.978	115.022	270	0.761	−0.11859
175	34.754	35.246			
200	25.177	4.823			
225	18.238	0.761			

TABLE 13.3 Calculations of the Second Residual Line

Time (min)	Log 2nd Extrap. Concn	2nd Extrap. Concn	1st Resid. Concn	2nd Resid. Concn	Log 2nd Resid. Concn
70	4.5100	32359.4	56.695	32302.7	4.50924
100	3.8050	6382.6	165.414	6217.2	3.79360
125	3.2175	1650.1	258.589	1391.5	3.14347
140	2.8650	732.8	233.778	499.0	2.69814
155	2.5125	325.5	195.424	130.0	2.11407

reported in Table 13.4. The following biexponential equation was fitted to the intravenous data:

$$C_p = 120e^{-4.145t} + 91.41e^{-0.4145t}$$

Determine the absorption rate constant by using the Loo–Riegelman method. The calculations involve the use of k_{12}, k_{21}, and k_{10} and the following general equations:

$$k_{21} = [(120 \times 0.4145) + (91.41 \times 4.145)]/(120 + 91.41) = 2.0275 \ \text{h}^{-1}$$

$$k_{10} = 1.7181/2.0275 = 0.8474 \ \text{h}^{-1}$$

$$k_{12} = 0.4145 + 4.145 - 2.0275 - 0.8474 = 1.6846 \ \text{h}^{-1}$$

$$C_{\text{total}} = (C_p)_{t_n} + (C_2)_{t_{n-1}} + \frac{k_{12}}{k_{21}}(C_p)_{t_{n-1}}[1 - e^{-k_{21}\Delta t}] + \frac{k_{12}}{2}\Delta C_{p_1}\Delta t + k_{10}\text{AUC}_0^{t_n}$$

$$(C_2)_{t_n} = (C_2)_{t_{n-1}}e^{-k_{21}\Delta t} + \frac{k_{12}}{k_{21}}(C_p)_{t_{n-1}}[1 - e^{-k_{21}\Delta t}] + \frac{k_{12}}{2}\Delta C_p\Delta t$$

TABLE 13.4 Data Related to Application 13.2

Time (h)	C_p (mg/L) Oral	C_p (mg/L) IV
0.10	1.000	166.979
0.20	12.000	136.516
0.30	28.000	115.326
0.40	46.000	100.306
0.60	56.000	81.262
0.75	59.700	72.345
1.00	60.000	62.293
2.00	40.000	39.929
3.00	26.200	26.361
4.00	17.500	17.415
5.00	11.500	11.506
6.00	7.580	7.602
10.00	1.400	1.448
14.00	0.268	0.276

TABLE 13.5 Calculations of Absorption Rate Constant of Application 13.2 Using Loo–Riegelman Method: Part 1

t_n	t_{n-1}	Δt	$(C_p)_{t_n}$	$(C_p)_{t_{n-1}}$	ΔC_p	$\dfrac{k_{12}}{2}\,\Delta C_p\,\Delta t$	$\dfrac{k_{12}}{k_{21}}\,(C_p)_{t_{n-1}}\,[1-e^{-k_{21}\Delta t}]$
0.10	0.0	0.10	1.000	0	1.000	0.0842	0.0000
0.20	0.10	0.10	12.000	1.000	11.000	0.9265	0.1525
0.30	0.10	0.10	28.000	12.000	16.000	1.3477	1.8298
0.40	0.10	0.10	46.000	28.000	18.000	1.5161	4.2694
0.60	0.10	0.20	56.000	46.000	10.000	1.6846	12.7410
0.75	0.20	0.15	59.700	56.000	3.700	0.4675	12.2014
1.00	0.15	0.25	60.000	59.700	0.300	0.0632	19.7235
2.00	0.25	1.00	40.000	60.000	−20.000	−16.8460	43.2887
3.00	1.00	1.00	26.200	40.000	−13.800	−11.6237	28.8592
4.00	1.00	1.00	17.500	26.200	−8.700	−7.3280	18.9027
5.00	1.00	1.00	11.500	17.500	−6.000	−5.0538	12.6259
6.00	1.00	1.00	7.580	11.500	−3.920	−3.3018	8.2970
10.00	1.00	4.00	1.400	7.580	−6.180	−20.8217	6.2961
14.00	4.00	4.00	0.268	1.400	−1.132	−3.8139	1.1629

279

TABLE 13.6 Calculations of Absorption Rate Constant of Application 13.2 Using Loo–Riegelman Method: Part 2

$(C_2)_{t_{n-1}}e^{-k_{21}\Delta t}$	$(C_2)_{t_n}$	$AUC_{t_{n-1}}^{t_n}$	$AUC_0^{t_n}$	$k_{10} \times AUC_0^{t_n}$	C_{total}
0	0.0842	0.050	0.050	0.042	1.127
0.0687	1.1477	0.650	0.700	0.593	13.741
0.9370	4.1145	2.000	2.700	2.288	34.402
3.3594	9.1449	3.700	6.400	5.423	60.568
7.4667	21.8923	10.200	16.600	14.067	91.959
14.5943	27.2632	8.677	25.277	21.420	108.383
20.1139	39.9006	14.962	40.239	34.099	133.999
24.0351	50.4778	50.000	90.239	76.469	166.946
6.6461	23.8816	33.100	123.339	104.517	154.599
3.1443	14.7190	21.850	145.189	123.033	155.252
1.9379	9.5100	14.500	159.689	135.320	156.330
1.2521	6.2473	9.540	169.229	143.405	157.232
0.8225	−13.7031	17.960	187.189	158.624	146.321
−4.1180	−6.7690	3.336	190.525	161.451	154.950

Average = 156

The stepwise calculations of the rate constant are presented in three parts in Tables 13.5, 13.6, and 13.7. The slope of $\log(100 - \%(A_{total}/FD)$ versus time $= -0.94 = -k_a/2.303$. Therefore, $k_a = 0.94 \times 2.303 = 2.165 \ h^{-1}$.

ASSIGNMENT (EXTRA CREDIT)
EC-13.1 Based on the following articles discuss the differences between the Wagner–Nelson method (Chapter 8) and the Loo–Riegelman method (Chapter 13) for calculation of absorption rate constants of drugs that follow a two-compartment model.

TABLE 13.7 Calculations of Absorption Rate Constant of Application 13.2 Using Loo–Riegelman Method: Part 3

$\dfrac{A_{total}}{FD} \times 100$	$100 - \% \dfrac{A_{total}}{FD}$	$\log\left(100 - \% \dfrac{A_{total}}{FD}\right)$
0.722	99.278	1.99685
8.808	91.192	1.95996
22.053	77.947	1.89180
38.826	61.174	1.78657
58.948	41.052	1.61333
69.476	30.524	1.48464
85.897	14.103	1.14931
107.017		
99.102		
99.521		
100.212		
100.790		
93.795		
99.327		

I. Loo JCK, Riegelman S. New method for calculating the intrinsic absorption rate of drugs. *J Pharm Sci* 1968;57:918–28.

II. Wagner JG. Application of the Wagner–Nelson absorption method to the two-compartment open model. *J Pharmacokinet Biopharm* 1974;2:469–86.

Include in your discussion the difference between $k_{10}\text{AUC}_0^{t_n}$ and $\beta \times \text{AUC}_0^{t_n}$ in calculation of k_a by the Loo–Riegelman method.

■ Repeat the calculations of reference I using the same plasma concentration and time points, assuming $\alpha = 1.37$ h^{-1}.

■ Using the following article discuss the influence of distribution and overall elimination rate constants on the calculations of absorption rate constant by the Loo–Riegelman method.

III. Zeng YL, Akkermans AAMD, Breimer DD. Factors affecting the error in the Loo–Riegelman method for estimating the rate of drug absorption. *Arzneimittel-Forschung* 1983;33:757–60.

EC-13.2 Read the following article and answer the questions for this assignment:

Katashima M, Yamada Y, Yamamoto K, Kotaki H, Sato H, Swada Y, Iga T. Analysis of antiplatelet effect of ticlopidine in humans: modeling based on irreversible inhibition of platelet precursors in bone marrow. *J Pharmacokinet Biopharm* 1999;27:283–96.

■ Discuss the pharmacodynamic parameter measured in the article.

■ What type of kinetics, zero- or first-order, is assumed for the biosynthesis rate of platelet precursor and the formation of platelets from platelet precursors in the blood?

■ Write the two-compartment pharmacokinetic equation of ticlopidine in terms of the estimated rate constants and parameters of the study.

■ Explain the hypothesis of the investigators for the long half-life of ticlopidine ($\approx$100 h) in a multiple-dosing regimen.

EC-13.3 Based on the data presented by Sharma et al, answer the questions for this assignment.

Sharma A, Slugg PH, Hammett JL, Jusko WJ. Estimation of oral bioavailability of a long half-life drug in healthy subjects. *Pharm Res* 1998;15:1782–6.

■ Do you consider the amounts of BMS-187745 and BMS-188494 eliminated during 30 minutes of infusion significant? Why?

■ Interpret the F values for patient 8.

■ How long would it take for either drug to be fully eliminated from the body?

■ Does the protein precipitation by methanol release the protein-bound drug and increase the concentration of free drug?

■ Explain why the plasma concentrations of both compounds increased following oral administration and then declined sharply to a lower level (Figure 2 of the article).

■ What are the possible reasons for the low apparent volume of distribution?

BIBLIOGRAPHY

1. Wagner JG. Application of the Wagner–Nelson absorption method to the two-compartment model. *J Pharmacokinet Biopharm* 1974;2:469.

2. Loo JCK, Riegelman S. New method for calculating the intrinsic absorption rate of drugs. *J Pharm Sci* 1968;57:918.

3. Wagner JG. Pharmacokinetic absorption plots from oral data or oral/intravenous data and an exact Loo–Riegelman equation. *J Pharm Sci* 1983;72:838.

4. Boxenbaum HG, Kaplan SA. Potential source of error in absorption rate calculations. *J Pharmacokinet Biopharm* 1975;3:257.

5. Ronfeld RA, Benet LZ. Interpretation of plasma concentration–time curves after oral dosing. *J Pharm Sci* 1977;66:178.

6. Curry SH. Theoretical considerations in calculation of terminal phase half times following oral doses: illustrated with model data. *Biopharm Drug Dispos* 1981;21:115.

7. Till AE, Benet LZ, Kwan KC. An integrated approach to the pharmacokinetic analysis of drug absorption. *J Pharmacokinet Biopharm* 1974;2:525.

8. Gerardin A, Wantiez D, Jaouen A. An incremental method for the study of the absorption of drug whose kinetics are described by a two-compartment model: Estimation of the microscopic rate constants. *J Pharmacokinet Biopharm* 1983;11:401.

CHAPTER 14

GENERAL APPROACHES TO DOSAGE ADJUSTMENT FOR PATIENTS WITH RENAL FAILURE

If you fixed them in your strong intelligence and gaze upon them propitiously with pure attention, these things will all be very much present to you all your life long and from them you will obtain many others. For these very things grow into each kind of character, depending on each person's nature.

HIPPOLYTUS (REFUTATION)

OBJECTIVES

■ To discuss general methodologies for adjusting the normal dosing regimen for patients with renal failure.

■ To estimate glomerular filtration rate based on endogenous and exogenous markers.

■ To discuss creatinine as a biomarker of renal impairment.

■ To review various relationships between serum creatinine and creatinine clearance.

■ To discuss the general pharmacokinetic equations for the adjustment of dosing regimens.

14.1 INTRODUCTION

Renal excretion is the major route of elimination of end products of protein metabolism such as urea, uric acid, and creatinine and wastes such as phenols and sulfates. It is also an important pathway for elimination of drugs and their water-soluble metabolites. In addition, renal excretion plays other important roles such as regulation of acid–base balance and control of body fluids that are secondary to the objectives of this chapter.

The excretory unit of the kidneys, the nephron, consists of segments: Bowman's capsule, the proximal tubule, Henle's loop, the distal tubule, the collecting duct, and finally the ducts of Bellini (Chapter 5, Figure 5.1). The cluster of arterial capillaries, which is engulfed by Bowman's capsule, is known as the glomerulus. The walls of these capillaries are more permeable than those of the capillaries in the body. There are about 1 million nephrons in both kidneys. The blood flow to both kidneys is approximately 1.2 L/min. The filtrate resulting from this flow, as was mentioned in Chapter 5, is roughly 125 mL/min or 180 L/d (ie, 125 mL/min × 60 min/h × 24 h × 1 L/1000 mL = 180 L/d). This rate is known as glomerular filtration rate. In renal impairment, because of the reduction of diffusion to or from different regions of nephrons, the volume of filtrate and the amount of solutes, endogenous or exogenous, are reduced significantly. This inability of the kidneys to remove the drugs and their metabolites significantly increases the accumulation of drug metabolites in the body, the area under the plasma concentration–time curve, and the likelihood of toxicity. In this pathologic condition the pharmacokinetic profile of any compound in the body, which for elimination relies on the kidney, is altered significantly. Thus, dosing regimens for drugs that are recommended for individuals with normal renal function are not appropriate for patients with renal failure and modified dosing regimens must be designed for these patients.

14.2 ADJUSTMENT OF DOSING REGIMEN

The major concern in the management of drug therapy of patients with renal failure is with drugs given on a continuous basis for the purpose of achieving a consistent therapeutic outcome. Therefore, the adjustment is mostly for intravenous infusion and multiple-dosing administration. As was discussed in Chapter 10 (Section 10.4), if the half-life of a drug increases because of renal failure, the steady-state plasma level increases and may surpass the maximum effective concentration of the therapeutic range (Figure 14.1). Therefore, the objective of dosage adjustment for these patients is to achieve plasma concentrations of free drug (eg, $(C_{pss})_{infusion}$, $(C_{pave})_{ss}$, $(C_{pmin})_{ss}$, and $(C_{pmax})_{ss}$) comparable to those associated with the optimum response in patients with normal renal function. To present a simple and general method for the adjustment of dosing regimens for patients with renal impairment we make the following assumptions:

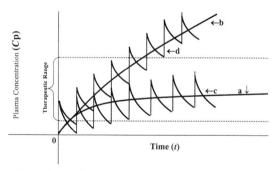

FIGURE 14.1 Comparison of the effect of renal impairment on the plasma concentration of drug following intravenous infusion and multiple-dosing regimen: (a) infusion of drug with the recommended standard rate to patients with normal renal function; (b) infusion at the standard rate to patients with renal failure; (c) multiple-dosing fluctuation in patients with normal renal function receiving a standard regimen; (d) multiple-dosing fluctuation in patients with renal impairment receiving the standard regimen.

1. The renal failure is the only alteration in the elimination of drug.

2. Hepatic metabolism remains unchanged and follows first-order kinetics.

3. The disposition of drug follows linear pharmacokinetics.

On the basis of these assumptions the dosing adjustment can be accomplished in three steps:

> Step I: Determination of the degree of renal impairment by estimation of the glomerular filtration rate (GFR).
>
> Step II: Estimation of the overall elimination rate constant or disposition rate constant of the drug in patients with renal impairment based on the calculated GFR from Step I.
>
> Step III: Utilization of appropriate pharmacokinetic equations such as the average steady-state plasma concentration to modify the standard dosing regimen according to the estimated rate constant from Step II. For multiple-dosing therapy the adjustment is achieved by:
>> i. Changing the standard dosing interval and keeping the normal dose unchanged.
>>
>> ii. Reducing the normal dose and keeping the standard dosing interval the same.
>>
>> iii. Changing both the normal dose and the dosing interval.

Obviously the therapeutic range of a drug plays an important role in dosage adjustment. For drugs with a narrow therapeutic range caution must be exercised when the dose or dosing interval is changed, and regardless of the method of adjustment, the fluctuation of plasma concentration should be checked to determine if it remains within the therapeutic range. For intravenous infusion, because the rate of input is continuous, the adjustment is made only on the rate of infusion.

14.3 STEP I: ESTIMATION OF GLOMERULAR FILTRATION RATE

Various endogenous and exogenous markers can be used to estimate the glomerular filtration rate. Among the endogenous biomarkers, creatinine is used routinely and urea nitrogen is often mentioned as a biomarker of renal function. It should, however, be noted that urea might not be a reliable marker of GFR. It undergoes substantial reabsorption following glomerular filtration and its clearance depends on urine flow and various pathologic and medication factors that modify blood urea nitrogen (BUN).

Various exogenous markers are used to estimate different aspects of renal function and most of these molecules are radiolabeled. For example, the following are used to determine GFR: inulin (labeled with ^{3}H or ^{14}C); ^{125}I-Na iothalmate; ^{131}I-Na diatrizoate; ^{51}Cr-EDTA; ^{140}La-, ^{99m}Tc-, ^{113m}In-, or ^{169}Yr-DTPA; ^{57}Co-vitamin B$_{12}$. Other markers are used to determine blood flow and plasma flow to the kidney that should not be mistaken with the above markers. For example, a marker that is used to determine renal plasma flow is radiolabeled *para*-aminohippuric acid (^{3}H- or ^{14}C-PAH) or the marker for blood flow is ^{125}I- or ^{131}I-human serum albumin (HSA).

14.3.1 Creatinine Clearance

The serum level of creatinine and the clearance of creatinine by the kidney have been used universally in conventional clinical practice as indicators of renal function, roughly reflecting the glomerular filtration rate. Creatinine is a secondary amino acid and anhydride of creatine. It has long been clear that the body is capable of synthesizing whatever creatine, a primary amino acid, it needs because its excretory product, creatinine, appears in constant amounts in the urine even when the diet contains no creatine. Creatinine biosynthesis in mammalian systems requires three enzymes: an amidinotransferase (L-arginine: glycine amidinotransferase), an N-methyltransferase (S-adenosylmethionine:guanidoacetate N-methyltransferase), and creatine phosphokinase. The overall synthesis of creatinine in the body is presented in the diagram of Figure 14.2. The loss of creatine as such is limited. It is assumed that following glomerular filtration, creatine is reabsorbed and secreted into the tubules by active transport. Approximately 98% of all creatine in the body is normally accumulated within skeletal muscle. The major loss of creatine from the body occurs through nonenzymatic formation of creatinine and subsequent urinary excretion. Hence, creatinine excretion is a function of lean body mass in normal individuals and shows little or no response to dietary changes or alteration in electrolyte balance. Creat-

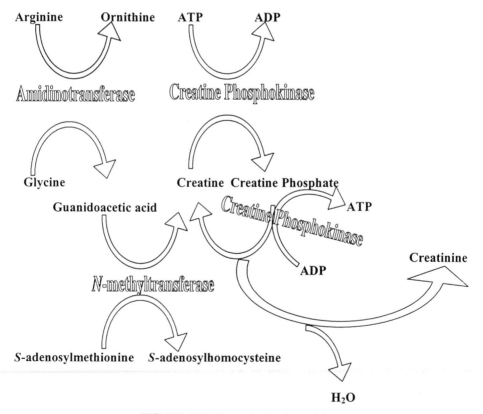

FIGURE 14.2 Biosynthesis of creatinine.

inine leaves the body after biosynthesis and apparently has no physiologic or biochemical role in the body. The serum concentration and daily urinary excretion are relatively constant because of the zero-order rate of formation in the body, and creatinine clearance unquestionably provides an informative approximation of GFR. Creatinine in the filtrate is not reabsorbed; however, it is weakly secreted.

Creatinine clearance, C_{cr}, can be measured directly by collecting 24-hour urine and a serum sample or it can be estimated from the serum concentration by using various empirical equations or nomograms.

14.3.1.1 Direct Measurement from 24-Hour Urine Sample: This method requires complete collection of urine during this period. After the total amount of creatinine excreted in 24 hours is measured, the rate of excretion is determined by dividing the amount of creatinine by 1440 minutes or 24 hours. By dividing this rate of excretion by the serum concentration of creatinine (S_{cr}) in units of milligram percent (ie, mg/dL). the creatinine clearance can be estimated. Because the clearance of creatinine reflects the filtration of the molecule in Bowman's capsules, it represents the GFR:

$$C_{cr}(mL/min) = \frac{(amount)_{24\,h} \div 1440}{S_{cr}(mg\%)} \tag{14.1}$$

Equation 14.1 assumes zero-order production of creatinine and a steady-state serum level. The equation is based on a concept discussed in previous chapters: clearance can be estimated as rate/concentration. A similar equation was used in Chapter 7 (Equation 7.7), for determination of clearance. There are several disadvantages to measuring creatinine clearance using 24-hour urine sample. The complete collection of urine is laborious and sometimes interferes with other diagnostic studies, and the inconvenience involved for outpatients is substantial.

Numerous investigators and clinicians have sought an appropriate mathematical transformation of the data that would result in a linear relationship between creatinine clearance and serum creatinine so that the value of clearance could be predicted from the plasma concentration. Among all published equations the following have been selected for their historical and practical significance.

14.3.1.2 Empirical Equations of Estimating Creatinine Clearance from Serum:

1. Equations that take only gender into consideration (Jelliffe et al.):

$$\text{For men:} \quad C_{cr} = \frac{100}{S_{cr}(mg\%)} - 12 \tag{14.2}$$

$$\text{For women:} \quad C_{cr} = \frac{80}{S_{cr}(mg\%)} - 7 \tag{14.3}$$

To take advantage of the role played by the daily rise and fall of serum creatinine, and to extend the estimation of creatinine clearance to situations where serum creatinine levels are unstable, the following equation was suggested:

$$\text{TBW}(S_{cr_1} - S_{cr_2}) = P - 100 \times S_{cr_{ave}} \times C_{cr} \times 1440 \tag{14.4}$$

Here TBW = total body water (in hundreds of milliliters), taken as 40% of body weight; S_{cr_2} = today's serum creatinine level (mg%); S_{cr_1} = yesterday's serum creatinine level; $S_{cr_{ave}}$ = the average of S_{cr_1} and S_{cr_2}; and P = creatinine production (mg/d) calculated with the following equations:

$$\text{For men:} \quad P(\text{mg/d}) = \text{body weight (kg)} \times (29.3 - (0.203 \times \text{age}))$$

$$\text{For women:} \quad P(\text{mg/d}) = \text{body weight (kg)} \times (25.3 - (0.175 \times \text{age}))$$

2. Equations that take gender and age into consideration (Jelliffe et al.):

$$\text{For men:} \quad C_{cr} = \frac{98 - \left(16\left(\dfrac{\text{age} - 20}{20}\right)\right)}{S_{cr}(\text{mg\%})} = \frac{98 - 0.8(\text{age} - 20)}{S_{cr}(\text{mg\%})} \tag{14.6}$$

$$\text{For women:} \quad C_{cr} = 0.9\left[\frac{98 - 0.8(\text{age} - 20)}{S_{cr}(\text{mg\%})}\right] \tag{14.7}$$

3. Equations that take gender, age, and weight into consideration (Cockcroft and Gault):

$$\text{For men:} \quad C_{cr} = \frac{(140 - \text{Age})(\text{weight(kg)})}{72 \times S_{cr}(\text{mg\%})} \tag{14.8}$$

$$\text{For women:} \quad C_{cr} = 0.85\left[\frac{(140 - \text{age})(\text{weight(kg)})}{72 \times S_{cr}(\text{mg\%})}\right] \tag{14.9}$$

The advantages of using these equations are the ease and convenience of taking one blood sample for determination of serum creatinine. These equations are empirical and are based mostly on stepwise multiple regression analysis of serum creatinine and creatinine clearance measured in selected populations of patients in the clinic/hospital of the investigator. As the ages of individuals in most of these investigations were in range 18 to 70, use of these equations in children younger than 18 years is not recommended. An example of an equation that may be used for pediatric patients is

$$C_{cr} = \frac{0.48 \times \text{height(cm)}}{S_{cr}(\text{mg/dL})}\left(\frac{\text{BSA}}{1.73 \text{ m}^2}\right) \tag{14.10}$$

where BSA is body surface area, which can be estimated with the following allometric equation:

$$\text{BSA} = \text{weight}^{0.425} \times \text{height}^{0.725} \times 71.84 \tag{14.11}$$

Patients with marked obesity or ascites usually excrete less creatinine per kilogram body weight than usually expected. Under these conditions the ideal body weight (IBW) should be used in the above equations. IBW is calculated as follows:

For men: IBW(kg) = 50 kg + 2.3 kg for each inch over 5 ft   (14.12)

For women: IBW(kg) = 45 + 2.3 kg for each inch over 5 ft   (14.13)

Prediction of creatinine clearance from serum creatinine is not accurate unless renal function and serum creatinine are at the steady state. For example, prediction of creatinine clearance can be greatly overestimated from serum creatinine in the early phase of acute renal failure before the serum creatinine has risen significantly.

14.3.2 Inulin Clearance

An exogenous marker of GFR is a polysaccharide (polymer of fructose) with a molecular weight of 5200 known as inulin. Inulin is small enough to pass through glomerulus freely. It is neither secreted nor reabsorbed by the tubules of the kidney. To determine the GFR, inulin is infused over a long enough period to attain a steady-state level. The half-life of excretion is less than 2 hours. Inulin is not metabolized in the body and is excreted only in urine. Therefore, with use of Equation 7.5 (Chapter 7), the inulin clearance can be estimated and is equal to the GFR. For example, if the steady-state plasma concentration of inulin is 100 mg/dL and the volume of urine collected over 3 hours is 270 mL with a concentration of 80 mg/L, the GFR can then be estimated as

$$(C_{p_{ss}})_{inulin} = \frac{k_0}{(Cl_t)_{inulin}} = \frac{KA}{GFR}$$

$$KA = (270 \text{ mL/3 h}) \times 80 \text{ mg/mL} = 7200 \text{ mg/h}$$

$$GFR = (7200 \text{ mg/h})/(100 \text{ mg/dL}) = 72 \text{ dL/h} = 120 \text{ mL/min} \qquad (14.14)$$

The disadvantage of using inulin for determination of GFR is that although this marker provides accurate information, it can be used only for hospitalized patients. Another application of inulin clearance is determining whether a drug is being secreted from or reabsorbed into the tubules. This is determined by estimating the ratio of clearance of drug to clearance of inulin. A ratio greater than one would be indicative of tubular secretion of the drug. A ratio less than one would indicate that the drug is being reabsorbed. And a ratio of one indicates that the drug is eliminated only by glomerular filtration.

14.3.3 Radiolabeled Markers

Radioisotope-labeled markers are popular because of their use for simultaneous evaluation of function and structure of the kidney. The well-known techniques of scintiscanning and renography are based on the use of these markers. Clearance of these markers is determined similarly to radiolabeled inulin as described above.

14.4 STEP II: ESTIMATION OF THE OVERALL ELIMINATION RATE CONSTANT OR HALF-LIFE OF DRUG IN PATIENTS WITH RENAL FAILURE BASED ON THE ESTIMATED RATE OF GLOMERULAR FILTRATION

The main assumption in determining the overall elimination rate constant of drugs for patients with renal impairment is that the metabolic rate constant remains unaffected by renal failure. Thus, the equation of the rate constant can be presented as

$$\overline{K} = \overline{k}_e + k_m \quad \text{(one-compartment model)} \tag{14.15}$$

$$\overline{k}_{10} = \overline{k}_e + k_m \quad \text{(two-compartment model)} \tag{14.16}$$

Note that this assumption may not be true for all therapeutic agents. There are drugs that because of the increase in their free concentrations in plasma, have accelerated or decelerated phase I and/or phase II metabolism. The simple methodology explained in this section, however, is suitable for a number of drugs that maintain their linear pharmacokinetic characteristics in renal impairment. A discussion of the names and categories of drugs is beyond the scope of this text and the reader is referred to books on therapeutic drug monitoring and clinical pharmacology.

To estimate $\overline{K}$ for a drug in a patient with renal impairment we have two options. The first option is to inject a dose, collect blood samples at different intervals, and estimate $\overline{K}$ directly from the decline in plasma concentration of the drug. Obviously the inconvenience of this option for the patient is excessive and unnecessary. Furthermore much time is required to collect blood samples, measure concentrations, and analyze data. The second option, which is the focus of this section, is to determine the GFR by measuring the serum creatinine and then estimate creatinine clearance with the empirical equations discussed in Section 14.3.1.2. The estimated creatinine clearance, which reflects the GFR of the patient, is then used to calculate $\overline{K}$ from normal values of K or half-life. As $K = k_e + k_m$ and its magnitude depends on the contribution of renal excretion and metabolism, we may classify the drugs into three groups.

- First group: those drugs that are eliminated entirely by the renal route of elimination and glomerular filtration.
- Second group: those drugs removed from the body completely by nonrenal elimination such as metabolism and biliary elimination.
- Third group: those drugs removed by renal and nonrenal routes of elimination.

14.4.1 Drugs of the First Group

$$K = k_e \tag{14.17}$$

The rate of elimination is equal to the rate of excretion:

$$\frac{dA}{dt} = \frac{dA_e}{dt} = -KA = -k_e A = Cl_t C_p = Cl_r C_p \tag{14.18}$$

Therefore, $Cl_t = Cl_r$,

$$K = \frac{dA_e/dt}{A} = \frac{dA_e/dt}{C_p V_d} = \frac{Cl_t}{V_d} \qquad (14.19)$$

$$Cl_t = \frac{dA_e/dt}{C_p} \qquad (14.20)$$

14.4.1.1 Wagner's Method: If we set

$$I = \frac{Cl_t}{C_{cr}} \qquad (14.21)$$

$$Cl_t = IC_{cr} \qquad (14.22)$$

Therefore,

$$\frac{dA_e}{dt} = IC_{cr}C_p = Cl_tC_p = KV_dC_p \qquad (14.23)$$

$$K = \frac{I}{V_d} C_{cr} \qquad (14.24)$$

Equation 14.24 indicates that for drugs in the first group, a plot of K versus C_{cr} yields a straight line through the origin with a slope of I/V_d (Figure 14.3). To determine $\overline{K}$ the creatinine clearance of patients with renal impairment is multiplied by the slope:

$$\overline{K} = \left(\frac{I}{V_d}\right)\overline{C}_{cr} \qquad (14.25)$$

14.4.1.2 Dettli's Method: In this method k_e is assumed to be proportional to GFR or C_{cr}:

$$k_e = K = aC_{cr} \qquad (14.26)$$

Similar to Wagner's method a plot of K versus C_{cr} yields a straight line with slope of a, which is equal to:

$$a = K/C_{cr} \qquad (14.27)$$

Therefore, $\overline{K}$ is calculated as

$$\overline{K} = K \frac{\overline{C}_{cr}}{C_{cr}} \qquad (14.28)$$

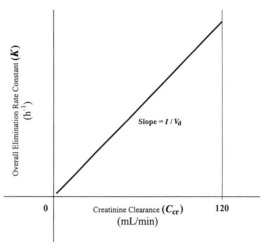

FIGURE 14.3 A plot of K versus C_{cr} yields a straight line that passes through the origin with a slope of I/V_d, where $I = Cl_t/C_{cr}$ (Wagner plot).

Equations 14.25 and 14.28 are the same:

$$\overline{K} = K \frac{\overline{C}_{cr}}{C_{cr}} = \frac{I}{V_d} \overline{C}_{cr} = \frac{Cl_t/C_{cr}}{V_d} \overline{C}_{cr} \tag{14.29}$$

14.4.1.3 Giusti's Method: According to Giusti's method the excretion rate constant of patients with renal failure can be defined in terms of the normal excretion rate constant with the ratio $\overline{C}_{cr}/C_{cr}$ as the correction factor:

$$\overline{K} = \overline{k}_e = k_e \frac{\overline{C}_{cr}}{C_{cr}} \tag{14.30}$$

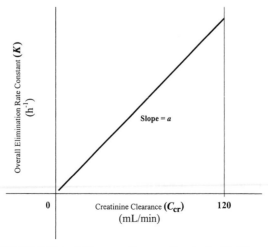

FIGURE 14.4 Plot of K versus C_{cr} according to the Dettli equation.

Dividing both sides of Equation 14.30 by K yields

$$\frac{\overline{K}}{K} = f_e \frac{\overline{C}_{cr}}{C_{cr}}$$ (14.31)

Because for the first group, $f_e = 1$, Equation 14.31 is the same as Equation 14.28.

14.4.2 Drugs of the Second Group

The overall elimination rate constant is independent of renal function and dependent on the activity of drug-metabolizing enzyme systems, the concentrations of these drugs in the systemic circulation and biliary elimination. Therefore, unless there is a change in the linearity of pharmacokinetics of the drug, no adjustment in dosage regimen is needed. For these drugs, the plot of K versus C_{cr} is parallel to the x axis.

14.4.3 Drugs of the Third Group

Most therapeutic agents that are eliminated by renal excretion and metabolism belong to the third group. By including the first-order metabolic rate constant in Equations 14.25, 14.28, and 14.30 we obtain the following relationships.

14.4.3.1 Wagner's Method:

$$\overline{K} = k_m + \left(\frac{I}{V_d}\right)\overline{C}_{cr}$$ (14.32)

14.4.3.2 Dettli's Method:

$$K = aC_{cr} + k_m$$ (14.33)

Therefore,

$$a = \frac{K - k_m}{C_{cr}}$$ (14.34)

The slope of the line, a, is calculated with the equation $(y_2 - y_1)/(x_2 - x_1)$, where $y_2 - y_1 = K - k_m$ and $x_2 - x_1 = C_{cr} = 120$ mL/min.

Substituting Equation 14.34 into Equation 14.33 and solving for $\overline{K}$ yield the following equation that can be used to determine the overall elimination rate constant of a drug for a patient with renal impairment by measuring the serum creatinine of the patient and estimating the creatinine clearance and by knowing the normal half-life and metabolic rate constant:

$$\overline{K} = \frac{K - k_m}{C_{cr}}\overline{C}_{cr} + k_m$$ (14.35)

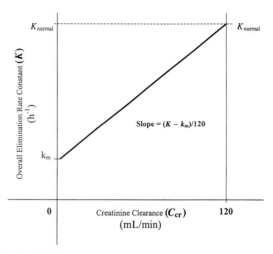

FIGURE 14.5 Plot of K versus C_{cr} according to Equation 14.35.

Equations 14.32 and 14.35 represent a similar plot as is shown in Figure 14.5, which indicates that when creatinine clearance is zero, at the origin of the graph, no renal function exists, a situation similar to that of end-stage uremic or anuric or anephric patients, and the y intercept equals k_m. Thus, the only route of elimination at $C_{cr} = 0$ is metabolism. When the clearance of creatinine is normal, that is, $C_{cr} = 120$ mL/min, which reflects the normal GFR, the overall elimination rate constant is normal, that is, $0.693/T_{1/2}$. Therefore, as renal failure progresses and C_{cr} decreases, the overall elimination rate constant also decreases whereas the half-life, $T_{1/2}$, increases.

14.4.3.3 Giusti's Method: Modifying Equation 14.30 to include the metabolic rate constant yields

$$\overline{K} = k_e \frac{\overline{C_{cr}}}{C_{cr}} + k_m \tag{14.36}$$

Dividing both sides of Equation 14.36 by K produces a relationship in terms of fraction of dose excreted unchanged:

$$\frac{\overline{K}}{K} = \frac{k_e}{K} \frac{\overline{C_{cr}}}{C_{cr}} + \frac{k_m}{K}$$

$$\frac{\overline{K}}{K} = f_e \frac{\overline{C_{cr}}}{C_{cr}} + 1 - f_e$$

Therefore,

$$\frac{\overline{K}}{K} = 1 - \left(f_e \left(1 - \frac{\overline{C_{cr}}}{C_{cr}} \right) \right) \tag{14.37}$$

or

$$\overline{K} = K \left[1 - \left(f_e \left(1 - \frac{\overline{C_{cr}}}{C_{cr}} \right) \right) \right] \tag{14.38}$$

Basically all these methods are the same and should provide exactly the same answer for the overall elimination rate constant of patients with renal failure.

In general, a few pitfalls are associated with the methods of estimation of $\overline{K}$ based on creatinine clearance, for example, when the serum creatinine concentration fluctuates and the measured value does not represent the steady-state concentration of creatinine, or the increase in the plasma concentration of free drug causes capacity-limited metabolism and changes the linear pharmacokinetics to dose-dependent (nonlinear) pharmacokinetics.

14.5 STEP III: ADJUSTMENT OF STANDARD DOSING REGIMEN FOR PATIENTS WITH RENAL FAILURE

For patients with renal impairment, because the rate of output is reduced significantly, the rate of input should be adjusted accordingly. The rate of input for an intravenous infusion is k_0, and in multiple dosing it is D/τ. The objective of adjusting a dosing regimen is then to modify k_0, D, and/or τ such that the accumulation of a drug in the body of patients with renal impairment becomes equal to the recommended level for patients with normal renal function. Mathematically we may define this as to set

$$(\overline{A}_{ave})_{ss} = (A_{ave})_{ss} \quad \text{or} \quad \overline{A}_{ss} = A_{ss} \tag{14.39}$$

For oral absorption, assuming bioavailability remains the same, Equation 14.39 can be expressed as

$$\frac{F\overline{D}}{\overline{K}\overline{\tau}} = \frac{FD}{K\tau}$$

$$\overline{D} = \frac{D\overline{K}\overline{\tau}}{K\tau} \tag{14.40}$$

For an intravenous infusion,

$$\frac{\overline{k}_0}{\overline{K}} = \frac{k_0}{K} \quad \text{or} \quad \frac{\overline{k}_0}{\overline{Cl}_t} = \frac{k_0}{Cl_t}$$

$$\overline{k}_0 = k_0 \frac{\overline{K}}{K} = k_0 \frac{\overline{Cl}_t}{Cl_t} \tag{14.41}$$

For an intravenous bolus one-compartment model,

$$\frac{\overline{D}}{\overline{K}\overline{\tau}} = \frac{D}{K\tau}$$

$$\overline{D} = \frac{D\overline{K}\overline{\tau}}{K\tau} \tag{14.42}$$

For an intravenous bolus injection two-compartment model,

$$\frac{\overline{D}}{\overline{k_{10}\overline{\tau}}} = \frac{D}{k_{10}\tau}$$

$$\overline{D} = \frac{\overline{k_{10}}\overline{\tau}}{k_{10}\tau} \qquad (14.43)$$

These equations are used to adjust the dosing regimen by one of the following approaches.

14.5.1 Adjustment of Dosing Regimen with Respect to Normal Dose and/or Dosing Interval

1. We may keep the dosing interval the same as standard and change the dose:

$$\overline{\tau} = \tau, \quad \overline{D} = D\,\frac{\overline{K}}{K} \qquad (14.44)$$

2. We may keep the dose the same as standard and change the dosing interval:

$$\overline{D} = D, \quad \overline{\tau} = \tau\,\frac{K}{\overline{K}} \qquad (14.45)$$

3. We may change both the dose and dosing interval. Because there will be two unknowns in the formula depending on considerations such as patient compliance and strength of the marketed dosage form, we set one of the unknowns equal to a convenient value and solve for the other. For example, if the standard dose is given four times daily, we may decide to set the dosing interval equal to 8 hours and calculate the new dose based on a three-times-daily schedule. Therefore, we set the dosing interval equal to λ, where λ is a known value (eg, 8 hours) different from τ (eg, 6 hours) and calculate the dose:

$$\overline{\tau} = \lambda, \quad \overline{D} = \frac{D\overline{K}\lambda}{K\tau} \qquad (14.46)$$

Or, if the dose can be set different from the standard regimen, the dosing interval can be estimated as

$$\overline{D} = \text{dose}, \quad \overline{\tau} = \frac{\text{dose} \times K\tau}{D\overline{K}} \qquad (14.47)$$

where "dose" is a known value that is different from standard D. Equations 14.44 to 14.47 are based on the assumption that the fraction of dose absorbed and the volume of distribution of patients with renal impairment are the same as those for patients with normal renal function. If the volume of distribution of a drug changes because of renal impairment one option would be to adjust the dosing interval according to the area under the plasma concentration–time curve at steady state and adjust the dose according to total body clearance:

$$\overline{C}_{p_{ave}} = C_{p_{ave}}$$

$$\frac{\overline{AUC}}{\overline{\tau}} = \frac{AUC}{\tau} \tag{14.48}$$

$$\overline{\tau} = \tau \frac{\overline{(AUC)}_\tau}{(AUC)_\tau} \tag{14.49}$$

$$\overline{D} = \frac{\overline{\tau} D \times \overline{Cl}_t}{\tau \times Cl_t} \tag{14.50}$$

14.5.2 Adjustment of Dosing Regimen with Respect to the Normal Amount of Accumulation

A different approach to adjusting the dosing regimen for patients with renal failure is to modify the dose and/or dosing interval based on the normal average amount of accumulation in the body at steady state. This approach, also known as the accumulation ratio method, can be carried out according to the following steps:

1. Estimate the average amount of accumulation in the body of patients with normal renal function. This calculated value should correspond to the optimum response for patients with normal renal function. For example, for multiple oral doses the equation is

$$(A_{ave})_{ss} = \frac{FD}{K\tau} = \frac{1.44 T_{1/2} FD}{\tau} \tag{14.51}$$

2. Using the same equation, include $(A_{ave})_{ss}$ and $\overline{T}_{1/2}$ or $\overline{K}$ and solve for a new regimen by changing the dose, dosing interval, or both as follows:
   a. Solve for a new dose by keeping the dosing interval the same as in the standard regimen:

$$\overline{D} = \frac{(A_{ave})_{ss}\overline{K}\tau}{F} = \frac{(A_{ave})_{ss}\tau}{1.44\overline{T}_{1/2}F} \tag{14.52}$$

   b. Solve for a new dosing interval by keeping the dose the same as in the standard regimen:

$$\overline{\tau} = \frac{FD}{K(A_{ave})_{ss}} = \frac{1.44\overline{T}_{1/2}FD}{(A_{ave})_{ss}} \tag{14.53}$$

c. Change both the dose and dosing interval:

$$\overline{D} = \frac{(A_{ave})_{ss}\overline{K}\overline{\tau}}{F} = \frac{(A_{ave})_{ss}\overline{\tau}}{1.44\overline{T}_{1/2}F} \tag{14.54}$$

Because there are two unknowns in Equation 14.54, we set one of them equal to an acceptable value and solve for the other.

We may use a similar approach to adjust the infusion rate of a drug for patients with renal impairment:

a. $\quad A_{ss} = \dfrac{k_0}{K} = 1.44T_{1/2}k_0 \tag{14.55}$

b. $\quad \overline{k}_0 = \dfrac{A_{ss}}{1.44\overline{T}_{1/2}} \tag{14.56}$

14.5.3 Adjustment of Dosing Regimen with Respect to Peak and Trough Levels

We may also use the equations of peak or trough levels to adjust the standard dosing regimen:

1. Calculate the normal maximum amount of drug in the body, then adjust the regimen with one of the following choices (a–c):

$$(A_{max})_{ss} = \frac{D}{1 - e^{-K\tau}} = \frac{D}{(f_{el})_{\tau}} \tag{14.57}$$

a. Estimate the dose by keeping the dosing interval the same as standard:

$$\overline{D} = (A_{max})_{ss}(1 - e^{-\overline{K}\tau}) \tag{14.58}$$

b. Estimate the dosing interval if giving the normal dose:

$$\overline{\tau} = \frac{2.303}{\overline{K}} \log \frac{(A_{max})_{ss}}{(A_{max})_{ss} - D} \tag{14.59}$$

c. To change both $\overline{\tau}$ and $\overline{D}$ we may use either Equation 14.58 or 14.59 depending on which of the two unknowns we select to set equal to a known value.
2. To use the trough level we follow the same procedure as for the maximum amount in the body, that is, first estimate the normal minimum amount and then select which method of adjustment to use:

$$(A_{min})_{ss} = \frac{De^{-K\tau}}{1 - e^{-K\tau}} \tag{14.60}$$

a. Estimate the dose by keeping the dosing interval the same:

$$\overline{D} = \frac{(A_{min})_{ss}(1 - e^{-\overline{K}\tau})}{e^{-\overline{K}\tau}} \tag{14.61}$$

b. Estimate the dosing interval by giving the standard dose:

$$\overline{\tau} = \frac{2.303}{\overline{K}} \log \frac{D - (A_{min})_{ss}}{(A_{min})_{ss}} \tag{14.62}$$

c. To change both $\overline{\tau}$ and $\overline{D}$ we may use either Equation 14.60 or 14.61 depending on which of the two unknown we select to set equal to a known value.

APPLICATION

14.1 A 42-year-old male weighing 70 kg is to be treated with an antibiotic for a serious infection. The patient has a serum creatinine of 3.0 mg/100 mL.

1. Using equations 14.6 and 14.8 estimate the creatinine clearance of this patient.

$$\overline{C}_{cr} = \frac{98 - 16\left(\dfrac{42 - 20}{20}\right)}{3 \text{ mg/dL}} = 26.8 \text{ mL/min}$$

$$\overline{C}_{cr} = \frac{(140 - 42)(70)}{72 \times 3} = 31.76 \text{ mL/min}$$

2. Using Equation 13.35 calculate the amount of drug in this patient if $K = 0.3 \text{ h}^{-1}$ and $k_m = 0.02 \text{ h}^{-1}$.

$$\overline{K} = a\overline{C}_{cr} + k_m$$

$$\text{slope} = a = (0.3 - 0.02)/100 = 0.0028$$

$$\overline{K} = 0.02 + 0.0028\overline{C}_{cr} = 0.02 + 0.0028(26.8) = 0.095 \text{ h}^{-1}$$

$$\overline{T}_{1/2} = 0.693/0.095 = 7.29 \text{ h}$$

14.2 A 50-year-old female weighing 70 kg is to be treated for a serious infection with an antibiotic. The patient has impaired renal function as indicated by a serum creatinine level of 4 mg/100 mL.

1. Estimate the creatinine clearance by using the Crokroft and Gault equation.

$$\overline{C}_{cr} = 0.85 \times \frac{(140 - 50)(70)}{72 \times 4} = 18.6 \text{ mL/min}$$

2. If the normal and anuric elimination rate constants of this drug are 1.4 and 0.06 h^{-1}, respectively, calculate the overall elimination rate constant for the patient.

$$\overline{K} = \left(\left(\frac{1.4 - 0.06}{120 \text{ mL/min}}\right)18.6 \text{ mL/min}\right) + 0.06 = 0.2677 \text{ h}^{-1}$$

$$\overline{T}_{1/2} = 2.59 \text{ h}$$

3. If the normal IV dosing regimen is 1 g every 6 hours for patients with normal renal function, recommend a new dosage regimen for this patient by changing the dosing interval.

$$\overline{\tau} = \tau\left(\frac{K}{\overline{K}}\right) = 6 \times \left(\frac{1.4}{0.2677}\right) = 31.37 \text{ h}$$

Using the accumulation ratio method,

$$(A_{\text{ave}})_{\text{ss}} = \frac{1.44 \times 1 \text{ g} \times 0.495 \text{ h}}{6 \text{ h}} = 0.119 \text{ g} = 119 \text{ mg}$$

$$\overline{\tau} = \frac{1.44 \times 1 \text{ g} \times 2.59 \text{ h}}{0.119 \text{ g}} = 31.34 \text{ h}$$

4. Calculate the dose if the drug is to be given twice a day.

$$\overline{D} = \frac{D\overline{K}\overline{\tau}}{K\tau} = \frac{1 \text{ g} \times 0.2677 \text{ h}^{-1} \times 12}{1.4 \times 6 \text{ h}} = 0.382 \text{ mg}$$

Using the accumulation ratio method,

$$\overline{D} = \frac{(A_{\text{ave}})_{\text{ss}}\tau}{1.44\overline{T}_{1/2}} = \frac{119 \text{ mg} \times 12}{1.44 \times 2.59} = 382.9 \text{ mg}$$

14.3 For patients with normal renal function who suffer from urinary tract infections, an IV dose of 15 to 30 mg/kg body weight of a new cephalosporin is recommended every 6 to 8 hours. For patients with chronic renal insufficiency, dosage depends not only on the type of infection but also on the degree of renal impairment. Generally, the elimination half-life for this drug increases with decreasing renal function, ranging from 48 minutes in patients with normal renal function to 22 hours in patients with chronic end-stage renal function (ie, $C_{\text{cr}} = 0$). Adjust the dosage regimen of 15 mg/kg q.i.d. for the patients listed in Table 14.1.

TABLE 14.1 Patient Information Related to Application 14.3

Patient	Sex	Ideal Body Weight (kg)	C_{cr} (mL/min)
MW	F	60	60
JS	M	75	20
JB	F	55	0

1. Patient MW using Giusti's method for calculation of $\overline{K}$

$$K = 0.693/0.8 \text{ h} = 0.866 \text{ h}^{-1}$$

$$k_m = 0.693/22 \text{ h} = 0.0315 \text{ h}^{-1}$$

$$f_e = (0.866 - 0.0315)/0.866 = 0.963$$

$$\frac{\overline{K}}{K} = 1 - \left(0.963\left(1 - \frac{60}{120}\right)\right) = 0.52$$

$$\overline{K} = 0.52 \times 0.866 = 0.45 \text{ h}^{-1}$$

2. Patient MW using Dettli's method for calculation of $\overline{K}$

$$\overline{K} = \left(\frac{0.866 - 0.0315}{120 \text{ mL/min}}\right)60 \text{ mL/min} + 0.0315 = 0.448 \text{ h}^{-1}$$

3. Dosage adjustment for Patient MW by keeping dosing interval the same

$$\overline{D} = (15 \text{ mg/kg})(0.52) = 7.8 \text{ mg/kg q.i.d. } (468 \text{ mg q.i.d.})$$

or

$$\overline{D} = D(\overline{K}/K) = 15 \text{ mg/kg } (0.448/0.866) = 7.76 \text{ mg/kg}$$

4. Dosage adjustment for Patient MW by keeping dosing interval the same and using accumulation ratio method

$$(A_{ave})_{ss} = \frac{1.44 \times 0.8 \text{ h} \times 15 \text{ mg/kg} \times 60 \text{ kg}}{6 \text{ h}} = 172.8 \text{ mg}$$

$$\overline{D} = \frac{172.8 \text{ mg} \times 6 \text{ h}}{1.44 \times (0.693/0.45)} = 467.53 \text{ mg}$$

5. Calculations for Patient JS using Dettli's method for calculation of $\overline{K}$ and the accumulation ratio method for calculation of $\overline{D}$ given every 6 hours

$$\overline{K} = \left(\frac{0.866 - 0.0315}{120 \text{ mL/min}} \right) \times 20 \text{ mL/min} + 0.0315 = 0.170 \text{ h}^{-1}$$

$$\overline{T_{1/2}} = 0.693/0.170 = 4 \text{ h}$$

$$(A_{\text{ave}})_{\text{ss}} = (172.8)(75/60) = 216 \text{ mg}$$

$$\overline{D} = \frac{216 \times 6}{1.44 \times 4} = 225 \text{ mg q.i.d.}$$

6. Calculations of $\overline{K}$ and $\overline{D}$ for Patient JB

$$\overline{K} = k_{\text{m}} = 0.0315 \text{ h}^{-1}$$

$$\overline{T_{1/2}} = 22 \text{ h}$$

$$\overline{D} = 15 \text{ mg/kg } (0.0315/0.866) = 0.545 \text{ mg/kg} \times 55 \text{ kg} = 30 \text{ mg q.i.d.}$$

$$(A_{\text{ave}})_{\text{ss}} = (172.8 \text{ mg/kg})(55/60 \text{ kg}) = 158.4 \text{ mg}$$

$$\overline{D} = (158.4(6))/(1.44(22)) = 30 \text{ mg q.i.d.}$$

ASSIGNMENT

14.1 The half-life of a drug is 2.3 hours and its volume of distribution is 20 L. The total body clearance of this drug in patients with normal renal function is 6 L/h and that for anephric patients is 0.4 L/h.

    14.1.1 The recommended dosing regimen for this drug is 3 mg/kg per day in three equal IV doses. Adjust this regimen for a 70-year-old man with a serum creatinine of 4 mg% and ideal body weight of 176 lb.

    14.1.2 Adjust the dose if the drug is given twice a day.

    14.1.3 If the apparent volume of distribution remains the same, what would be the peak and trough levels when the dose is given every 8 hours? Every 12 hours?

    14.1.4 What dosing interval would you recommend if the dose remains the same?

    14.1.5 What would be the dose if the drug is given once a day?

14.2 A 30-year-old female is scheduled to begin a course of therapy with an antibiotic. Her height is 5 ft 11 inches. Her serum creatinine is 30 μg/mL. The drug has an overall elimination rate constant of 0.12 h^{-1} and metabolic rate constant of 0.003 h^{-1}. Using Giusti's method determine the overall elimination rate constant of the drug for this patient.

14.3 Adjust the standard dosing regimen of 600 mg b.i.d. of drug X with $K = 0.15$ and $k_{\text{m}} = 0.06$ for the patient listed in Table 14.2.

    14.3.1 Use a dosing interval of 12 hours.

    14.3.2 Use a dosing interval of 8 hours.

TABLE 14.2 Patient Information Related to Assignment 14.3

Name	Sex	Weight	Height	Age	S_{cr} (mg%)
JJ	F	80 kg	5'4"	70	8.96

14.4 A 50-year-old, 60-kg female with congestive heart failure has been maintained on Drug Z 0.25 mg daily for the past 8 weeks. Her serum level of the drug and serum creatinine concentration 8 weeks ago were 1.6 μg/L and 1 mg%, respectively. Her serum creatinine today is 4 mg/dL.

14.4.1 Estimate the creatinine clearance of this patient by using the Cockroft and Gault method.

14.4.2 The normal overall elimination and metabolic rate constants are 0.017 and 0.08 h^{-1}, respectively. Determine the overall elimination rate constant of the drug for this patient.

14.4.3 What would be the dosing interval if the dose were decreased to 0.125 mg?

14.4.4 Determine the dose if the drug is to be given once a day.

BIBLIOGRAPHY

1. Bjornsson TD. Use of serum creatinine concentrations to determine renal function. *Clin Pharmacokinet* 1979;4:200.
2. Boroujerdi M, Mattocks AM. Kinetics of creatinine. *J Pharmacokinet Biopharm* 1979;7:291.
3. Boroujerdi M. The comparability of pharmacokinetics of creatinine in rabbit and man: a mathematical approach. *J Theor Biol* 1982;95:369.
4. Boroujerdi M, Mattocks AM. Metabolism of creatinine *in vivo*. *Clin Chem* 1983;29:1363.
5. Burton ME, Vasko MR, Brater DC. Comparison of drug dosing methods. *Clin Pharmacokinet* 1985;10:1.
6. Chiou WL, Hsu FH. A new simple and rapid method to monitor the renal function based on pharmacokinetic consideration of endogenous creatinine. *Res Commun Chem Pathol. Pharmacol* 1975;10:315.
7. Chrymko M, Schentag J. Creatinine clearance predictions in acutely ill patients. *Am J Hosp Pharm* 1981;38:837.
8. Chrzanowski FA, Niebergall PJ, Magock RL, Taubin JM, Sugita ET. Kinetics of intravenous theophyllin. *Clin Pharmacol Ther* 1977;22:188.
9. Cockcroft DW, Gault MH. Prediction of creatinine clearance from serum creatinine. *Nephron* 1976;16:31.
10. DeSanto N, Anastasio P, Cirillo M, Santoro D, Spitali L, Mansi L, Celantano L, Capodicaso D, Cirillo E, Del Vecchio E, Pascale C, Capasso G. Measurement of glomerular filtration rate by the ^{99m}Tc-DTPA renogram is less precise than measured and predicted creatinine clearance. *Nephron* 1999;81:136.
11. Dettli L. Elimination kinetics and dosage adjustment of drugs in patients with kidney disease. In: Grobecker H, et al, editors. *Progress in pharmacology.* New York: Gustav Fisher Verlag, 1977: vol. 1.
12. DeVane CL, Jusko WJ. Dosage regimen design. *Pharmacol Ther* 1982;17:143.

13. Drusano GL, Plaisance KI, Forrest A, Standiford HC. Dose ranging study and constant infusion evaluation of ciprofloxacin. *Antimicrob Agents Chemother* 1986;30:440.

14. Jelliffe RW. Estimation of creatinine clearance when urine cannot be collected. *Lancet* 1971; 975–976.

15. Jelliffe RW. Creatinine clearance: bedside estimate: *Ann Intern Med* 1973;79:604.

16. Giusti DL, Hayton WL. Dosage regimen adjustment in renal impairment. *Drug Intell Clin Pharm* 1973;7:382.

17. Levy G. Pharmacokinetics in renal disease. *Am J Med* 1977;62:461.

18. Richter O, Reinhardt D. Methods for evaluating optimal dosage regimens and their application to theophylline. *Int J Clin Pharmacol Ther Toxicol* 1982;20:564.

19. Ritschel WA. A simple method for dosage regimen adjustment. *Methods Find Exp Clin Pharmacol* 1983;5:407.

20. Slatlery JT, Gibaldi M, Koup JR. Prediction of maintenance dose required to attain a desired drug concentration at steady state from a single determination of concentration after an initial dose. *Clin Pharmacokinet* 1980;5:377.

21. Van Dalen R, Vree TB, Baars AM, Termond E. Dosage adjustment for ceftazidine in patients with impaired renal function. *Eur J Clin Pharmacol* 1986;30:597.

22. Wagner JG. Fundamentals of clinical pharmacokinetics. Hamilton, IL: *Drug Intelligence,* 1975: 374.

23. Wagner JG, Northam JI, Always CD, Carpenter OS. Blood levels of drug at the equilibrium state after multiple dosing. *Nature* 1965;207:1301.

CHAPTER 15

EFFECT OF DIALYSIS ON PHARMACOKINETICS OF DRUGS

Best for a person is to live his life being as cheerful and as little distressed as possible.
This will occur if he does not make his pleasure in mortal things.
STOBAEUS (SELECTIONS)

OBJECTIVES

■ To present the application of pharmacokinetic principles in therapeutic management of patients with chronic severe renal impairment who use dialytic procedures.

■ To discuss briefly the principles of hemodialysis and peritoneal dialysis.

■ To introduce the general methodologies for adjusting the standard dosing regimen for patients on dialysis.

■ To discuss the general pharmacokinetic equations for adjustment of the dosing regimen.

15.1 INTRODUCTION

Patients with chronic severe renal impairment usually accumulate water and endogenous and exogenous wastes. To restore the normal dynamic equilibrium between plasma and extracellular fluid and to remove the waste products, they are usually subjected to various dialytic procedures. The process of elimination in these patients during dialysis is a combination of metabolism, dialytic removal of drug, and the residual renal elimination plus other negligible routes of elimination. The two different dialytic procedures most commonly used for the treatment of the symptoms of chronic renal failure are hemodialysis and peritoneal dialysis. The fundamental principle in both procedures is the removal of solutes and wastes from the systemic circulation via diffusion across a semipermeable membrane based on concentration gradient into a dialysis solution known as dialysate. The process is similar to glomerular filtration, but without the physiologic selectivity of the kidney. Dialytic treatments remove the drug from the systemic circulation and reduce the concentration of drug in plasma. The plasma concentration is much lower during dialysis than in the interdialytic period. Therefore, a patient on dialysis who receives any therapeutic agent(s), particularly one with a narrow therapeutic range, may require a maintenance dose to maintain the plasma concentration at the therapeutic level.

Biochemical criteria are considered before initiating dialysis:

- C_{cr} or GFR $\cong$ 5 mL/min
- BUN/S_{cr} $\cong$ 3.5
- S_{cr} $\cong$ 10–20 mg/dL
- High serum uric acid
- High serum inorganic phosphorus
- Presence of toxins such as guanidosuccinic acid, methyl guanidine, methyl histidine, and phenolic acids in the blood

15.2 HEMODIALYSIS

Hemodialysis is carried out by use of a hemodialyzer, also known as an artificial kidney. The procedure is valuable for the management of advanced renal failure. Various types of commercially available hemodialyzers provide the semipermeable membrane for removal. These units that are used in the so-called kidney machine may fall into one of the following categories:

1. Disposable coil dialyzer
2. Disposable fiber dialyzer
3. Disposable flat plate dialyzer
4. Nondisposable flat plate dialyzer

The following is a brief description of the procedure to provide enough background for the discussion of kinetics. For more detailed and specialized information the reader may consult related books and publications in nephrology.

The procedure involves the aseptic insertion of one catheter each into an artery and a vein. Sometimes the catheters are inserted into femoral vein approximately 2 inches apart. After placement of the catheters, a dialyzer, for example, a coil dialyzer, is connected to the machine, and dialysate is added to a container of water at 37°C. The dilution provides a solution similar to extracellular fluid. After the unit is primed with heparinized saline, the inlet and outlet of the unit are connected to the arterial and venous catheters, respectively. The blood flow rate is usually maintained at 12 L/h. In long-term dialysis, the dialysate is changed every 2 to 3 hours and dialysis is usually carried out for 6 to 8 hours.

15.3 PERITONEAL DIALYSIS

The patient's peritoneum serves as the dialysis membrane. The procedure involves the aseptic insertion into the peritoneal cavity of a nylon catheter, approximately 3 mm in diameter and 25 to 30 cm long, that has side perforations and is attached to a metal stylet. The catheter is inserted through a small incision, about one-third the distance from the umbilicus to the pubic bone. The skin of the abdomen is prepared as for any surgery. There are times that the bladder should be emptied prior to insertion of the catheter. The patient is positioned supine. Local anesthesia is administered around the insertion site. After the insertion the tip of the stylet is withdrawn and the catheter is inserted as far as it can penetrate on the right side of the pelvis. The dialysate, approximately 2 L for adults and 0.5 to 1 L for children, is infused by gravity for 5 to 10 minutes. After approximately 1 hour equilibrium is established between blood and dialysate and the abdomen is drained. The procedure may be repeated depending on the severity of renal impairment.

15.4 COMPOSITION OF DIALYSATE

Various dialysate formulations that generally contain electrolytes and hypertonic dextrose are commercially available. The composition of the dialysate is formulated to meet the patient's metabolic needs, serum osmolality, and potassium, sodium, and bicarbonate concentrations. The formulation in Table 15.1 is a typical dialysate composition. One of the shortcomings of this type of formulation is that it is physiologic with respect to only few electrolytes. Therefore, all other dialyzable compounds that should not be removed by dialysis, such as amino acids, are also removed. Obviously, such indiscriminate removal can become significant over time and may cause unwarranted side effects. The formulation presented in Table 15.1 contains the ionic compounds listed in Table 15.2.

There are other dialysate formulations containing superior ingredients that may prevent indiscriminate removal of endogenous compounds.

15.5 DIALYSIS CLEARANCE

Dialysis clearance is determined as an indicator of the dialyzability of a drug. The meaning of clearance is as described in previous chapters. It is the volume of plasma cleared of a drug per unit of time by a dialytic procedure:

$$\text{dialysis clearance} = (\text{extraction ratio})_{\text{dialysis}} \times \text{blood flow}$$

TABLE 15.1 Typical Ingredients of Dialysate Formulation

Compound	g/L
Sodium chloride	5.8
Sodium bicatbonate	4.5
Potassium chloride	0.15
Calcium chloride	0.18
Magnesium chloride	0.15
Glucose	2.00

TABLE 15.2 Concentrations of Ions in the Formulation in Table 15.1

Component	mEq/L
Na^+	132
K^+	2.0
Cl^-	105
HCO_3^-	33
Ca^{2+}	2.5
Mg^{2+}	1.5

or
$$\text{Cl}_{\text{dialysis}} = Q\left(\frac{C_{\text{in}} - C_{\text{out}}}{C_{\text{in}}}\right) \qquad (15.1)$$

where Q is the blood flow with units of volume per time, and C_{in} and C_{out} are the concentrations of drug in the blood entering and leaving the dialysis machine, respectively. Equation 15.1 is more practical for hemodialysis. For peritoneal dialysis, clearance is determined with the equation

$$\text{Cl}_{\text{dialysis}} = \frac{A_{\text{d}}}{tC_{\text{pmidpoint}}} \qquad (15.2)$$

where A is the total amount of drug removed by dialysis, t is the length of dialysis, and $C_{\text{pmidpoint}}$ is the arterial plasma level at the midpoint of peritoneal dialysis.

The extraction ratio of hemodialysis is also used to determine the efficiency of a hemodialyzer and is

$$\text{ER} = \frac{C_{\text{in}} - C_{\text{out}}}{C_{\text{in}}} = \frac{Q(C_{\text{in}} - C_{\text{out}})}{QC_{\text{in}}} \qquad (15.3)$$

where $Q(C_{\text{in}} - C_{\text{out}})$ is the rate of elimination by dialysis, and QC_{in} is the rate of input into the dialyzer.

As a general rule, drugs with a large volume of distribution tend to remain longer in the body and only a small fraction is cleared per unit of time by dialysis. As only free drug can pass through the membrane most clinicians use the ratio of percentage unbound to volume of distribution as an index of the dialyzability of a drug. According to some clinicians, when the ratio is greater than 80%, 6 hours of hemodialysis is sufficient to remove up to 50% of the drug. Obviously a lower ratio, for example, under 20%, would indicate that only a small amount of the drug would be removed during 6 hours of dialysis.

15.6 EFFECT OF DIALYSIS ON PHARMACOKINETIC PARAMETERS

The elimination of drug during dialysis depends on metabolism, dialysis, and residual renal elimination. As dialysis is based on a concentration gradient and simple diffusion through a semipermeable membrane, it is considered a first-order process with a rate constant of k_{d}. Therefore, the overall elimination rate constant of a drug in patients with severe chronic renal failure who are on dialysis can be expressed as

$$\ddot{K} = \bar{k}_{\text{e}} + k_{\text{m}} + k_{\text{d}} \quad \text{during dialysis} \qquad (15.4)$$

$$\overline{K} = \bar{k}_{\text{e}} + k_{\text{m}} \qquad \text{between dialyses} \qquad (15.5)$$

The effect of dialysis on the profile of the plasma concentration–time curve is illustrated in Figures 15.1 and 15.2. The amount of drug removed by dialysis depends on whether the procedure is initiated immediately after administration of the drug or sometime later.

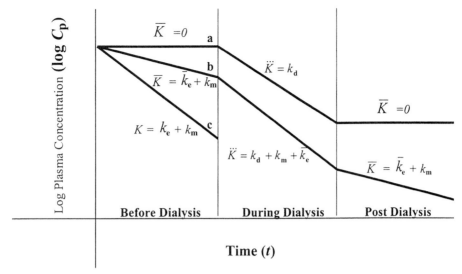

FIGURE 15.1 Change in the profile of log plasma concentration of drug following intravenous bolus injection before, during, and after dialysis: (a) when there is no elimination from the body; (b) when the drug is eliminated by metabolism and the residual kidney funciton; (c) when elimination is normal. The drug is assumed to follow a one-compartment model, where $\ddot{K}$ is the overall elimination rate constant during dialysis and k_d is the first-order dialysis rate constant.

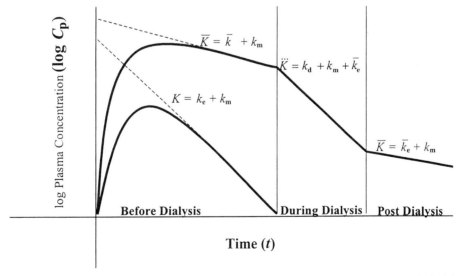

FIGURE 15.2 Change in the profile of log plasma concentration of drug following oral administration before, during, and after dialysis. The elimination before dialysis is by metabolism and residual kidney function ($\overline{K} = k_e + k_m$), and that during dialysis is by dialysis and the biological processes ($\ddot{K} = k_d + \overline{k}_e + k_m$). The normal decline in plasma concentration is represented by the overall elimination rate constant of $K = k_e + k_m$.

For a drug that follows a one-compartment model and is given by intravenous bolus injection, the fractions of dose excreted, metabolized, and removed by dialysis can be estimated individually with the following equations:

$$\bar{\bar{f}}_e = \frac{\bar{k}_e}{\bar{\bar{K}}} \tag{15.6}$$

$$\bar{\bar{f}}_m = \frac{k_m}{\bar{\bar{K}}} \tag{15.7}$$

$$f_d = \frac{k_d}{\bar{\bar{K}}} \tag{15.8}$$

The fraction removed by dialysis is also determined by dividing the total amount of unchanged drug removed by dialysis by the administered dose:

$$f_d = (\text{concentration of dialysate} \times \text{volume of dialysate})/\text{dose}$$

If the dose is injected during dialysis, the fraction of dose in the body and the fraction of dose eliminated at time t can be expressed as

$$\bar{\bar{f}}_b = e^{-\bar{\bar{K}}t} \tag{15.9}$$

$$\bar{\bar{f}}_{el} = 1 - e^{-\bar{\bar{K}}t} \tag{15.10}$$

The following equation can be employed to estimate what fraction of dose eliminated at time t is removed by dialysis:

$$(f_{el})_{\text{dialysis}} = \bar{\bar{f}}_{el} f_d \tag{15.11}$$

The plasma concentration of a drug during dialysis is

$$\ddot{C}_p = C_p^0 e^{-\ddot{K}t_{\text{dialysis}}} \tag{15.12}$$

where C_p^0 is the initial plasma concentration during dialysis. If the dialysis is initiated sometime after injection of the drug (Figure 15.1), the plasma concentration at anytime during dialysis is

$$\ddot{C}_p = (C_p^0 e^{-\bar{K}t}) e^{-\ddot{K}t_{\text{dialysis}}} \tag{15.13}$$

where $C_p^0 e^{-\bar{K}t}$ is the plasma concentration of drug at the start of dialysis, which is the initial plasma concentration for the steep decline during dialysis, t is the time between the injection and the start of dialysis, and t_{dialysis} is the time of dialysis.

A similar approach can be employed to estimate the plasma concentration at anytime after the end of dialysis:

$$C_p = ((C_p^0 e^{-\overline{K}t}) e^{-\overline{K}t_{\text{dialysis}}}) e^{-\overline{K}t_p} \tag{15.14}$$

t_p represents anytime during postdialysis period.

If the drug is administered orally, depending on the timing of the administration we may have the following cases:

1. Drug is administered before dialysis and dialysis is initiated during either the absorption phase or the postabsorption phase (Figure 15.2).
2. Drug is administered during dialysis (Figure 15.3).

To calculate the plasma concentrations of drugs administered during dialysis (Figure 15.3) we may use the following equation:

$$C_{p_{\text{during}}} = \widehat{C}_p^0 (e^{-\ddot{K}t_{\text{dialysis}}} - e^{-k_a t_{\text{dialysis}}}) \tag{15.15}$$

If dialysis is discontinued before total elimination of the drug, the plasma concentration in the postdialysis phase can be estimated as

$$C_{p_{\text{postdialysis}}} = (\widehat{C}_p^0 (e^{-\ddot{K}t_{\text{dialysis}}})) e^{-\overline{K}t} \tag{15.16}$$

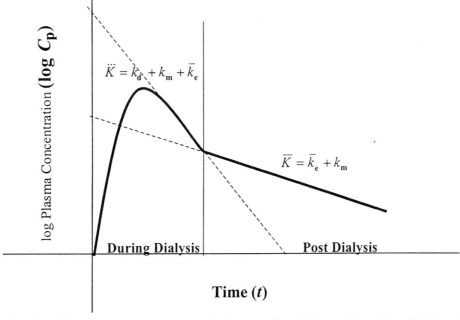

FIGURE 15.3 Decline in plasma concentration for an orally administered drug during dialysis and postdialysis.

To predict plasma concentration for a drug that is administered before the start of dialysis (Figure 15.2) the following equation can be used:

$$C_{p_{during}} = (\tilde{C}_p^0(e^{-\bar{K}t} - e^{-k_a t}))e^{-\ddot{K}t_{dialysis}} \tag{15.17}$$

Estimation of plasma concentration of drug during or after dialysis is mostly to determine whether the concentration is within the therapeutic range, and also to determine the maintenance dose required to achieve certain concentration. Assume that a case similar to Figure 15.1 is under consideration. The maintenance dose to be given at the end of dialysis to achieve, for instance, the initial plasma concentration would be

$$D_M = V_d(C_p^0 - C_{p_{end\ of\ dialysis}}) \tag{15.18}$$

Figure 15.4 depicts the effect of dialysis on plasma concentration of a multiple-dosing regimen. The maintenance dose required to achieve the maximum steady-state plasma concentration is

$$D_M = V_d[(C_{p_{max}})_{ss} - C_{p_{end\ of\ dialysis}}]$$

APPLICATION
15.1 A 45-year-old, 70-kg male patient with no kidney function undergoes 6 hours of hemodialysis every 48 hours. He receives an antibiotic intravenously three times daily. The

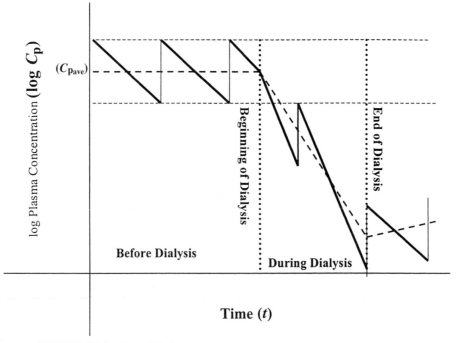

FIGURE 15.4 Effect of dialysis on plasma levels of a multiple-dosing regimen.

first dose with a peak concentration of 6 mg/L was given 2 hours before the dialysis. The apparent volume of distribution of the drug is estimated as 0.25 L/kg and the total body clearance is 0.35 L/h. The rate constant of dialysis is 0.103 h^{-1}. Calculate the following:

1. Plasma concentration just before the start of dialysis (predialysis concentration)

$$V_d = 0.25 \text{ L/kg} \times 70 \text{ kg} = 17.5 \text{ L}$$

$$\overline{K} = 0.35/17.5 = 0.02 \text{ h}^{-1}$$

$$C_{p_2 \text{ h}} = (6 \text{ mg/L})e^{-0.02 \times 2} = 5.76 \text{ mg/L}$$

2. Plasma concentration at the end of dialysis

$$\ddot{K} = 0.103 + 0.02 = 0.123 \text{ h}^{-1}$$

$$C_{p_{\text{end of dialysis}}} = 5.76e^{-0.123 \times 6} = 2.75 \text{ mg/L}$$

3. Replacement dose to restore plasma concentration to predialysis level

$$D_M = 17.5(5.7 - 2.75) = 52.675 \text{ mg}$$

4. Replacement dose to restore plasma concentration to initial level after injection

$$D_M = 17.5 \, (6 - 2.75) = 56.875 \text{ mg}$$

5. Original maintenance dose

$$D_M = 17.5 \times 6 = 105 \text{ mg}$$

6. Total amount removed by dialysis

$$\ddot{f}_{\text{el}} = 1 - e^{-0.123 \times 6} = 0.522$$

$$f_d = 0.103/0.123 = 0.837$$

total amount in body at start of dialysis $= 5.76 \times 17.5 = 100.8 \text{ mg}$

total amount eliminated by dialysis $= 100.8 \times 0.522 \times 0.837 = 44.04 \text{ mg}$

7. Peak and trough levels at steady state

$$(C_{p_{\text{max}}})_{\text{ss}} = \frac{6}{1 - e^{-0.02 \times 8}} = 40.58 \text{ mg/L}$$

$$(C_{p_{\text{min}}})_{\text{ss}} = 40.58e^{-0.02 \times 8} = 34.58 \text{ mg/L}$$

8. Trough level at steady state if dialysis was initiated 2 hours after injection and continued for 6 hours

$$C_{p_{2h}} = 40.58e^{-0.02 \times 2} = 38.98 \text{ mg/L}$$

$$C_{p_{\text{end of dialysis}}} = 38.98e^{-0.123 \times 6} = 18.63 \text{ mg/L}$$

ASSIGNMENT

15.1 A 20-year-old, 60-kg female patient with end-stage renal failure receives a 250-mg oral dose of Drug X twice daily. The elimination half-life of the drug for this patient is approximately 12 hours. The patient undergoes 6 hours of hemodialysis every week. The patient is advised to take the medication at 8 AM and 8 PM. The weekly dialysis starts at 12 noon and ends at 6 PM. The volume of distribution is 12 L, the absorption rate constant is 5.98 h^{-1}, and the bioavailability is 1. The rate constant of dialysis is 0.2 h^{-1}. Calculate the following:

   15.1.1 Peak and trough at steady state.
   15.1.2 Plasma concentration at 6 PM on the day of dialysis during steady state.
   15.1.3 Maintenance dose to attain the average steady-state concentration of 8 PM.

BIBLIOGRAPHY

1. Frost TH, Kerr DNS. Kinetics of hemodialysis: a theoretical study of the removal of solutes in chronic renal failure compared to normal health. *Kidney Int* 1977;12:41.
2. Parker PR, Parker WA. Pharmacokinetic consideration in hemodialysis of drugs. *J Clin Hosp Pharm* 1982;7:87.
3. Rostaing L, Chatelut E, Payen JL, Izopet J, Thalamas C, Ton-that H, Pascal JP, Durand D, Canal P. Pharmacokinetics of α1FN-2b in chronic hepatitis C virus patients undergoing chronic hemodialysis or with normal renal function: clinical implication. *J Am Soc Nephrol* 1998;9:2344.
4. Sprenger KBG, Kratz W, Lewis AE, Stadtmüller U. Kinetic modeling of hemodialysis, hemofiltration and hemodiafiltration. *Kidney Int* 1983;24:143.

CHAPTER 16

BIOAVAILABILITY AND BIOEQUIVALENCE EVALUATION

There is a capacity, called cleverness, which is such as to be able to do the actions that tend to promote whatever goal is assumed and to achieve it. If, then, the goal is fine, cleverness is praiseworthy, and if the goal is base, cleverness is unscrupulousness; hence both intelligent and unscrupulous people are called clever.
ARISTOTLE (NICOMACHEAN ETHICS)

OBJECTIVES

■ To define the related terminology

■ To discuss the significance of bioequivalence evaluation as it relates to therapeutic equivalence.

■ To discuss relevant pharmacokinetic parameters in bioavailability and bioequivalence evaluations.

■ To review the factors affecting bioavailability and bioequivalence.

■ To discuss various methods of determining bioavailability using plasma and urinary data.

16.1 INTRODUCTION

The discussion of bioavailability and bioequivalence in this chapter is centered on orally administered drug products and is an extension of Chapter 8. A discussion of the bioavailability and bioequivalence considerations of biotechnology products and specialized dosage forms is beyond the scope of this chapter.

Most regulatory decisions related to drug products may require bioavailability and bioequivalence data. For example, bioavailability data are considered an important part of supportive documentation for the following:

■ Submission of new drug applications (NDAs)
■ Abbreviated new drug applications (ANDAs)
■ Investigational new drug applications (INDs)
■ Decisions on the therapeutic equivalency of two products.

The regulatory guidelines related to bioavailability and bioequivalence studies are well described in the appropriate sections of Title 21 of the Code of Federal Regulations (21CFR 314.94, 21 CFR 320.1–36, 21 CFR 320.38, and 21CFR 320.63). These guidelines are related to such topics as:

- Criteria for waiver of an *in vivo* bioavailability or bioequivalence study
- Guidelines for conduct of *in vivo* bioavailability studies
- Guidelines on design of single-dose bioavailability studies
- Guidelines on design of multiple-dose *in vivo* bioavailability studies
- Analytical method for an *in vivo* bioavailability study

In addition, publications of the U.S. Department of Health and Human Services, Food and Drug Administration (FDA), Center for Drug Evaluation and Research (CDER) are valuable scientific documents that can help students to understand the interesting details of the guidelines. The careful selection of these guidelines as reading assignments for this chapter is highly encouraged. These regulatory guidelines are available on line and can be reached at http://www.access.gpo.gov/nara/cfr/index.html and http://www.fda.gov/.

16.2 TERMINOLOGY AND DEFINITIONS

The following definitions are taken from the Code of Federal Regulations or publications of the CDER:

16.2.1 Bioavailability

This term means the rate and extent to which active ingredient or active moiety is absorbed from a drug product and becomes available at the site of action. For drug products that are not intended to be absorbed into the bloodstream, bioavailability may be assessed by measurements intended to reflect the rate and extent to which the active ingredient or active moiety becomes available at the site of action. (21 CFR 320.1)

The rate represents how fast a drug is absorbed from an oral dosage form and the extent represents how much of the active ingredient of the dosage form reaches the systemic circulation.

16.2.2 Pharmaceutical Equivalents

Drug products that contain the same active ingredient(s), are of the same dosage form, route of administration and are identical in strength or concentration. (21 CFR 320.1)

In other words, two or more drug products with the same active ingredient(s) (ie, the same salt or ester of the same therapeutic moiety that have the same quality, purity, identity, and strength according to USP or other standards) are considered pharmaceutical equivalents. This indicates that pharmaceutical equivalents can be different in their inactive ingredients (excipients) including preservatives, coloring, and flavoring agents. They can also be different in release mechanism, expiration date, packaging and labeling (with some limitations), and shape.

16.2.3 Pharmaceutical Alternatives

Drug products are considered pharmaceutical alternatives if they contain the same therapeutic moiety, but are different salts, esters, or complexes of that moiety, or are different dosage forms or strength. (21 CFR 320.1)

Therefore, in contrast to pharmaceutical equivalents, pharmaceutical alternatives have different salts of the active ingredient(s) such as hydrochlorides, sulfates, and phosphates. They can also be of different strength in different dosage forms. Thus, controlled-release capsules and standard-release tablets are pharmaceutical alternatives.

16.2.4 Bioequivalence

The absence of a significant difference in the rate and extent to which the active ingredient or active moiety in pharmaceutical equivalents, or pharmaceutical alternatives, become available at the site of drug action when administered at the same molar dose under similar conditions in an appropriately designed study. (21 CFR 320.1)

Therefore, pharmaceutical equivalents or pharmaceutical alternatives that have the same bioavailability under the same experimental protocol are considered bioequivalents. Section 505(j)(7)(B) of the Federal Food, Drug, and Cosmetic Act describes the circumstances in which two formulations are considered bioequivalent drug products:

[T]he rate and extent of absorption of the test drug do not show a significant difference from the rate and extent of absorption of the reference drug when administered at the same molar dose of the therapeutic ingredient under similar experimental conditions in either a single dose or multiple doses; or

the extent of absorption of the test drug does not show a significant difference from the extent of absorption of the reference drug when administered at the same molar dose of the therapeutic ingredient under similar experimental conditions in either a single dose or multiple doses and the difference from the reference drug in the rate of absorption of the drug is intentional, is reflected in its proposed labeling, is not essential to the attainment of effective body drug concentrations on chronic use, and is considered medically insignificant for the drug.

The above definitions are intended for drug products that are absorbed into the systemic circulation.

16.2.5 Therapeutic Equivalents

Drug products are considered to be therapeutic equivalents only if they are pharmaceutical equivalents and if they can be expected to have the same clinical effect and safety profile when administered to patients under the conditions specified in the labeling. (21 CFR 320.1)

16.3 METHODS OF ESTIMATION OF BIOAVAILABILITY

In general, bioavailability of an oral dose represents the fraction of dose that reaches the systemic circulation in comparison to the same dosage form or different dosage form. This comparison provides significant information on the absorption of drug from the GI tract. A low bioavailability can be indicative of a number of events such as hepatic first-pass effect, presystemic metabolism by intestinal CYP450, influence of P-glycoprotein, simultaneous removal of drug from the site of absorption by chemical degradation, and instability of drug in the GI tract. Because intravenously injected drugs bypass the obstacles of absorption and are introduced completely into the systemic circulation, their bioavailability is considered 100% (ie, $F = 1$). The bioavailability of an oral dosage form compared with that of an intravenous injection is called *absolute bioavailability* (Figure 16.1). It represents the fraction of dose absorbed from an oral dosage form divided by 1 (ie, F_{oral}/F_{IV}, where F_{IV} is the fraction available after an intravenous dose and is equal to 1). Thus, absolute bioavailability cannot exceed 1. When it is 1, the drug is fully ab-

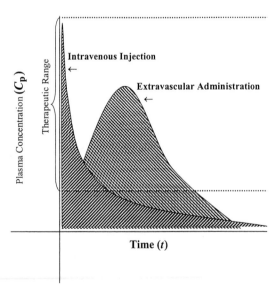

FIGURE 16.1 Schematic presentation of area under plasma concentration–time curve following intravenous and extravascular administration of a drug that is used for estimation of absolute bioavailability.

sorbed and totally bioavailable; however, the absorption may or may not be rapid. Obviously, an absolute bioavailability of 1 may not be attainable for a number of extravascular routes of administration including the oral route. As was discussed in Chapter 3, a number of factors can influence the rate and extent of absorption of an orally administered drug. Notable among them are physiologic factors associated with absorption, such as presystemic metabolism; influence of P-glycoprotein or other transporters; physicochemical characteristics of the drug; and formulation factors. The estimation of absolute bioavailability was discussed to some extent earlier in Chapter 8 (Equations 8.37 to 8.39). It can also be estimated according to the following relationships.

16.3.1 Estimation of Absolute Bioavailability from Plasma Data: Single Dose

By using the following model independent equations for oral administration and intravenous injection

$$\text{(oral)} \quad Cl_t = \frac{F \times \text{dose}}{\text{AUC}}$$

$$\text{(IV)} \quad Cl_t = \frac{\text{dose}}{\text{AUC}} \tag{16.1}$$

we obtain

$$\text{(oral)} \quad F = \frac{Cl_t \times \text{AUC}}{\text{dose}}$$

$$\text{(IV)} \quad 1 = \frac{Cl_t \times \text{AUC}}{\text{dose}} \tag{16.2}$$

Therefore, the absolute bioavailability can be estimated as

$$\frac{F}{1} = \frac{(Cl_t)_{\text{oral}} \times (\text{AUC})_{\text{oral}} \times (\text{dose})_{\text{IV}}}{(Cl_t)_{\text{IV}} \times (\text{AUC})_{\text{IV}} \times (\text{dose})_{\text{oral}}} \tag{16.3}$$

Because for drugs that follow linear pharmacokinetics clearance is considered a constant and independent of the amount of drug in the body or route of administration, $(Cl_t)_{\text{oral}}$ should be equal to $(Cl_t)_{\text{IV}}$. If equal doses are administered orally and intravenously then $(\text{dose})_{\text{oral}} = (\text{dose})_{\text{IV}}$; thus, Equation 16.3 will convert to

$$F = \frac{(\text{AUC})_{\text{oral}}}{(\text{AUC})_{\text{IV}}} \tag{16.4}$$

which is the same as Equation 8.39 in Chapter 8.

16.3.2 Estimation of Absolute Bioavailability from Total Amount Eliminated from the Body: Single Dose

Based on measurements of the total amount excreted unchanged and eliminated as metabolites the following relationships, contingent on the feasibility of the measurement, can be employed:

$$\text{(oral)} \quad F \times \text{dose} = A_e^\infty + A_m^\infty$$

$$\text{(IV)} \quad \text{dose} = A_e^\infty + A_m^\infty \tag{16.5}$$

or

$$\text{(oral)} \quad A_e^\infty = f_e \times F \times \text{dose}$$

$$\text{(IV)} \quad A_e^\infty = f_e \times \text{dose} \tag{16.6}$$

From Equation 16.5 we obtain two relationships:

$$F = \frac{A_e^\infty + A_m^\infty}{\text{dose}} \tag{16.7}$$

and

$$F = \frac{(A_e^\infty + A_m^\infty)_{\text{oral}} \times (\text{dose})_{\text{IV}}}{(A_e^\infty + A_m^\infty)_{\text{IV}} \times (\text{dose})_{\text{oral}}} \tag{16.8}$$

From Equation 16.6 we develop the following equations that may also be used to determine the absolute bioavailability:

$$F = \frac{A_e^\infty}{f_e \times \text{dose}} \tag{16.9}$$

$$F = \frac{(A_e^\infty)_{\text{oral}} \times (f_e \times \text{dose})_{\text{IV}}}{(A_e^\infty)_{\text{IV}} \times (f_e \times \text{dose})_{\text{oral}}} \tag{16.10}$$

16.3.3 Estimation of Relative Bioavailability from Plasma Data: Single Dose

The relative bioavailability is estimated by:

1. Comparison of a new formulation of a drug with its reference dosage form using the same or different route of administration. The intravenous injection usually is not included in this comparison.
2. Comparison of the effect(s) of different conditions such as fasting, exercise, and drug interaction on similar or different dosage forms intended for the same or different routes of administration.

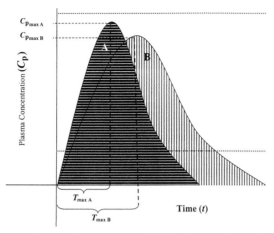

FIGURE 16.2 Schematic diagram of comparison of AUC, C_{pmax}, and T_{max} of plasma concentration–time curves of two orally administered dosage forms for the evaluation of relative bioavailability.

Relative bioavailability, in contrast to absolute bioavailability, can exceed 1. A relative bioavailability greater than one means that more of the active ingredient is absorbed from the test formulation, or the condition under investigation facilitates the absorption process. A value less than 1 indicates that absorption from the test formulation may not be comparable to that from the reference, or the condition under investigation hinders absorption of the drug (Figure 16.2). The related equation is similar to that for absolute bioavailability:

$$F = \frac{(\text{Cl}_{\text{t}})_{\text{test}} \times (\text{AUC})_{\text{test}} \times (\text{dose})_{\text{reference}}}{(\text{Cl}_{\text{t}})_{\text{reference}} \times (\text{AUC})_{\text{reference}} \times (\text{dose})_{\text{test}}} \tag{16.11}$$

16.3.4 Estimation of Relative Bioavailability from Total Amount Eliminated from the Body: Single Dose

The equations are similar to those used to estimate absolute bioavailability from the total amount eliminated from the body (Equations 16.5–16.10):

$$(\text{test}) \qquad F \times \text{dose} = A_{\text{e}}^{\infty} + A_{\text{m}}^{\infty}$$

$$(\text{reference}) \quad F \times \text{dose} = A_{\text{e}}^{\infty} + A_{\text{m}}^{\infty} \tag{16.12}$$

$$(\text{test}) \qquad A_{\text{e}}^{\infty} = f_{\text{e}} \times F \times \text{dose}$$

$$(\text{reference}) \quad A_{\text{e}}^{\infty} = f_{\text{e}} \times F \times \text{dose} \tag{16.13}$$

Therefore,

$$\frac{F_{\text{test}}}{F_{\text{reference}}} = \frac{(A_e^\infty + A_m^\infty)_{\text{test}} \times (\text{dose})_{\text{reference}}}{(A_e^\infty + A_m^\infty)_{\text{reference}} \times (\text{dose})_{\text{test}}} \tag{16.14}$$

$$\frac{F_{\text{test}}}{F_{\text{reference}}} = \frac{(A_e^\infty)_{\text{test}} \times (f_e \times \text{dose})_{\text{reference}}}{(A_e^\infty)_{\text{reference}} \times (f_e \times \text{dose})_{\text{test}}} \tag{16.15}$$

16.4 BIOAVAILABILITY AND LIVER FIRST-PASS METABOLISM

Drugs that are subjected to liver first-pass metabolism usually show very low absolute bioavailability. Theoretically the fraction that escapes metabolism is the bioavailable amount of drug and depends on the rate and extent of first-pass metabolism. One approach to estimating the bioavailability of such a drug is to determine the fraction that escapes first-pass metabolism:

$$\text{amount of drug that enters liver} = Q \times \text{AUC}_{\text{input}}$$

$$\text{amount that escapes first-pass metabolism} = Q \times \text{AUC}_{\text{output}}$$

$$\text{amount of drug that is metabolized} = \text{Cl}_m \times \text{AUC}_{\text{input}}$$

Q is the blood flow. Therefore, the fraction that is metabolized by the liver can be calculated as:

$$F_{\text{metab}} = \frac{\text{Cl}_m \times (\text{AUC})_{\text{input}}}{Q \times (\text{AUC})_{\text{input}}} = \frac{\text{Cl}_m}{Q}$$

which is the ratio of metabolic clearance to blood flow of the liver. Therefore, the fraction that escapes metabolism and represents the bioavailability of the drug can be calculated as:

$$F_{\text{escaped}} = 1 - F_{\text{metab}}$$

16.5 IMPORTANT PARAMETERS OF MULTIPLE DOSING FOR ESTIMATION OF RELATIVE AND ABSOLUTE BIOAVAILABILITY

To be confident that the behavior of the test drug following a multiple-dosing regimen remains the same as in a single-dose study, multiple-dosing parameters such as $(C_{\text{pave}})_{\text{ss}}$, C_{pmin}, C_{pmax}, $(\text{AUC})_\tau$ and accumulation index should also be compared. Depending on the drug, the multiple-dosing study may or may not require the steady-state condition. Various relationships have been suggested that involve parameters of multiple-dosing kinetics, for example,

$$\%PTF \text{ (peak–trough level fluctuation)} = \frac{(C_{p_{max}})_{ss} - (C_{p_{min}})_{ss}}{(C_{p_{ave}})_{ss}} \times 100$$

$$\%swing = \frac{(C_{p_{max}})_{ss} - (C_{p_{min}})_{ss}}{(C_{p_{min}})_{ss}} \times 100 \qquad (16.16)$$

For certain drugs the steady-state peak and trough levels cannot be predicted on the basis of a single-dose study. The common reason is that for certain drugs the linear pharmacokinetic characteristics observed after a single-dose administration may change during multiple dosing to dose-dependent or nonlinear pharmacokinetics. Obviously, prediction of the parameters of multiple dosing based on the constants and parameters of single-dose administration is very risky. Therefore, the data from a multiple-dosing study are necessary to provide a complete bioavailability evaluation. One approach would be to compare the area under the plasma concentration–time curve of the single dose from zero to infinity with the area under the plasma concentration–time curve of a maintenance dose during one dosing interval at steady state (Figure 16.3). For drugs that follow linear pharmacokinetics these two areas should be the same.

16.6 BIOEQUIVALENCE STUDY

The objective of a bioequivalence study is to compare the systemic exposure profile of a test drug with that of a reference drug in a meticulously designed experimental protocol. If both drugs demonstrate similar rates and extents of absorption under the experimental protocol they are considered bioequivalent drug products. In a typical bioequivalence study, the investigation is carried out in a crossover design. The subjects should be 18 years old

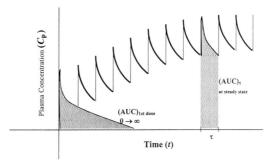

FIGURE 16.3 For drugs that follow linear pharmacokinetics, the area under the plasma concentration–time curve of the first dose from time zero to infinity is equal to the area under the plasma concentration–time curve of a maintenance dose at steady state. Under this condition the parameters of multiple-dosing kinetics can be estimated from parameters of single-dose administration.

or older and from different age groups and racial groups with a balance of men and women, unless the drugs are used by one gender. If the drugs are intended for children, similar diversity should be the goal in recruitment of young patients, if feasible. A bioequivalence study is usually based on single-dose administration; however, for certain drugs multiple-dosing needs to be evaluated. For most bioequivalence evaluations the preferred biologic sample is serum, plasma, or whole blood. Urine or tissue analysis may be required for special cases. The number of blood samples required ranges from 12 to 18 for each patient and each drug. Samples should be carefully timed so that $C_{p_{max}}$ and the terminal portion of the curve can be identified and estimated accurately. Drug or metabolites in the biological samples should be measured with validated procedure, equipment, and software as accurately, precisely, and reproducibly as possible.

Presently, the pharmacokinetic parameters required for evaluation of bioequivalence are AUC_0^t, AUC_0^∞, $C_{p_{max}}$, T_{max}, and (half-life)$_K$. These parameters are needed to define the systemic exposure profile. The equations and methods of estimation are described in Chapter 8, Section 8.6.

A recently drafted Guidance distributed by FDA recommends a change from the measurements of "rate and extent of absorption" to the measurements of parameters that collectively are called systemic exposure and are defined in terms of early exposure, peak exposure, and total exposure. Early exposure refers to the initial area between time zero and T_{max} (Figure 16.4). Peak exposure refers to the maximum plasma concentration that is measured directly in serum/plasma/whole blood, it is the highest concentration value of the raw data. Total exposure refers to the areas under the serum/plasma/whole blood concentration–time curves from time zero to t and from zero to infinity. Furthermore, the half-life of elimination should also be reported. If a multiple-dosing study is carried out, the areas under the serum/plasma/whole blood concentration–time curves for one dosing interval should also be compared.

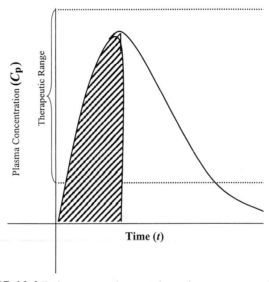

FIGURE 16.4 Early exposure (truncated area between zero and T_{max}).

At present, to determine if two drug products are considered bioequivalent, their rate and extent of absorption should differ by only −20% to +25% or less. In other words, for a number of drugs, a bioequivalence limit of 80 to 125% of the reference has been adopted as an average bioequivalence criterion, and outside this range, marketing of the test product is denied. This rule is based on medical judgment and clinical observation that a difference between −20 and +25% may not contribute significantly to the therapeutic outcome of the drug. To substantiate that the pharmacokinetic parameters of the test product are indeed within −20 to +25% of the reference product, appropriate statistical tests, such as two one-sided tests at the 0.05 level of significance using log-transformed data from the bioequivalence study, are required.

A discussion of the appropriate statistical models and analysis related to individual and population bioequivalence is beyond the scope of this textbook.

16.7 CODING SYSTEM OF THERAPEUTIC EQUIVALENCE: SIGNIFICANCE OF BIOEQUIVALENCE EVALUATION

The following coding system is designed by FDA to identify drug products that are therapeutically equivalent (Source: FDA–CDER Publication: Approved *Drug Products with Therapeutic Equivalence Evaluation*). The two major categories are A codes and B codes.

A Codes: The products that are placed under A code are considered therapeutically equivalent to other pharmaceutically equivalent products and are those for which actual or potential bioequivalence problems have been resolved. This category is subdivided:

- **AA**   Products in conventional dosage forms not presenting a bioequivalence problem.
- **AB**   Products meeting necessary bioequivalence requirements. These are products that have identical active ingredient(s), dosage form, and route(s) of administration and the same strength if a study is submitted demonstrating bioequivalence. In certain instances a number is added to the code (AB1, AB2, AB3, etc.). These three character codes are given when more than one reference listed drug of the same strength has been designated under the same heading.
- **AN**   Solutions and powders intended for aerosolization that are marketed for use in any of several delivery systems, which are pharmaceutically and therapeutically equivalent.
- **AO**   Injectable oil solutions that contain the same concentration of the same active ingredient and identical type of oil as vehicle. These products are pharmaceutically and therapeutically equivalent.
- **AP**   Injectable aqueous solutions and, in certain instances, intravenous nonaqueous solutions.
- **AT**   Topical drugs that are pharmaceutically and therapeutically equivalent and include all solutions and drug products for which a waiver of in vivo bioequivalence has been granted but the processes of formulation are adequate to demonstrate bioequivalence.

B Codes: Drugs that are placed under B codes are not considered therapeutically equivalent to other pharmaceutically equivalent dosage forms because they have actual or potential bioequivalence problems. These problems are related mostly to the dosage form rather than the active ingredient. This category is also subdivided:

- **B***   Products that require further investigation by FDA, which takes no position on the therapeutic equivalence of the products until the completion of the study and evaluation.
- **BC**   Extended-release dosage forms including capsules, injectables, and tablets. These products are not considered therapeutically equivalent unless the rates and extents of absorption of the products are demonstrated to be equivalent through a well-designed bioequivalence study.
- **BD**   Active ingredients and dosage forms with known and documented bioequivalence problems and for which sufficient data have not been submitted to demonstrate bioequivalence.
- **BE**   Delayed-release oral dosage forms such as enteric-coated dosage forms. Different dosage forms that have delayed-release characteristics usually have potential bioequivalence problems.
- **BN**   Products in aerosol–nebulizer drug delivery systems. For example, FDA does not consider different metered aerosol dosage forms containing the same active ingredient(s) in equal strength to be therapeutically equivalent unless they meet bioequivalence standards.
- **BP**   Active ingredients and dosage forms with potential bioequivalence problems. The criteria for identifying a trouble-causing ingredient is defined in 21CFR 320.33. Inclusion of any ingredient meeting these criteria in a dosage form is considered a potential bioequivalence problem unless sufficient data are submitted to demonstrate bioequivalence.
- **BR**   Suppositories or enemas that deliver drugs for systemic absorption. The bioavailability may vary significantly from product to product. They are not therapeutically equivalent unless evidence of bioequivalence is available.
- **BS**   Products having drug standard deficiencies. For example, if the standards allow a wide variation of pharmacologically active components of the active ingredient such that the pharmaceutical equivalence is in question all products containing that active ingredient in that dosage form are coded BS.
- **BT**   Topical products with bioequivalence issues. They may have acceptable clinical performance but are not bioequivalent.
- **BX**   Products for which the data submitted to FDA and reviewed by the Agency are considered inadequate to confirm therapeutic equivalence.

At the time of this writing, the draft of the new Guidance for evaluation of bioavailability and bioequivalence, representing current FDA thinking, was announced to the public for review and feedback.

ASSIGNMENT (EXTRA CREDIT)

EC-16.1 Read the following investigation by Bauer et al and answer the questions for this assignment:

Bauer KS, Kohn EC, Lush RM, Steinberg SM, Davies P, Kohler D, Reed E, Figg WD. Pharmacokinetics and relative bioavailability of caboxyamido-triazole (CAI) with respect to food and time of administration: use of a single mode for simultaneous determination of changing parameters. *J Pharmacokinet Biopharm* 1998;26:673–687.

■ Discuss the effect of food on the bioavailability of CAI.
■ Calculate T_{max} based on the median values of constants presented in Table IV. Compare your calculated values of T_{max} with the median observed values of T_{max} reported in Tables II and III.
■ In our opinion why is the bioavailability low?

EC-16.2 Based on the paper by Johnson et al answer the questions for this assignment:
Johnson JA, Akers WS, Herring VL, Wolf MS, Sullivan JM. Gender differences in labetalol kinetics: importance of determining stereoisomers kinetics for racemic drugs. *Pharmacotherapy* 2000; 20:622–628.

■ Explain the hypothesis of the investigators regarding the gender differences in plasma concentration, AUC, and $C_{p_{max}}$ of labetalol.
■ According to this study why do women require a higher concentration of the drug to achieve an antihypertensive effect comparable to that of men?
■ What is the significance of determining individual stereoisomer concentrations in a bioavailability study? Use labetalol as an example.

EC-16.3 Answer the questions of this assignment based on the paper by Daley-Yates et al:
Daley-Yates PT, Gregory AJ, Brooks CD. Pharmacokinetic and pharmacodynamic assessment of bioavailability for two prodrugs of methylprednisolone. *Br J Clin Pharmacol* 1997;43:593–601.

■ Describe the objectives of the study.
■ What are the differences between a single-blind, randomized, crossover design and a double-blind, randomized, parallel design.
■ Determine the relative bioavailability of methylprednisolone (MP) suleptanate and MP succinate.
■ Write the pharmacokinetic equation for plasma concentration of methylprednisolone in terms of data presented in Table 2 of the article.
■ What is the assumption of the paper concerning the absolute bioavailability of MP suleptanate and MP succinate? Can *F* be calculated from the data? Would you consider the intramuscular injection of drugs the same as their intravenous bolus injection?
■ Are the two compounds therapeutically equivalent?
■ By using the mean values of the absorption and elimination rate constants, calculate T_{max}. Compare your answer with the reported values.

EC-16.4 Two different formulations of capecitabine tablets are compared with respect to bioequivalence and in the article by Cassidy et al. Based on the information provided in the paper answer the questions:
Cassidy J, Twelves C, Cameron D, Steward W, O'Byrne K, Jordell D, Banken L, Goggin T, Jones D, Roos B, Bush E, Weidekamm E, Reigner B. Bioequivalence of two tablet formulations of capecitabine and exploration of age, gender, body surface area, and creatinine clearance as factors influencing systemic exposure in cancer patients. *Cancer Chemother Pharmacol* 1999;44: 453–460.

■ What are the differences between the two formulations?
■ The authors selected AUC but not $C_{p_{max}}$ as the primary parameter for assessment of bioequivalence. Why?

- In your opinion are the differences between the pharmacokinetic parameters of formulations A and B related to the inactive ingredients or other factors?
- Figure 6 of the article is based on geometric mean and geometric standard deviation. What are geometric mean and standard deviation and their significance?
- Calculate the relative bioavailability of the two formulations.
- Is the effect of gender on the AUC of capecitabine and its metabolites statistically and clinically significant?
- What was the purpose of using BSA as a parameter for correlation?
- Calculate the total body clearance and apparent volume of distribution of the parent compound for both formulations.
- What is the rate of absorption of the drug at T_{max} from both formulations?

EC-16.5 Review the article by Marathe et al and answer the questions for this assignment.
Marathe PH, Greene DS, Kollia GD, Barbhaiya RH. Evaluation of the effect of food on the pharmacokinetics of avitriptan. *Biopharm Drug Dispos* 1998;19:381–394.

- Discuss the food-related decrease in bioavailability of avitriptan.
- How would you explain the effect of ranitidine on the bioavailability of avitriptan?
- Calculate the relative bioavailability of a 150-mg capsule and a 150-mg solution of avitriptan (use the data in Table 5 of the article) in fasting subjects and subjects fed a standard high-fat meal.
- Did the timing of the meal influence the bioavailability of the drug?

EC-16.6 In the following paper Weidkamm et al have assessed the bioequivalence of two dosage forms. The data indicate a lack of equivalency between the two formulations. Review the article and summarize the data that represent the bioequivalence of the two dosage forms and comment on the clinical ramification of this type of bioequivalency.
Weidekamm E, Rüsing G, Caplain H, Sörgel F, Crevoisier C. Lack of bioequivalence of a generic mefloquine tablet with the standard product. *Eur J Clin Pharmacol* 1998;54:615–619.

BIBLIOGRAPHY

1. Anderson S, Hauk WW. Consideration of individual bioequivalence. *J Pharmacokinetic Biopharm* 1990;18:259.
2. Colburn WA, Gibson DM, Rodriguez LC, Bugge CJL, Blumenthal HP. Effect of meals on the kinetics of etretinate. *J Clin Pharmacol* 1985;25:583.
3. Colburn WA, Welling PG. Relative bioavailability: what reference? *J Pharm Sci* 1986;75:921.
4. Cutler DJ. Drug availability to noneliminating tissues and sites of action following an intravenous dose. *J Pharm Sci* 1986;75:1141.
5. Diletti E, Hauschke D, Steinijous VW. Sample size determination: extended tables for the multiplicative model and bioequivalence ranges of 0.9 to 1.11 and 0.7 to 1.43. *Int J Clin Pharmacol Ther Toxicol* 1992;30(suppl 1):S59.
6. *Drug bioequivalence: a report of the Office of Technology Assessment*—Drug Bioequivalence Study Panel, 1974.
7. Farolfi M, Powers JD, Rescigno A. On the determination of bioequivalence. *Pharmacol Res* 1999;39(1).

8. FDA Center for Drug Evaluation and Research. *Guidance for industry—extended release oral dosage forms: development, evaluation, and application of* in vitro/in vivo *correlation.* Rockville, MD: FDA, 1997.

9. FDA Center for Drug Evaluation and Research. Guidance for industry—average, population and individual approaches to establishing bioequivalence. Rockville, MD: FDA, 1999.

10. FDA Center for Drug Evaluation and Research. Guidance for Industry—BA and BE studies for orally administered drug products: general consideration. Rockville, MD: FDA, 1999.

11. FDA. *Code of Federal Regulations: Food and Drug,* 1988.

12. Feldman EB. How grapefruit juice potentiates drug bioavailability. *Nutr Rev* 1999;55:398.

13. Francisco GE, Honigberg IL, Stewart JT, Kotzan JA, Brown WJ. *In vitro* and *in vivo* bioequivalence of commercial prednisolone tablets. *Biopharm Drug Dispos* 1984;5:335.

14. Gibaldi M, Boyes RN, Feldman S. Influence of first-pass effect on availability of drugs on oral administration. *J Pharm Sci* 1971;60:1338.

15. Kwan KC. Oral bioavailability and first-pass effects. *Drug Metab Dispos* 1997;25:1329.

16. Ritschel WA. Aspects for bioavailability and bioequivalence revision: possible implication on clinical pharmacology. *Methods Find Exp Clin Pharmacol* 1987;9:453.

17. Rowland M. Influence of route of administration on drug availability. *J Pharm Sci* 1972;61:70.

18. Scheuplein RJ, Shaaf SE, Brown RN. Role of pharmacokinetics in safety evaluation and regulatory consideration. *Annu Rev Pharmacol Toxicol* 1990;30:197.

19. Steinijans VW, Hauschke D, Jonkman JHG. Controversies in bioequivalence studies. *Clin Pharmacokinet* 1992;22:247.

CHAPTER 17

NONCOMPARTMENTAL APPROACH IN PHARMACOKINETICS BASED ON STATISTICAL MOMENTS

Among our intellectual states that grasp the truth, some—knowledge and understanding—are always true, whereas others—for example, belief and reasoning— admit of being false; and the understanding is the only sort of state that is more exact than knowledge. Since the principles of demonstration are better known "than the conclusions derived from them," and since all knowledge requires an account, it follows that we can have no knowledge of the principles. Since only understanding can be truer than knowledge, we must have understanding of the principles.
ARISTOTLE (POSTERIOR ANALYTICS—BOOK II)

OBJECTIVES

- To discuss noncompartmental analysis and contrast it with compartmental or physiologic modeling.
- To learn about the parameters of noncompartmental analysis such as mean residence time, mean absorption time, clearance, area under the moment curve, and volume of distribution
- To understand the utility of the approach and possible limitations in pharmacokinetic analysis.

17.1 INTRODUCTION

The principle of noncompartmental analysis is based on application of the statistical theory called the moments of a random variable. This theory is useful because the passage of a drug through the body can be considered a stochastic process subject to some random fluctuation. These random fluctuations cause the measurements of the variable, for example, plasma concentration of a drug, to be basically repeatable from dose to dose, but the measurements vary from one dose to another. In other words, if the dependent variable is the change in plasma concentration of a drug with time, that change is a function of the independent variables "time" and a variable that indexes a particular measurement, known as the *random variable.*

In statistics, the parameters *mean* and *standard deviations* are meaningful numerical descriptive measures that identify the center and spread of a set of observations and their distribution; however, these parameters may not characterize the observations and the related distribution in a unique manner. We may have different sets of observations that are very different but possess the same mean and standard deviation. In theory a set of plasma concentration–time data may be considered a statistical distribution. In statistics, the equation of observations that defines the distribution is called the probability density function, and a probability density function is characterized by the moments of the function. A major use of moments is to approximate the probability distribution of a random variable. We can estimate the moments about the origin or about the mean. The general equation of moments about the origin is

$$\mu_r = \int_{-\infty}^{+\infty} x^r f(x)dx = E(X^r) \tag{17.1}$$

where $f(x)$ is the probability density function, E refers to the "expected value," and X is a random variable. When $r = 0$, μ_0, is equal to the integral of $f(x)$ and the expected value of X, $E(X) = 1$. When $r = 1$, $\mu_1 = E(X)$, which is the expected value of X, and so on. The general equation of moments about the mean of a random variable is

$$\mu_r = \int_{-\infty}^{+\infty} (x - \bar{x})^r f(x)dx = E[(X - \bar{x})^r] \tag{17.2}$$

When $r = 0$, $\mu_0 = 1$; however, for $r = 1$, $\mu_1 = 0$. The second moment about the mean, μ_2, is called the variance of the distribution of X and reflects the spread of the distribution of a random variable. The third moment determines the symmetry or skewness (lack of symmetry) of the distribution, and the fourth moment determines the kurtosis (the extent to which a distribution is peaked or flat) of the distribution.

Parallel to the statistical equations of moments, the following equations have been developed for the statistical moments of plasma concentration–time curves. The assumption, as was mentioned earlier, is to consider the time course of plasma data as a statistical distribution curve that can be defined by a probability density function. The formulas are based on moments about the origin within the interval of observation (ie, from 0 to ∞)

$$\mu_0 = \int_0^\infty C_p dt = \text{AUC}_0^\infty \tag{17.3}$$

$$\mu_1 = \int_0^\infty t C_p dt = \text{AUMC}_0^\infty \tag{17.4}$$

$$\mu_2 = \int_0^\infty t^2 C_p dt = \text{AUM}_2\text{C}_0^\infty \tag{17.5}$$

AUC_0^∞ is the area under the plasma concentration–time curve or the area under the zero-moment curve. It is calculated according to the trapezoidal rule as described in Chapter 1. AUMC_0^∞ represents the area under the first-moment curve. The method of estimation is the trapezoidal rule. The observed plasma concentrations are multiplied by the corresponding time points and plotted against the same time points. The terminal area of AUMC is calculated as

$$\text{(terminal area)}_{\text{AUMC}} = \frac{C_{p_n} t_n}{K} + \frac{C_p}{K^2} \tag{17.6}$$

C_{p_n} and t_n are the last plasma concentration and time point, respectively. $\text{AUM}_2\text{C}_0^\infty$ is the area under the second moment curve, which is constructed by multiplying the plasma concentrations by the square of time points and then plotting against time.

17.2 MEAN RESIDENCE TIME AND MEAN INPUT TIME

If we normalize the first and second moments (Equations 17.4 and 17.5) with respect to zero moment (Equation 17.3), the following normalized moments about the origin are generated:

$$\text{MRT} = \frac{\mu_1}{\mu_0} = \frac{\text{AUMC}_0^\infty}{\text{AUC}_0^\infty} \tag{17.7}$$

$$\text{VRT} = \frac{\mu_2}{\mu_0} = \frac{\text{AUM}_2\text{C}_0^\infty}{\text{AUC}_0^\infty} \tag{17.8}$$

where MRT stands for mean residence time and VRT is the variance of the residence time, which may reflect the magnitude of the random error. For drugs that are given by bolus injection and follow a one-compartment model, Equation 17.7 can be presented as

$$\text{MRT} = \frac{C_p^0/K^2}{C_p^0/K} = \frac{1}{K} = 1.44 T_{1/2} \tag{17.9}$$

Therefore, the mean residence time for drugs that follow a one-compatment model is equal to the time constant or turnover time that was discussed in Chapter 6 (Equations 6.12 and 6.13). A different version of MRT is obtained by multiplying and dividing Equation 17.9 by the initial plasma concentration:

$$\text{MRT} = \frac{\text{AUC}_0^\infty}{C_p^0} \tag{17.10}$$

For drugs that follow a two-compartment model the MRT equation can be written as

$$\text{MRT} = \frac{a/\alpha^2 + b/\beta^2}{a/\alpha + b/\beta} \tag{17.11}$$

When $\alpha \gg \beta$,

$$\text{MRT} \cong \frac{1}{\beta} = 1.44(T_{1/2})_\beta \tag{17.12}$$

If the system and data are considered linear and dose independent, the mean residence time would represent the time required for 63.3% of the dose to be eliminated via all routes of elimination. Because in linear systems AUC is equal to dose/Cl_t, Equation 17.7 can also be written as

$$MRT = \frac{AUMC \times Cl_t}{dose} \tag{17.13}$$

For instantaneous input such as bolus injection, the mean residence time is estimated according to Equations 17.7 and 17.9. When the input is not instantaneous such as in zero-order infusion or first-order absorption, the mean residence time is equal to the mean residence time of the bolus injection plus the mean input time (MIPT), that is, mean infusion time or mean absorption time:

$$MRT_{infusion} = MRT_{bolus} + \frac{T}{2} \tag{17.14}$$

where T represents the time of infusion and $0.5T$ is the mean infusion time (MIT).

$$MRT_{oral} = MRT_{bolus} + 1/k_a \tag{17.15}$$

where k_a is the absorption rate constant and $1/k_a$ represents the mean absorption time (MAT). Therefore, MAT can be estimated as

$$MAT = MRT_{oral} - MRT_{bolus} = 1/k_a = 1.44(T_{1/2})_{absorption} \tag{17.16}$$

When the absolute bioavailability is close to one, the value of MAT estimated by Equation 17.16 represents the true value of the mean absorption time. If the bioavailability is low because of presystemic metabolism or decomposition of the drug at the site of absorption, the value of MAT is considered only an apparent value. In general, for routes of administration such as the oral route where bioavailability is an issue, the MRT should be estimated as

$$MRT_{oral} = MRT_{bolus} \times \frac{(AUC_0^\infty)_{oral}}{F(AUC_0^\infty)_{bolus}} + MIPT \tag{17.17}$$

17.3 TOTAL BODY CLEARANCE AND APPARENT VOLUME OF DISTRIBUTION

The total body clearance in noncompartmental analysis is estimated by the model-independent equation that, as we discussed in previous chapters, is also useful in compartmental analysis:

$$(Cl_t)_{bolus} = \frac{dose}{AUC_0^\infty} \quad and \quad (Cl_t)_{oral} = \frac{F \times dose}{AUC_0^\infty} \tag{17.18}$$

Substituting AUC_0^∞ from Equation 17.7 yields the following relationship for total body clearance:

$$(\text{Cl}_t)_{\text{bolus}} = \frac{\text{dose} \times \text{MRT}}{\text{AUMC}} \tag{17.19}$$

The apparent volume of distribution is estimated from the relationship between total body clearance and mean residence time and is denoted $(V_d)_{ss}$:

$$(V_d)_{ss} = \text{Cl}_t \times \text{MRT} \tag{17.20}$$

By substitution of the equations of Cl_t and MRT in Equation 17.20 the following relationship for the apparent volume of distribution is obtained:

$$(V_d)_{ss} = (\text{dose}/\text{AUC})(\text{AUMC}/\text{AUC})$$

$$(V_d)_{ss} = \frac{\text{dose} \times \text{AUMC}}{\text{AUC}^2} \tag{17.21}$$

Equations 17.20 and 17.21 are used for drugs that are given intravenously regardless of the disposition profile (ie, the drug may follow a one- or two-compartment model).

Substituting Equations 17.17 and 17.18 into Equation 17.20 provides the volume of distribution of a drug administered by noninstantaneous input eg oral absorption:

$$V_{d_{ss}} = \frac{F \times \text{dose}}{(\text{AUC}_0^\infty)_{\text{oral}}} \left[\text{MRT}_{\text{bolus}} \times \frac{(\text{AUC}_0^\infty)_{\text{oral}}}{F \times (\text{AUC}_0^\infty)_{\text{bolus}}} + \text{MIPT} \right]$$

Therefore,

$$V_{d_{ss}} = \frac{\text{dose} \times \text{MRT}_{\text{bolus}}}{\text{AUC}_{\text{bolus}}} + \frac{F \times \text{dose} \times \text{MIPT}}{\text{AUC}_{\text{oral}}} \tag{17.22}$$

The volume of distribution for drugs administered by short-term infusion is defined as

$$V_{d_{ss}} = \frac{A_{\text{infused}} \times \text{AUMC}}{\text{AUC}^2} - \frac{A_{\text{infused}} T}{2 \times \text{AUC}} \tag{17.23}$$

where A_{infused} is the total amount administered to the patient and can be expressed as $A_{\text{infused}} = k_0 T$, that is, the rate of infusion multiplied by the time of infusion. Therefore, Equation 17.23 can also be written as

$$V_{d_{ss}} = \frac{k_0 T \times \text{AUMC}}{\text{AUC}^2} - \frac{k_0 T^2}{2 \times \text{AUC}} \tag{17.24}$$

17.4 MULTIPLE-DOSING RELATIONSHIPS

The equation describing the average steady-state plasma concentration is the same as discussed in Chapter 10:

$$(C_{p_{ave}})_{ss} = \frac{(AUC)_\tau}{\tau} \tag{17.25}$$

The average amount at steady state following intravenous or oral multiple dosing in terms of MRT is

$$\text{oral} \quad (A_{ave})_{ss} = \frac{MRT \times F \times \text{dose}}{\tau},$$

$$\text{Bolus} \quad (A_{ave})_{ss} = \frac{MRT \times \text{dose}}{\tau} \tag{17.26}$$

MRT represents the overall mean residence time of a drug.

A suggested equation for calculation of the mean residence time of multiple dosing is

$$MRT = \frac{AUMC_{ss}|_0^\tau + (\tau \times AUC_{ss}|_{n\tau}^\infty)}{AUC_{ss}|_0^\tau} \tag{17.27}$$

$AUMC_{ss}|_0^\tau$ is the area under the first-moment curve at steady state; $AUC_{ss}|_{n\tau}^\infty$ is the area under the zero-moment curve of the last dose to infinity, which requires a correct assessment of the terminal slope for the estimation of terminal area; $AUC_{ss}|_0^\tau$ is the area under the zero-moment curve of one dosing interval at steady state.

Because of the dependence of Equation 17.27 on the value of the terminal slope of the last dose, an alternative relationship has been suggested that relies on the area under the zero-moment curve from time zero to the end of the nth dosing interval.

$$MRT = \frac{AUMC_{ss}|_0^\tau + (n\tau \times AUC_{ss}|_0^\tau) - \left(\tau \int_0^{n\tau} C_p dt\right)}{AUC_{ss}|_0^\tau} \tag{17.28}$$

$\int_0^{n\tau} C_p dt$ is the area from zero to the last dosing interval, $n\tau$. The corresponding equations for calculation of the volume of distribution are

$$V_{d_{ss}} = \frac{\text{dose} \times (AUMC_{ss}|_0^\tau + \tau \times AUC_{ss}|_{n\tau}^\infty)}{(AUC_{ss}|_0^\tau)^2} \tag{17.29}$$

$$V_{d_{ss}} = \frac{\text{dose} \times \left[AUMC_{ss}|_0^\tau + (n\tau \times AUC_{ss}|_0^\tau) - \tau \int_0^{n\tau} C_p dt\right]}{(AUC_{ss}|_0^\tau)^2} \tag{17.30}$$

The definitions of the terms of Equation 17.29 are the same as described before. Equation 17.29 also depends on an accurate assessment of the area under the last dose to infinity. The alternative equation is Equation 17.30.

17.5 OTHER USEFUL CONCEPTS

Based on the area under the zero-moment curve of a single dose of a drug we can estimate the fraction of dose in the body at time t:

$$f_b = \frac{\text{AUC}_0^\infty - \text{AUC}_0^t}{\text{AUC}_0^\infty} = 1 - \frac{\text{AUC}_0^t}{\text{AUC}_0^\infty} \tag{17.31}$$

or the fraction of dose eliminated from the body at time t:

$$f_{el} = 1 - \left(\frac{\text{AUC}_0^\infty - \text{AUC}_0^t}{\text{AUC}_0^\infty} \right) = \frac{\text{AUC}_0^t}{\text{AUC}_0^\infty} \tag{17.32}$$

If the concentration of the metabolite(s) can be measured accurately, the fraction of dose metabolized can also be estimated based on the area under the zero-moment curve of the metabolite and parent compound. Obviously the fractions of dose excreted unchanged or eliminated as metabolites can still be calculated from the measurement of A_e^∞ in urine if the unchanged drug is excreted only in urine (Chapter 9).

Using the urinary data we can approximate the MRT of drug or its metabolites. A suggested equation that is based on the first-moment curve of the amount excreted unchanged is:

$$\text{MRT} = \frac{1}{\text{dose}} \int_0^\infty t dA_e \cong \frac{1}{\text{dose}} \times \sum_{i=1}^\infty t_{\text{midpoint}_i} \Delta A_{e_i} \tag{17.33}$$

APPLICATION

17.1 Two grams of a new drug was administered orally and intravenously in a crossover design with a washout period of 2 days to a 70-kg healthy volunteer. The concentration of the drug in plasma was measured at different time points and the results are summarized Table 17.1. Calculate the following:

1. Mean residence time of both treatments

$$(\text{AUC}_0^{7\,h})_{\text{IV}} = 391.38 \text{ mg h/L}$$

$$(\text{AUC}_0^{7\,h})_{\text{oral}} = 241.95 \text{ mg h/L}$$

$$(\text{terminal area})_{\text{IV}} = 6.039/0.5 = 12.078 \text{ mg h/L}$$

$$(\text{terminal area})_{\text{oral}} = 4.529/0.5 = 9.058 \text{ mg h/L}$$

TABLE 17.1 Data Related to Application 17.1

IV Bolus		Oral Dose	
Time (h)	C_p (mg/L)	Time (h)	C_p (mg/L)
0.00	200.00	0.00	0.00
0.10	190.246	0.17	47.702
0.25	176.499	0.25	61.519
0.50	155.760	0.33	71.447
0.75	137.458	0.50	83.350
1.00	121.306	0.75	87.283
1.50	94.473	1.00	83.511
2.00	73.576	1.50	69.188
3.00	44.626	2.00	54.810
4.00	27.067	3.00	33.451
5.00	16.417	4.00	20.299
6.00	9.957	5.00	12.312
7.00	6.039	6.00	7.468
		7.00	4.529

$$(\text{AUC}_0^\infty)_{\text{IV}} = 391.38 + 12.078 = 403.46 \text{ mg h/L}$$

$$(\text{AUC}_0^\infty)_{\text{oral}} = 241.95 + 9.058 = 251.00 \text{ mg h/L}$$

$$(\text{AUMC}_0^{7\text{ h}})_{\text{IV}} = 637.26 \text{ mg h}^2/\text{L}$$

$$(\text{AUMC}_{7\text{ h}}^\infty)_{\text{IV}} = 108.70 \text{ mg h}^2/\text{L}$$

$$(\text{AUMC}_0^\infty)_{\text{IV}} = 833.52 \text{ mg h}^2/\text{L}$$

$$(\text{AUMC}_0^{7\text{ h}})_{\text{oral}} = 499.50 \text{ mg h}^2/\text{L}$$

$$(\text{AUMC}_{7\text{ h}}^\infty)_{\text{oral}} = 65.52 \text{ mg h}^2/\text{L}$$

$$(\text{AUMC}_0^\infty)_{\text{oral}} = 565.02 \text{ mg h}^2/\text{L}$$

$$\text{MRT}_{\text{IV}} = \frac{833.52}{403.46} = 2.06 \text{ h}$$

$$\text{MRT}_{\text{oral}} = \frac{565.02}{251.01} = 2.25 \text{ h}$$

2. Mean absorption time

$$\text{MAT} = 2.25 - 2.06 = 0.19 \text{ h}$$

3. Total body clearance

$$Cl_t = \frac{2000 \text{ mg}}{403.46 \text{ mg h/L}} = 4.96 \text{ L/h}$$

or

$$Cl_t = \frac{(251/403.46) \times 2000}{251} = 4.96 \text{ L/h}$$

4. Apparent volume of distribution

From IV data,

$$V_{d_{ss}} = 4.96 \times 2.06 = 10.21 \text{ L}$$

From oral data,

$$V_{d_{ss}} = \frac{2000 \times 2.06}{403.46} \times \frac{0.622 \times 2000 \times 0.19}{251} = 9.616 \text{ L}$$

5. Fraction of dose in the body at $t = 7$ hours for both treatments

$$(f_b)_{IV} = 1 - \frac{391.38}{403.46} = 0.03$$

$$(f_b)_{oral} = 1 - \frac{241.95}{251} = 0.036$$

6. Amount in the body at $t = 7$ hours for both treatments

$$(A_{7\,h})_{IV} = 2000 \text{ mg} \times 0.03 = 60 \text{ mg}$$

$$(A_{7\,h})_{oral} = 0.622 \times 2000 \times 0.036 = 44.78 \text{ mg}$$

ASSIGNMENT

17.1 A single oral dose of an analgesic (250 mg) with absolute bioavailability of 0.85 was given to a patient. Blood samples were taken periodically and the serum concentrations were determined as reported in Table 17.2. Calculate the following:

  17.1.1 Mean residence time.
  17.1.2 Total body clearance.
  17.1.3 Fraction of dose in the body at $t = 4$ hours.

TABLE 17.2 Data Related to Assignment 17.1

C_p (mg/L)	0	0.7	1.2	1.4	1.4	1.1	0.8	0.6	0.5	0.3
Time (h)	0	1	2	3	4	6	8	10	12	16

ASSIGNMENT (EXTRA CREDIT)

EC-17.1 Read the article by Chouchane et al,

Chouchane N, Barre J, Toumi A, Tillement JP, Benakis A. Bioequivalence study of two pharmaceutical forms of rifampin capsules in man. *Eur J Drug Metab Pharmacokinet* 1995;20:315–320.

- Calculate the terminal area of the mean plasma concentrations.
- Calculate the relative bioavailability by using AUC_0^∞ and $AUC_0^{10\ h}$.
- Calculate the mean residence time.
- To which of the following factors would you attribute the interindividual variations? (Your answer should include adequate explanation based on recent publications.)

  Inconsistency of absorption
  Gender differences
  Genetic differences
  Weight differences and dose differences
  Other

EC-17.2 Review the paper by Eradiri et al, and answer the questions.

Eradiri O, Midha KK. Use of parent drug and metabolite data in bioavailability assessment of a novel diltiazem HCl once-daily product. *Pharm Res* 1995;12:2071–2074.

- Based on the data presented in Table I and Figure 1-A of the article, determine which product, Cardizen or Triazac, has a slower rate of absorption.
- Approximate the amount of drug in the body just before administration of the second dose of Cardizen.
- Compare the last 28 hours of study (ie, 20 to 48 hours) of the two drugs and comment on the amount of drug present in the body and whether the concentration remains within the therapeutic range.

EC-17.3 Review the article by Fischer et al, and answer the questions.

Fischer JD, Song MH, Futtle AB, Heizer WD, Burns CB, Vargo DL, Brouwer KLR. Comparison of zafirlukast (Accolate®) after oral and clonic administration in humans. *Pharm Res* 2000;17:154–159.

- Discuss the significance and practical application of oroenteric administration of drugs.
- What parameter or constant would be needed to determine the mean absorption time (MAT) of zafirlukast (Accolate®) after oral administration. Can the MAT be estimated from the reported data?

- What conclusion can be made, if any, from the comparison of $(T_{max})_{oral}$ and $(T_{max})_{distal\ Ileum}$?
- Considering the extent of availability of the drug after oral administration $AUC_{\%\ extent}$ and AUC_0^t, would you expect a significant portion of the oral dose to reach the distal portion of ileum?
- Can gut flora influence the bioavailability of the drug in colonic absorption?

EC-17.4 The questions of this assignment are related to the following article.
Nolting A, Abramowitz W. Lack of interaction between citalopram and the CYP3A4 substrate triazolam. *Pharmacotherapy* 2000;20:750–755.

- Based on the data provided in the paper would you expect a change in the rate of absorption of triazolam on day 33? Why?
- Can the MAT be estimated from the data? If the answer is yes, how? If it is no, why?
- How would you explain the large standard deviations of Cl/F and V_{dss}/F? Can they be attributed to the influence of ethnicity and/or gender differences on F, the bioavailability factor?

EC-17.5 Read the article by Keung et al before answering the questions of this assignment.
Keung ACF, Eller MG, Weir SJ. Single-dose pharmacokinetics of rifapentine in women. *J Pharmacokinet Biopharm* 1998;26:75–85.

- Compare the chemical structures of rifapentine, rifampin, and rifabutin.
- What is the major route of elimination of rifapentine in the body? Is the biliary elimination of the drug significant?
- Name the enzyme system involved in the formation of 25-desacetyl-rifamentine.
- Would you expect gender related differences in the pharmacokinetics of rifapentine and rifampin?
- Estimate the apparent volume of distribution and mean residence time for male and female.

BIBLIOGRAPHY

1. Benet LZ, Galaezzi RL. Noncompartmental determination of steady-state volume of distribution. *J Pharm Sci* 1979;68:1071.
2. Benet LZ. Mean residence time in the body versus mean residence time in the central compartment. *J Pharmacokinet Biopharm* 1985;13:555.
3. Bialer M, Look ZM, Silber M, Yacobi A. The relationship between drug input and mean residence time in the body. *Biopharm Drug Dispos* 1986;7:577.
4. Chan KKH, Gibaldi M. Estimation of statistical moments and steady-state volume of distribution for a drug given by intravenous infusion. *J Pharmacokinet Biopharm* 1982;10:551.
5. Chanter DO. The determination of mean residence time using statistical moments: is it correct? *J Pharmacokinet Biopharm* 1985;13:93.
6. Cheng H, Jusko WJ. Noncompartmental determination of the mean residence time and steady-state volume of distribution during multiple dosing. *J Pharm Sci* 1991;80:202.

7. Cheng H, Jusko WJ. Mean residence time of drugs in pharmacokinetic systems with linear distribution, linear or nonlinear elimination, and noninstantaneous input. *J Pharm Sci* 1991;80:1005.

8. Cutler DJ. Definition of mean residence times in pharmacokinetics. *Biopharm Drug Dispos* 1987;8:87.

9. Cutler DJ. Theory of mean absorption time, an adjunct to conventional bioavailability studies. *J Pharm Pharmacol* 1978;30:476.

10. Kasuya Y, Hirayama H, Kubota N, Pang S. Interpretation and estimates of mean residence time with statistical moment theory. *Biopharm Drug Dispos* 1987;8:223.

11. Landaw EM, Katz D. Comments on mean residence time determination. *J Pharmacokinet Biopharm* 1985;13:543.

12. Nüesch EA. Noncompartmental approach in pharmacokinetics using moments. *Drug Metab Rev* 1984;15:103.

13. Perrier D, Gibaldi M. General derivation of the equation for time to reach a certain fraction of steady state. *J Pharm Sci* 1982;71:474.

14. Riegelman S, Collier P. The application of statistical moment theory to the evaluation of *in vivo* dissolution time and absorption time. *J Pharmacokinet Biopharm* 1980;8:509.

15. Smith IL, Schentag JJ. Noncompartmental determination of the steady-state volume of distribution during multiple dosing. *J Pharm Sci* 1984;73:281.

16. Yamaoka K, Nakagawa T, Uno T. Statistical moment in pharmacokinetics. *J Pharmacokinet Biopharm* 1978;6:547.

CHAPTER 18

PHARMACOKINETIC-PHARMACODYNAMIC MODELING

Well, then, my good people: Since it has been shown that our salvation in life depends on the right choice of pleasures and pains, be they more or fewer, lesser or greater, farther or nearer, then doesn't our salvation seem primarily to be the art of measurement, which is the study of relative excess and deficiency and equality? It must be. Since it is measurement, it must definitely be an art, and knowledge.

SOCRATES VS PROTAGORAS

OBJECTIVES

■ To define the dose–response relationship.

■ To discuss various pharmacodynamic models.

■ To relate pharmacokinetic parameters to pharmacodynamic parameters.

■ To investigate pharmacokinetic–pharmacodynamic models.

18.1 INTRODUCTION

In the preceding chapters we studied the time course of plasma concentration of drug in the body as a function of the biologic processes of absorption, distribution, metabolism, and excretion (ADME). In reality we were exploring the manner in which the body handles a foreign substance following single or multiple administration via different routes, which is the definition of pharmacokinetics. Obviously, depending on the physicochemical characteristics of a compound and physiologic factors, we expect to observe different profiles among different xenobiotics. Throughout the preceding chapters we were mindful of the ultimate objective of drug therapy and why the plasma concentration of a drug must be maintained within the therapeutic range to achieve the desired therapeutic outcome. We are also aware that the desired therapeutic outcome can be achieved only if an optimum amount of a particular molecule of drug with a specific property and functional group(s) is administered to interact with a particular receptor site, which will then provide the pharmacologic response or therapeutic outcome. The quantitative evaluation of the interaction of a drug with its receptor site that provides the pharmacologic action of the drug is known as pharmacodynamics. Similar to any other dynamic process, such as thermodynamics, time is not a factor in pharmacodynamic evaluation. In other words, at the initial phase of evaluation when the concentration of drug is zero no response is anticipated, when the concentration is optimum the desired outcome is obtained, and when the concentration is high the toxic response is expected. The outcome is a function only of the amount or concentration of a drug and the affinity of the drug for the receptor. In most *in vitro* systems, such as cell culture, the interaction of drug with receptor site is direct and rather rapid and the concentration of the drug can be kept constant for a specific observation. Under *in vivo* conditions, however, the concentration of a drug at the receptor site or biophase is a function of time and physiologic processes such as ADME. Therefore, the *in vivo* pharmacodynamic observation is a function of the pharmacokinetic profile of the drug and it seems more logical to predict the overall therapeutic outcome of a drug based on pharmacokinetic–pharmacodynamic modeling rather than just pharmacodynamic analysis. It can also be stated that under *in vivo* conditions, the response is a function not only of concentration but also of time. The main objective of this chapter is to introduce the routine approaches in this type of modeling.

18.2 THE DOSE–RESPONSE RELATIONSHIP

The main factor in any dose–response relationship is whether the response can be measured directly or indirectly. Examples of direct responses are measurable physiologic changes such as reduction of blood pressure, reduction of intraoccular pressure, and change in the coagulation time of blood. Examples of indirect responses are changes in the serum levels of specific biomarkers such as creatine kinase MB, lactate dehydrogenase, troponin T, and endothelin 1 in cardiomyopathy evaluation. In a time-independent dose–response relationship, when the dose is zero the response is zero, and as the magnitude of dose increases the magnitude of response increases until no further increase in response can be observed with increasing the dose. This maximum response is denoted E_{max} and the dose that corresponds to half of E_{max} is D_{50}. (Figure 18.1). The scenario is analogous to the kinetics of drug metabolism discussed in Chapter 5, Section 5.6.3. In Figure 18.1 both ordinate (y axis) and abscissa (x axis) are linear. If we calibrate the abscissa logarithmically, the plot of response versus logarithm of dose will be sigmoidal as presented in Figure 18.2. The dose–response curves can also be presented as response versus concentration or logarithm of concentration.

18.2.1 Efficacy, Potency, and Affinity

The height of any point on the curve (Figure 18.1) that represents a desired pharmacologic response is a measure of the efficacy of a drug, and the width of the point from left to right is a measure of the potency the drug. Therefore, two compounds that produce the same pharmacologic response can have different efficacy and/or potency (Figures 18.3, 18.4, and 18.5). It is crucial to distinguish between "efficacy" and "potency." The term *efficacy* refers to the ability of a drug to produce a desired pharmacologic response. Therefore, it represents drug action, which is clinically significant and useful for therapeutic purposes. *Potency*, on the other hand, is related to the amount of drug required to produce a response. For example, if we are comparing two drugs, the drug that elicits the response

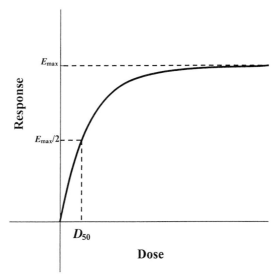

FIGURE 18.1 Hyperbolic dose–response curve. The plateau effect corresponds to maximum response, and the dose at half-maximum effect is identified as D_{50}.

with a smaller dose is considered more potent (Figure 18.6). Thus, the lower the dose necessary to create a response, the higher the potency of the drug. The physiologic processes ADME do not change the nature of the interaction of a drug with its receptor site; however, they can influence the potency of drugs significantly.

From the dose–response curves, in addition to determining the efficacy and potency of drugs, we can also assess the affinity of a drug for its receptor site. In Figures 18.5 and

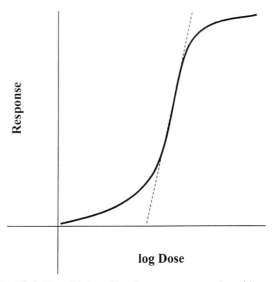

FIGURE 18.2 Sigmoidal profile of response versus logarithm of dose.

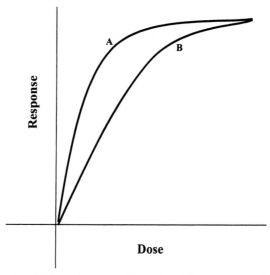

FIGURE 18.3 Drugs A and B have the same efficacy but different potency. Drug A has the greater potency.

18.6, drug A has a higher affinity and drug B has a lower affinity for the receptor site. In other words, the interaction of drug A with the receptor site, because of its shape and functional group(s), is chemically or thermodynamically more favorable than the interaction of drug B with the site. Therefore, affinity may be defined as a measure of favorable interaction between a drug and its receptor site.

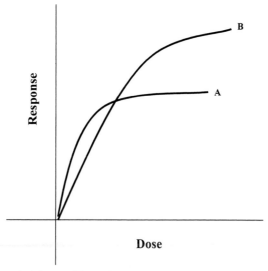

FIGURE 18.4 Drug A has lower efficacy but greater potency, whereas Drug B has greater efficacy and lower potency.

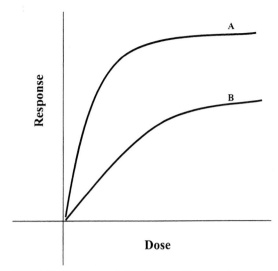

FIGURE 18.5 Drug B has lower efficacy and potency.

18.2.2 Intrinsic Activity and Antagonism

When the favorable affinity of a drug for its receptor site produces the maximum response, it is considered to have intrinsic activity and is known as an agonist. Drugs that have high affinity for a receptor site and produce drug–receptor complexes without eliciting the maximum response are known as partial agonists. Therefore, intrinsic activity represents the pharmacologic effectiveness of a drug.

Compounds that reduce or terminate the response of the agonist are known as antagonists. The antagonism can be pharmacologic or physiologic.

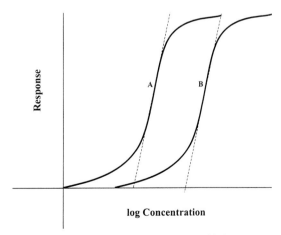

FIGURE 18.6 Both drugs, A and B, have the same E_{max}, but a higher concentration of B is needed to produce an effect comparable to that of drug A. Both drugs have similar efficacy but different potency.

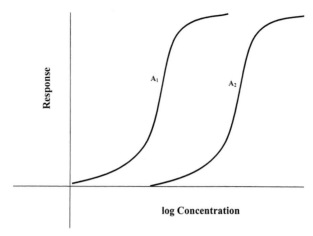

FIGURE 18.7 Competitive antagonism: A_1 represents the dose–response curve of agonist by itself. A_2 represents the full restoration of agonist in the presence of antagonist by increasing the concentration of agonist.

■ Pharmacologic antagonists are those compounds that have affinity for the receptor site of the agonist and competitively bind with little or no intrinsic activity. In other words, they occupy the receptor site without initiating any activity while preventing the agonist from binding to the site. The interaction of antagonist with the receptor site can be reversible or irreversible. The reversible interaction is competitive and can be fully overcome by increasing the concentration of the agonist (Figure 18.7). Irreversible binding is noncompetitive and increasing the concentration of agonist does not reestablish the full effect (Figure 18.8).

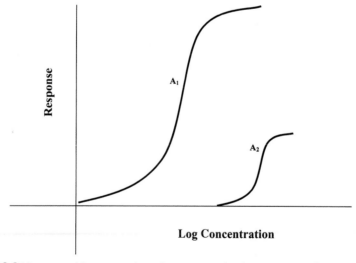

FIGURE 18.8 Noncompetitive antagonism: A_1 represents the dose response of agonist by itself. A_2 represents the effect of the noncompetitive antagonist. Increasing the concentration has no effect on restoration of the agonist's full effect.

■ Physiologic antagonists interact with receptor sites different from the agonist sites, but the interaction generates activity that antagonizes the effect of agonist. The dose–response curve of physiologic antagonism is similar to that of noncompetitive and irreversible binding (Figure 18.8). Increasing the concentration of agonist does not overcome the activity of physiologic antagonists.

18.3 DRUG–RECEPTOR INTERACTION AND THE LAW OF MASS ACTION

The interaction of drug with free receptor can be presented by the relationships

receptor [R] + drug [D] $\underset{\longleftarrow}{\longrightarrow}$ receptor–drug complex [RD] $\longrightarrow$ effect [E]

where [R] is the concentration of free receptors, [D] is the concentration of free drug in the environs of the receptor, and [RD] is the concentration of drug–receptor complex. This equation is a typical complexation reaction with the following assumptions:

1. The drug and receptor interact rather rapidly to form a drug–receptor complex.
2. Only a single molecule of drug interacts with a single receptor site.
3. Receptor, drug, and drug–receptor complex are at equilibrium.
4. The interaction is reversible.

According to the law of mass action the velocity of a reaction is proportional to the active masses of reacting substances. Based on this definition, we can define two useful constants: the association constant, K_A, and the dissociation constant, K_D, also known as the equilibrium constant:

$$K_A = \frac{[RD]}{[R][D]}$$

$$K_D = \frac{[R][D]}{[RD]} \tag{18.1}$$

If we designate the total concentration of all receptors, free and bound, as $[R_T]$, the free concentration of receptors can be defined as

$$[R] = [R_T] - [RD] \tag{18.2}$$

By substituting Equation 18.2 into Equation 18.1, we obtain the following relationships:

$$K_D = \frac{([R_T] - [RD]) \times [D]}{[RD]} = \frac{[R_T][D] - [RD][D]}{[RD]} \tag{18.3}$$

Therefore, $$[RD](K_D + [D]) = [R_T][D] \tag{18.4}$$

$$[RD] = \frac{[R_T][D]}{K_D + [D]} \tag{18.5}$$

Equation 18.5 indicates that the amount of drug bound to the receptor, [RD], is directly proportional to the concentration of free drug, [D], in the environs of the receptor. This is the same concept we followed in the previous chapters in developing equations of different models in terms of the plasma concentration of free drug. The tacit assumption was that the concentration of free drug in plasma is the same as the concentration of free drug in the environs of the receptor. If the concentration at the environs of the receptor is the same as the plasma concentration, Equation 18.5 can be written as

$$[RC_p] = \frac{[R_T][C_p]}{K_D + [C_p]} \qquad (18.6)$$

Another important assumption that is useful in defining Equations 18.5 and 18.6 is the so-called "occupancy theory." According to this theory when the molecules of drug bind to the receptor the response is initiated, and therefore the magnitude of response is proportional to the drug–receptor complex, [RD]. Furthermore, if all receptor sites, [R_T], were occupied by drug, the maximum response would be attained. Thus, the maximum response is proportional to [R_T] and Equation 18.5 can be written as

$$E = \frac{E_{max} \times [D]}{K_D + [D]} \qquad (18.7)$$

Equation 18.5 corresponds to Figure 18.1. As indicated earlier the interaction of a drug with its receptor site and the relationship between the response and the concentration of drug is similar to the interaction of drug and enzyme in drug metabolism (Chapter 5, Equation 5.19). Therefore, it can also be presented as linear relationships similar to Equations 5.29–5.31. Among the linear conversions of Equation 18.7, the following equation has wider acceptance:

$$\log \left(\frac{E}{E_{max} - E} \right) = \log[D] - \log K_D \qquad (18.8)$$

Thus, a plot of $(\log[E/(E_{max} - E])$ versus [D] is a straight line with slope of 1 and y intercept of $\log K_D$. E stands for effect, and E_{max}, the maximum effect. According to Equation 18.5 or 18.6 and Figure 18.1, when 50% of the receptor sites are occupied, that is, when $E = E_{max}/2$, the equilibrium constant K_D is equal to the drug concentration that corresponds to 50% of the maximum response, i.e.

$$\frac{E_{max}}{2} = \frac{E_{max}[D]_{50}}{K_D + [D]_{50}} \quad \text{or} \quad \frac{E_{max}}{2} = \frac{E_{max}C_{p_{50}}}{K_D + C_{p_{50}}} \qquad (18.9)$$

$$K_D = [D]_{50} = C_{p_{50}} = E_{50} \qquad (18.10)$$

18.4 PHARMACODYNAMIC MODELS OF PLASMA CONCENTRATION AND RESPONSE

Equation 18.5 and 18.6 represent the interaction of drug with receptor at the environs of the receptor and are useful for *in vitro* and *in vivo* evaluations of pharmacologic response.

Furthermore, when the response is measured as the overall therapeutic outcome, such as reduction of sugar level or blood pressure or gastric acidity, the magnitude of the outcome can also be linked to the plasma concentration of drug through other linear or nonlinear relationships. In this section we review some of these approaches, which are known as pharmacodynamic models.

18.4.1 Linear Pharmacodynamic Model

The relationship between response and plasma concentration is assumed to be linear,

$$E = mC_{\mathrm{p}} + b \tag{18.11}$$

where b is the response at time zero; that is, $b = E_0$ and when it is equal to zero, the equation changes to $E = mC_{\mathrm{p}}$. According to this model the receptor sites are never saturated. It assumes that the higher concentrations provide greater responses. This model can be useful for the correlation of response with the low concentrations of drug present when receptor sites are not fully occupied (Figure 18.9).

18.4.2 Log-linear Pharmacodynamic Model

This model is considered more practical than the linear model. It is based on the assumption that the relationship between response and logarithm of plasma concentration is linear:

$$E = m \log C_{\mathrm{p}} + b \tag{18.12}$$

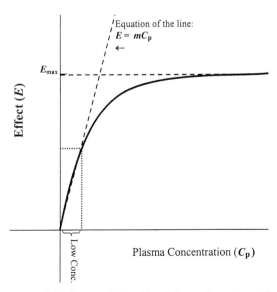

FIGURE 18.9 Divergence of the linear relationship of $E = mC_{\mathrm{p}}$ or $E = mC_{\mathrm{p}} + b$ from the hyperbolic curve of interaction of drug with receptor. The area of low concentration is the range within which the model is valid.

Equation 18.12 defines the midlinear segment of the sigmoidal curve presented in Figure 18.2. It follows that the response at time zero corresponds to the initial plasma concentration of the drug:

$$E_0 = m \log C_p^0 + b \qquad (18.13)$$

Solving for $\log C_p$ and $\log C_p^0$ provides the relationship

$$\log C_p = \frac{E - b}{m} \qquad (18.14)$$

$$\log C_p^0 = \frac{E_0 - b}{m} \qquad (18.15)$$

Substituting Equations 18.14 and 18.15 in the pharmacokinetic model with instantaneous input and first-order output (Chapter 6, Equation 6.6: $\log C_p = \log C_p^0 - Kt/2.303$), where $C_p^0 > C_p > C_{P_{MEC}}$, yields

$$\frac{E - b}{m} = \frac{E_0 - b}{m} - \frac{Kt}{2.303} \qquad (18.16)$$

Therefore,
$$E = E_0 - \frac{Ktm}{2.303} \qquad (18.17)$$

Equation 18.17 represents the time course of response as a function of the slope of the log plasma concentration–time curve $(-K/2.303)$ and slope of response (E)-versus-log C_p curve (m). By comparison of Equations 18.17 and 6.6 we can conclude that the decline in maximum response with respect to time follows zero-order kinetics, whereas the decline in plasma concentration versus time obeys first-order kinetics. Similar relationships can also be developed for an orally administered dose if only the decline in maximum response is considered. In other words, according to Equation 18.2 the maximum response can be achieved when the plasma concentration is at the highest level. As $C_{p_{max}}$ is the highest concentration after an orally administered dosage form (Chapter 8, Equation 8.28), the decline in maximum plasma concentration and maximum response between T_{max} and the time point that represents the end of duration of action is as follows:

$$\log C_p = \log C_{p_{max}} - \frac{Kt}{2.303} \qquad (18.18)$$

where $C_{p_{max}} > C_p > C_{P_{MEC}}$ and t represents any time point within the time interval of duration of action minus T_{max} (ie, $t_d - T_{max}$). Therefore,

$$E = E_{max} - \frac{Ktm}{2.303} \qquad (18.19)$$

The concept of the maximum response occurring at the maximum concentration of drug in plasma and both declining with time according to Equation 18.12 can also be used for other routes of administration when the decline in concentration is from a high to a low effective level. For example, during intravenous infusion, as long as the plasma concentration remains at steady state and within the therapeutic range, a consistent response is obtained (E_{ss}), which is independent of time; however, when the infusion is stopped and the plasma level declines, the response in the postinfusion period is defined by Equation 18.19, in which case $E_{max} = E_{ss}$.

18.4.3 E_{max} Pharmacodynamic Model

This model is based on the hyperbolic relationship of drug–receptor interaction developed by the law of mass action and presented by Equation 18.7, which in terms of concentration and assumption of Equation 18.10 can be written as

$$E = \frac{E_{max}C_p}{E_{50} + C_p} \tag{18.20}$$

An obvious characteristic of this model, as presented in Figure 18.1, is that the rise in the magnitude of response, E, versus concentration of drug occurs at certain concentrations that are less than E_{50}, and at high concentration the response reaches a plateau. The slope of this gradual increase in response as a function of concentration is determined as follows.

Because $e^{\ln C_p} = C_p$, Equation 18.20 can also be written as

$$E = \frac{E_{max}e^{\ln C_p}}{E_{50} + e^{\ln C_p}} \tag{18.21}$$

Thus, the change in response as a function of $\ln C_p$ is

$$\frac{dE}{d \ln C_p} = \frac{E_{max}C_p(E_{50} + C_p) - E_{max}C_p^2}{(E_{50} + C_p)^2} = \frac{E_{max}E_{50}C_p}{(E_{50} + C_p)^2} \tag{18.22}$$

By setting C_p equal to E_{50}, Equation 18.22 changes to

$$\frac{dE}{d \ln C_p} = \frac{E_{max}E_{50}^2}{(2E_{50})} = \frac{E_{max}E_{50}^2}{4E_{50}^2} = \frac{E_{max}}{4} \tag{18.23}$$

Thus, the slope of the rise in response as a function of $\ln C_p$ is directly proportional to the magnitude of E_{max}.

The E_{max} model can also be presented as the following logarithmic model, which is similar to Equation 18.8:

$$\log\left(\frac{E}{E_{max} - E}\right) = \log C_p - \log E_{50} \tag{18.24}$$

Similar to the Michaelis–Menten equation, at low concentrations of drug when $E_{50} \gg C_p$, the relationship between E and C_p becomes linear with a slope of E_{max}/E_{50}:

$$E = \frac{E_{max}}{E_{50}} C_p \tag{18.25}$$

Equation 18.25 corresponds to the initial linear segment of the hyperbolic curve of E versus C_p (Figure 18.1). At high concentrations of plasma, that is, when $C_p \gg E_{50}$, $E = E_{max}$, which represents the plateau line of the hyperbolic curve that is parallel to the x axis.

18.4.4 Sigmoidal E_{max} Pharmacodynamic Model

When more than one molecule of drug binds to a receptor site, the interaction between the drug molecules and receptor can be presented as

receptor [R] + drug [nD] $\rightleftharpoons$ receptor–drug complex [D_nR] $\longrightarrow$ effect [E]

The equilibrium constant, K_D, under this condition would be

$$K_D = \frac{[R][D]^n}{[D_nR]} \tag{18.26}$$

Mathematical manipulations similar to those in Equations 18.3 to 18.5 yield the equations

$$[D_nR] = \frac{[R_T] \times [D]^n}{K_D + [D]^n} \tag{18.27}$$

$$E = \frac{E_{max} \times [D]^n}{K_D + [D]^n} = \frac{E_{max} \times C_p^n}{E_{50}^n + C_p^n} \tag{18.28}$$

Equation 18.28 represents the sigmoidal curve of response versus concentration of drug. It can also be used for the curve-fitting of dose–response curves that are not visibly sigmoidal. In this case, the value of n may no longer represent the number of molecules reacting with the receptor site, but rather an element of convenience for the purpose of curve-fitting. The value of n influences the slope of the linear segment of the curve. Similar to Equation 18.23, the slope of the rise in response as a function of $\ln C_p$ is defined as

$$\frac{dE}{d \ln C_p} = \frac{n E_{max}}{4} \tag{18.29}$$

Therefore, a larger n corresponds to a sharper slope, making the linear segment of the curve more perpendicular.

Equation 18.28 can be changed into a linear relationship, similar to Equation 18.24, through the following steps:

$$\frac{E}{E_{max}} = \frac{[D]^n}{K_D + [D]^n}$$

$$[D]^n(E_{max} - E) = E \times K_D$$

$$K_D = \frac{[D]^n(E_{max} - E)}{E}$$

Taking the logarithm of both sides yields

$$\log K_D = n \log[D] + \log \frac{E_{max} - E}{E}$$

$$-\log \frac{E_{max} - E}{E} = -\log K_D + n \log D$$

Therefore,

$$\log \frac{E}{E_{max} - E} = n \log[D] - \log K_D \qquad (18.30)$$

Thus, a plot of $\log E/(E_{max} - E)$ versus $\log[D]$ provides a linear relationship with slope of n and y intercept of $\log K_D$. When $E = (E_{max})/2$, $E/(E_{max} - E) = 1$, and $\log 1 = 0$, $n \log[D] = \log K_D$; that is, $\log K_D = n \log E_{50}$, or $K_D = E_{50}^n$.

18.5 PHARMACOKINETIC–PHARMACODYNAMIC MODELING

In the preceding chapters we discussed equations related to pharmacokinetic (PK) models that essentially define the time course of plasma concentration of drugs. In this chapter we have discussed some of the pharmacodynamic (PD) models that represent the relationship between the response and plasma concentration. PK–PD linking provides useful information such as the relationship between the half-life of a drug and the duration of response. The linkage between PK and PD models is based on the assumption that was stated for linear pharmacokinetic models: "the concentration of free drug in plasma is proportional to the concentration at the receptor site." If the response fluctuates in parallel with the rise and fall of plasma concentration, the linkage between the two models is direct and often as simple as the correlation between the measured plasma concentration and the magnitude of response. The accuracy of the direct correlation depends on simultaneous measurements of plasma concentration and response. When simultaneous measurements are not feasible, the linkage may be achieved directly by substituting the calculated plasma concentration at various times of measurement of response into PD models. The calculated plasma concentration is determined with the use of PK equations. The tacit assumption in substitution of calculated plasma concentration in PD models is that the concentration at the receptor site is the same as the plasma concentration. If the concentration of drug in the receptor environs is proportional to but not the same as the plasma concentration, a separate compartment is needed to define the amount/concentration in the receptor environs. This separate compartment is known as the effect compartment. We discuss both approaches in the following sections.

18.6 CONNECTING THE E_{max} MODEL TO PHARMACOKINETIC MODELS BY DIRECT SUBSTITUTION

This type of linkage is similar to the approach presented in Section 18.4.2, Equations 18.12 to 18.19, for a log-linear pharmacodynamic model. The assumption that concentration at the receptor sites is the same as plasma concentration enables us to write the following relationships for one- and multicompartment models. In the case of a one-compartment model, the receptor sites or biophase is assumed to be associated with the systemic circulation (Figure 18.10). In the case of a two-compartment model, the biophase can be associated with the central or peripheral compartment (Figure 18.11). This type of PK–PD modeling may be used to predict the response from the calculated or observed plasma concentration.

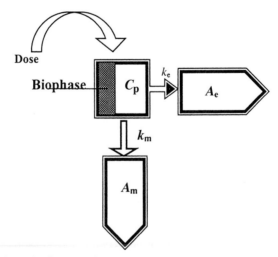

FIGURE 18.10 Schematic diagram of biophase as being associated with the systemic circulation of a one-compartment model.

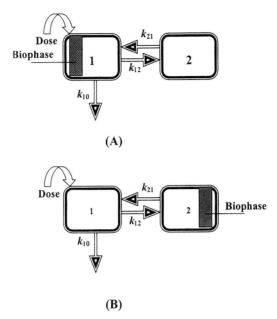

FIGURE 18.11 Schematic diagram of biophase as being associated with the central compartment (A) or peripheral compartment (B) of a two-compartment model.

18.6.1 Connecting the E_{max} Model to the One-compartment Model

18.6.1.1 Intravenous Bolus Injection

$$E = \frac{E_{max}C_p^0 e^{-Kt}}{E_{50} + C_p^0 e^{-Kt}} \tag{18.31}$$

Dividing the numerator and denominator of Equation 18.31 by C_p^0 yields

$$E = \frac{E_{max}e^{-Kt}}{E_{50}/C_p^0 + e^{-Kt}} = \frac{E_{max}f_b}{f_{b_{50}} + f_b} \tag{18.32}$$

where $f_{b_{50}}$ is the fraction of administered dose in the body that provides an effect equal to 50% of E_{max}. It represents the potency of the drug. A smaller $f_{b_{50}}$ is indicative of a more potent drug. From Equation 18.32 it can be concluded that 50% of the response may not correspond to 50% of the dose in the body. The only time that it may is when $f_{b_{50}} = 0.5$.

18.6.1.2 Intravenous Infusion: Substituting the equations of intravenous infusion (Chapter 7, Equations 7.4 and 7.5) for the concentration term in the E_{max} model gives the following relationships. Before achieving steady-state level,

$$E = \frac{E_{max}C_{p_{ss}}(1 - e^{-Kt})}{E_{50} + C_{p_{ss}}(1 - e^{-Kt})} = \frac{E_{max}(1 - e^{-Kt})}{E_{50}/C_{p_{ss}} + (1 - e^{-Kt})} = \frac{E_{max}(f_{ss})}{f_{ss_{50}} + f_{ss}} \tag{18.33}$$

At steady state,

$$E = \frac{E_{max}}{f_{ss50} + 1} \tag{18.34}$$

where f_{ss50} is the fraction of the steady-state plasma concentration that produces an effect equal to 50% of E_{max}.

18.6.1.3 Oral Administration: The E_{max} model after replacing C_p with the equation of oral administration (Chapter 8, Equation 8.20) is

$$E = \frac{E_{max}(\tilde{C}_p^0(e^{-Kt} - e^{-k_a t}))}{E_{50} + \tilde{C}_p^0(e^{-Kt} - e^{-k_a t})} = \frac{E_{max}(e^{-Kt} - e^{-k_a t})}{E_{50}/\tilde{C}_p^0 + (e^{-Kt} - e^{-k_a t})} \tag{18.35}$$

Equation 18.35 determines the time course of effect during the absorption process. When the absorption is complete the term $e^{-k_a t} \rightarrow 0$ and the equation changes to

$$E = \frac{E_{max}e^{-Kt}}{E_{50}/\tilde{C}_p^0 + e^{-Kt}} \tag{18.36}$$

The response, which is related to the maximum plasma concentration, can be estimated as

$$E = \frac{E_{max}(FD/V_d)e^{-KT_{max}}}{E_{50} + (FD/V_d)e^{-KT_{max}}} = \frac{E_{max}FDe^{-KT_{max}}}{(E_{50}V_d) + FDe^{-KT_{max}}} \tag{18.37}$$

According to Equation 18.37 the only time the maximum response can be associated with the maximum plasma concentration is when $C_{p_{max}} \gg E_{50}$, and when $E_{50} = C_{p_{max}}$, $E = E_{max}/2$.

18.6.1.4 Multiple Dosing: To estimate the responses that are associated with the peak and trough levels of a multiple-dosing regimen and to predict the fluctuation of response, equations 10.11 and 10.12 were substituted in Equation 18.20 to obtain the relationships

$$E_{peak} = \frac{E_{max} \times \dfrac{C_p^0}{1 - e^{-K\tau}}}{E_{50} + \dfrac{C_p^0}{1 - e^{-K\tau}}} = \frac{E_{max}C_p^0}{E_{50}(1 - e^{-K\tau}) + C_p^0} = \frac{E_{max}C_p^0}{E_{50}(f_{el})_\tau + C_p^0} \tag{18.38}$$

where $(f_{el})_\tau$, as described in Equation 10.19, is the fraction of dose eliminated in one dosing interval at steady state and C_p^0 is the initial plasma concentration of a maintenance dose.

$$E_{trough} = \frac{E_{max} \dfrac{C_p^0 e^{-K\tau}}{1 - e^{-K\tau}}}{E_{50} + \dfrac{C_p^0 e^{-K\tau}}{1 - e^{-K\tau}}} = \frac{E_{max}C_p^0}{E_{50}\left(\dfrac{1 - e^{-K\tau}}{e^{-K\tau}}\right) + C_p^0} = \frac{E_{max}C_p^0}{\left(\dfrac{E_{50}}{e^{-K\tau}} - 1\right) + C_p^0} \tag{18.39}$$

Therefore, the fluctuation of the response at steady state caused by giving a maintenance dose is

$$E_{\text{fluctuation}} = E_{\text{peak}} - E_{\text{trough}} \tag{18.40}$$

The average response at steady state can be determined by replacing C_p in Equation 18.20 with Equation 10.17 (Chapter 10):

$$E_{\text{ave}} = \frac{E_{\max}\dfrac{C_p^0}{K\tau}}{E_{50} + \dfrac{C_p^0}{K\tau}} = \frac{E_{\max} \times C_p^0}{E_{50}(K\tau) + C_p^0} = \frac{E_{\max} \times \text{AUC}}{E_{50}(\tau) + \text{AUC}} = \frac{E_{\max}D}{E_{50}(\text{Cl}_t\tau) + D} \tag{18.41}$$

Equations of response from multiple oral administration are similar to Equations 18.38 to 18.41.

18.6.2 Connecting the $E_{\max}$ Model to the Two-compartment Model

18.6.2.1 Single-dose IV Bolus: Central Compartment: By substituting equation 11.6 for C_p in Equation 18.20 we obtain

$$E = \frac{E_{\max} \times (ae^{-\alpha t} + be^{-\beta t})}{E_{50} + (ae^{-\alpha t} + be^{-\beta t})} \tag{18.42}$$

The response in the postdistributive phase can be predicted by

$$E = \frac{E_{\max}be^{-\beta t}}{E_{50} + be^{-\beta t}} \tag{18.43}$$

18.6.2.2 Multiple-dosing Two-compartment Model: Central Compartment: Equations for prediction of response during steady state for a drug that follows a two-compartment model are

$$E_{\text{peak}} = \frac{E_{\max}(C_{p_{\max}})_{\text{ss}}}{E_{50} + (C_{p_{\max}})_{\text{ss}}} \tag{18.44}$$

where, as presented in Equation 12.11,

$$(C_{p_{\max}}) = \frac{a}{1 - e^{-\alpha\tau}} + \frac{b}{1 - e^{-\beta\tau}}$$

$$E_{\text{trough}} = \frac{E_{\max}(C_{p_{\min}})_{\text{ss}}}{E_{50} + (C_{p_{\min}})_{\text{ss}}} \tag{18.45}$$

where $(C_{p\min})_{ss}$ is, as defined in Equation 12.12,

$$(C_{p\min})_{ss} = \frac{ae^{-\alpha\tau}}{1 - e^{-\alpha\tau}} + \frac{be^{-\beta\tau}}{1 - e^{-\beta\tau}}$$

18.6.2.3 Single-dose IV Bolus: Peripheral Compartment

When the receptor sites are considered to be associated with the peripheral compartment the equation of the model can be presented as

$$E = \frac{E_{\max}\left(\dfrac{k_{12}D}{\alpha - \beta}(e^{-\beta t} - e^{-\alpha})\right)}{E_{50} + \left(\dfrac{k_{12}D}{\alpha - \beta}(e^{-\beta t} - e^{-\alpha})\right)} \qquad (18.46)$$

18.7 CONNECTING THE SIGMOIDAL $E_{\max}$ MODEL TO PHARMACOKINETIC MODELS BY DIRECT SUBSTITUTION

18.7.1 One-compartment Model

Equations similar to Equations 18.31 to 18.45 can be developed for the sigmoidal $E_{\max}$ model:

18.7.1.1 IV Bolus Injection:

$$E = \frac{E_{\max} f_{b}^{n}}{f_{b\,50}^{n} + f_{b}^{n}} \qquad (18.47)$$

18.7.1.2 IV Infusion: Before achieving steady-state level,

$$E = \frac{E_{\max} f_{ss}^{n}}{f_{ss50}^{n} + f_{ss}^{n}} \qquad (18.48)$$

At steady state,

$$E = \frac{E_{\max}}{f_{ss50}^{n} + 1} \qquad (18.49)$$

18.7.1.3 Oral Administration:

$$E = \frac{E_{\max}(e^{-Kt} - e^{-k_a t})^{n}}{(E_{50}/C_{p}^{0})^{n} + (e^{-Kt} - e^{-k_a t})^{n}} \qquad (18.50)$$

In the postabsorptive phase,

$$E = \frac{E_{\max}(e^{-Kt})^n}{(E_{50}/\tilde{C}_p^0)^n + (e^{-Kt})^n} \tag{18.51}$$

At maximum plasma concentration,

$$E = \frac{E_{\max}(FDe^{-KT_{\max}})^n}{(E_{50}V_d)^n + (FDe^{-KT_{\max}})^n} \tag{18.52}$$

18.7.1.4 Multiple Dosing:

$$E_{\text{peak}} = \frac{E_{\max}(C_p^0)^n}{(E_{50}(f_{el})_\tau)^n + (C_p^0)^n} \tag{18.53}$$

$$E_{\text{trough}} = \frac{E_{\max}(C_p^0)^n}{(E_{50}/e^{-K\tau} - 1)^n + (C_p^0)^n} \tag{18.54}$$

$$E_{\text{fluctuation}} = E_{\text{peak}} - E_{\text{trough}} \tag{18.55}$$

$$E_{\text{ave}} = \frac{E_{\max}(C_p^0)^n}{(E_{50}K\tau)^n + (C_p^0)^n} = \frac{E_{\max} \times (\text{AUC})^n}{(E_{50}\tau)^n + (\text{AUC})^n} = \frac{E_{\max}D^n}{(E_{50}\text{Cl}_t\tau)^n + D^n} \tag{18.56}$$

18.7.2 Connecting the Sigmoidal $E_{\max}$ Model to the Two-compartment Model

18.7.2.1 Single-dose IV Bolus:

$$E = \frac{E_{\max} \times (ae^{-\alpha t} + be^{-\beta t})^n}{(E_{50})^n + (ae^{-\alpha t} + be^{-\beta t})^n} \tag{18.57}$$

In the postdistributive phase,

$$E = \frac{E_{\max} \times (be^{-\beta t})^n}{(E_{50})^n + (be^{-\beta t})^n} \tag{18.58}$$

18.7.2.2 Multiple Dosing: Two-compartment Model:

$$E_{\text{peak}} = \frac{E_{\max}(C_{p_{\max}})_{ss}^n}{(E_{50})^n + (C_{p_{\max}})_{ss}^n} \tag{18.59}$$

where

$$(C_{p_{\max}})_{ss} = \frac{a}{1 - e^{-\alpha\tau}} + \frac{b}{1 - e^{-\beta\tau}}$$

$$E_{\text{trough}} = \frac{E_{\max}(C_{p_{\min}})_{ss}^n}{(E_{50})^n + (C_{p_{\min}})_{ss}^n} \tag{18.60}$$

where

$$(C_{p_{min}})_{ss} = \frac{ae^{-\alpha\tau}}{1 - e^{-\alpha\tau}} + \frac{be^{-\beta\tau}}{1 - e^{-\beta\tau}}$$

18.7.2.3 IV Bolus Injection: Peripheral Compartment:

$$E = \frac{E_{max}\left(\dfrac{k_{12}D}{\alpha - \beta} \left(e^{-\beta t} - e^{-\alpha}\right)\right)^n}{(E_{50})^n + \left(\dfrac{k_{12}D}{\alpha - \beta} \left(e^{-\beta t} - e^{-\alpha}\right)\right)^n} \tag{18.61}$$

18.8 PK–PD MODELING: EFFECT COMPARTMENT

In the above discussion it was assumed that the concentration of drug at the receptor site is the same as the plasma concentration. This means that the drug in the receptor environs can reach rapid equilibrium with the plasma concentration. There are, however, receptor environs that do not reach rapid equilibrium with plasma, such as receptors in regions separated from plasma by a physiologic barrier or associated with the intracellular environment or located in the regions in which blood perfusion is poor. For this type of receptor the direct method of substitution may not be pertinent. One of the reasons is that the interaction of drug with this type of receptor occurs after a lag time or a threshold of response, which the direct method of substitution cannot predict. Thus, a different approach based on determining the amount or concentration of drug at the receptor site is needed. An interesting and accepted approach is to consider a hypothetical effect compartment as representing the receptor environs with the following assumptions (Figures 18.12 and 18.13):

- The effect compartment is in contact with the systemic circulation.
- The transfer of drug from the systemic circulation to the effect compartment is governed by a first-order process.
- The first-order rate constant of drug transfer from the systemic circulation to the effect compartment and the amount in the effect compartment are negligible with respect to the overall disposition of drug in the body.

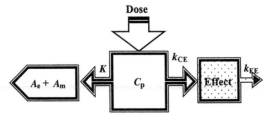

FIGURE 18.12 PK–PD one-compartment model: The effect compartment is presented as a separate compartment associated with the systemic circulation with input rate constant k_{CE} and exit rate constant k_{EE}. Dose is given by any route of administration. K is the overall elimination rate constant.

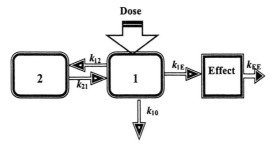

FIGURE 18.13 PK–PD two-compartment model. The effect compartment is associated with the central compartment. k_{12} and k_{21} are the first-order distribution rate constants, k_{10} is the overall elimination rate constant, and k_{1E} and k_{EE} are the input and exit rate constants of the effect compartment. Dose is by any route of administration.

- At steady state the concentration of drug in the effect compartment is the same as in systemic circulation.
- The effect compartment has a first-order exit rate constant that is also small and considered a negligible value.

The concentration of drug in the effect compartment can then be substituted in PD models.

Based on the diagram presented in Figures 18.12 and 18.13, the rates of change of amount of drug in the systemic circulation and the effect compartment can be presented in five categories.

18.8.1 IV Bolus Dose

$$\frac{dA}{dt} = -KA$$

$$\frac{dA_E}{dt} = k_{CE}A - k_{EE}A_E \tag{18.62}$$

Solving the two differential equations by the method of Laplace transforms (Chapter 1) yields the integrated equations

$$A = De^{-Kt}$$

$$A_E = \frac{k_{CE}D}{k_{EE} - K}\ (e^{-Kt} - e^{-k_{EE}t}) \tag{18.63}$$

A_E is the amount of drug in the effect compartment at time t, K is the overall elimination rate constant, and k_{CE} and k_{EE} are the input and exit rate constants of the effect compartment, respectively.

Calculation of the concentration of drug in the effect compartment requires knowledge of its apparent volume of distribution. Because at steady state the concentration of drug in the effect compartment is assumed to be equal to plasma concentration, one approach would be to determine a relevant proportionality constant between the apparent volume of distribution of drug in plasma and the volume of the effect compartment.

At steady state rate of input = rate of output or $k_{CE}C_pV_d = k_{EE}C_EV_E$. Therefore,

$$V_E = V_d \frac{k_{CE}C_p}{k_{EE}C_E}$$

As $C_p = C_E$

$$V_E = V_d \frac{k_{CE}}{k_{EE}} \qquad (18.64)$$

Thus, the concentration of drug in the effect compartment can be estimated as

$$C_E = A_E/V_E$$

18.8.2 Zero-order Infusion

Before steady-state level is achieved,

$$C_p = \frac{k_0}{KV_d}(1 - e^{-Kt})$$

$$A_E = \frac{k_{CE}k_0}{K(k_{EE} - K)}(1 - e^{-Kt}) + \frac{k_{CE}k_0}{k_{EE}(K - k_{EE})}(1 - e^{-k_{EE}t}) \qquad (18.65)$$

After infusion is stopped,

$$C_p = \frac{k_0}{KV_d}(1 - e^{-Kt})e^{-Kt'}$$

$$A_E = \frac{k_{CE}k_0}{K(k_{EE} - K)}(1 - e^{-Kt})e^{-Kt'} + \frac{k_{CE}k_0}{k_{EE}(K - k_{EE})}(1 - e^{-k_{EE}t})e^{-k_{EE}t'} \qquad (18.66)$$

At steady state,

$$C_{p_{ss}} = \frac{k_0}{KV_d}$$

$$A_E = \frac{k_{CE}k_0}{K(k_{EE} - K)} + \frac{k_{CE}k_0}{k_{EE}(K - k_{EE})} \qquad (18.67)$$

18.8.3 First-order Input

$$C_p = \frac{k_a FD}{V_d(k_a - K)} (e^{-Kt} - e^{-k_a t})$$

$$A_e = \frac{k_{CE} k_a FD}{(K - k_a)(k_{EE} - k_a)} e^{-k_a t} + \frac{k_{CE} k_a FD}{(k_a - K)(k_{EE} - K)} e^{-Kt} + \frac{k_{CE} k_a FD}{(k_a - k_{EE})(K - k_{EE})} e^{-k_{EE} t}$$

(18.68)

18.8.4 Multiple IV Injections

At steady-state peak level,

$$(C_{p_{max}})_{ss} = \frac{D}{V_d} \left(\frac{1}{1 - e^{-K\tau}} \right)$$

$$A_E = \frac{k_{CE} D}{(k_{EE} - K)} \left(\frac{1}{1 - e^{-K\tau}} - \frac{1}{1 - e^{-k_{EE}\tau}} \right)$$

(18.69)

At steady-state trough level,

$$(C_{p_{min}})_{ss} = \frac{D}{V_d} \left(\frac{e^{-K\tau}}{1 - e^{-K\tau}} \right)$$

$$A_E = \frac{k_{CE} D}{(k_{EE} - K)} \left(\frac{e^{-K\tau}}{1 - e^{-K\tau}} - \frac{e^{-k_{EE}\tau}}{1 - e^{-k_{EE}\tau}} \right)$$

(18.70)

At steady state at any point,

$$(C_{p_{min}})_{ss} = \frac{D}{V_d} \left(\frac{e^{-Kt}}{1 - e^{-K\tau}} \right)$$

$$A_E = \frac{k_{CE} D}{(k_{EE} - K)} \left(\frac{e^{-Kt}}{1 - e^{-K\tau}} - \frac{e^{-k_{EE}\tau}}{1 - e^{-k_{EE}\tau}} \right)$$

(18.71)

18.8.5 Two-compartment Model: IV Injection

$$C_p = Ae^{-\alpha t} + Be^{-\beta t}$$

$$A_E = \frac{k_{CE}}{(k_{EE} - \alpha)} Ae^{-\alpha t} + \frac{k_{CE}}{(k_{EE} - \beta)} Be^{-\beta t} + \frac{k_{CE} D(k_{21} - k_{EE})}{(\alpha - k_{EE})(\beta - k_{EE})} e^{-k_{EE} t}$$

(18.72)

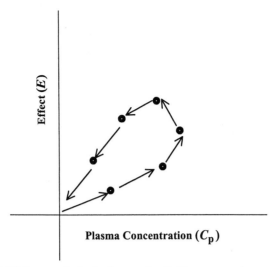

FIGURE 18.14 Counterclockwise hysteresis of effect versus plasma concentration.

Equations 18.63 to 18.72 are used to estimate the amount of drug in the effect compartment. Once the apparent volume of distribution of the effect compartment is calculated, the amount of drug in the compartment, A_E, can be converted to concentration, C_E, which can then be substituted for the concentration term in the pharmacodynamic models. The pharmacokinetic parameters of the plasma concentration, effect compartment, and pharmacodynamic E_{max} model can be estimated simultaneously only with appropriate software of nonlinear regression analysis.

18.9 HYSTERESIS CURVE

PK–PD models attempt to relate the plasma concentration to the magnitude of response. When the response is plotted against plasma concentration according to their time order a loop with a clockwise or counterclockwise direction can be obtained (Figure 18.14). The direction of the loop determines the latency of the pharmacologic response. A counterclockwise direction is usually associated with the delay or threshold of response. The delay of response can be indicative of slow equilibration of plasma concentration with the receptor environs or increase in the concentration of receptor or its activity. Theoretically, failure of the hysteresis of E versus C_p to collapse on plotting E versus concentration of effect compartment, C_E, may indicate that the delay in the pharmacologic response is related to the upregulation of receptors.

BIBLIOGRAPHY

1. Colburn WA. Simultaneous pharmacokinetic and pharmacodynamic modeling. *J Pharmacokinet Biopharm* 1981;9:367.
2. Fuseau E, Sheiner LB. Simultaneous modeling of pharmacokinetics and pharmacodynamics with a nonparametric pharmacodynamic model. *Clin Pharmacol Ther* 1984;35:733.

3. Hochhaus G, Derendorf H. Dose optimization based on pharmacokinetic–pharmacodynamic modeling. In: Derendorf H, Hochhaus G, editors. *Pharmacokinetic/pharmacodynamic correlation.* Boca Raton, FL: CRC Press, 1995: ch 4.

4. Holford NHG, Scheiner LB. Understanding the dose–effect relationship: clinical application of pharmacokinetic–pharmacodynamic models. *Clin Pharmacokinet* 1981;6:429.

5. Hull CJ, Van Beem HBH, McLeod K, Sibbald A, Watson MJ. A pharmacodynamic model for pancuronium. *Br J Anaesthesiol* 1978;50:1113.

6. Lalonde RL. Pharmacokinetic–pharmacodynamic relationships of cardiovascular drugs. In: Derendorf H, Hochhaus G, editors. *Pharmacokinetic/pharmacodynamic correlation.* Boca Raton, FL: CRC Press, 1995: ch 9.

7. Segre G. Kinetics of interaction between drugs and biological systems. *Farmaco* 1968;23:906.

8. Sheiner LB, Stanski DR, Vozeh S, Miller RD, Ham J. Simultaneous modeling of pharmacokinetics and pharmacodynamics: application to D-tubocurarine. *Clin Pharmacol Ther* 1979; 25:358.

9. Tallardia RJ, Jacob LS. *The dose–response relation in pharmacology.* New York: Springer-Verlag, 1979: 1–17.

10. Unadkat JD, Bartha F, Sheiner LB. Simultaneous modeling of pharmacokinetics and pharmacodynamics with nonparametric kinetics and dynamic model. *Clin Pharmacol Ther* 1980;40:86.

11. Vaidyanathan S, Boroujerdi M. Effect of tamoxifen pretreatment on the pharmacokinetics, metabolism and cardiotoxicity of doxorubicin in female rats. *Cancer Chemother Pharmacol* 2000; 46:185.

12. Venitz J. Pharmacokinetic–pharmacodynamic modeling of reversible drug effects. In Derendorf H, Hochhaus G, editors. *Pharmacokinetic/pharmacodynamic Correlation.* Boca Raton, FL: CRC Press, 1995: ch 1.

13. Verotta D, Sheiner LB. Simultaneous modeling of pharmacokinetics and pharmacodynamics: an improved algorithm, *Comput Appl Biosci* 1987;3:345.

14. Vora J, Boroujerdi M. Pharmacokinetic–toxicodynamic relationship of adriamycin in rat: prediction of a phenolic antioxidant mediated reduction in anthracycline cardiotoxicity. *J Pharm Pharmacol* 1996;48:1264.

15. Wada DR. Closed-loop stability of pharmacokinetic–pharmacodynamic models. *Math Biosci* 1997;146:75.

16. Wagner JG. Kinetics of pharmacological response. I. Proposed relationships between response and drug concentration in the intact animal and man. *J Theor Biol* 1968;20:173.

ASSIGNMENT ANSWERS

CHAPTER ONE

1. $Y = (20 \times 0.2)\, e^{(3+4)} = 4e^7$
2. $Y = 10e^{-(0.5+0.9)} = 10e^{0.4}$
3. $Y = e^{(5-7)} = e^{-2} = 1/e^2$
4. $Y = (e^{-5})^{-2}/(e^{-3})^{-2} = e^{10}/e^6 = e^4$
5. $Y = e^{-4} = 1/e^4$
6. $Y = (2e^0)^{-3} = 2^{-3} = \frac{1}{2}^3 = 1/8$
7. $Y = (15 \times 0.2)\, e^{(0.8+0.1)} = 3e^{0.3}$
8. $Y = e^{0.6}/e^{0.2} = e^{0.4}$
9. $Y = (e^{1/3})^2 = (e^2)^{1/3}$
10. $Y = \frac{1}{2}\,(1 - e^{-0.2}) = \frac{1}{2} - 1/(2e^{0.2})$
11. $16 = 4^4$
12. $2 = 4^{1/2}$
13. $1/9 = 3^{-2}$
14. $x = 10^3$
15. $x = 10^6$
16. $x = e^{0.2}$
17. $x = e^{-0.3}$
18. $x = 10^{-0.2}$
19. $x = (10^{0.2}) - 1 = 0.584$
20. $x = e^{0.6} - 2 = -0.177$
21. $\log_4 64 = 3$
22. $\log_2(1/8) = -3$
23. $\log Y = 5$
24. $\log Y = -2$
25. $\log Y = -(0.5/2.303)$
26. $\log Y = \log 10 - (0.1/2.303)$
27. $\log Y = \log 5 - (4.5/2.3030)$
28. $\log Y = -2/2.303$
29. $\log Y = \log 200 - (2.2/2.303)$
30. $\log Y = \log 50 + (1.6/2.303)$
31. $dy/dx = 2x/(x^2 - 1)$
32. $dy/dx = 3(\ln x)^2/x$

33. $dy/dx = 4/x$

34. $dy/dx = -2x \exp(-x^2)$

35. $dy/dx = -3e^{-x}$

36. $dy/dx = -12e^{-3x}$

37. $dy/dx = 40e^{-2t} - 4e^{-0.2t}$

38. $dy/dx = 3e^{3x-2}$

39. $dy/dx = 18x^2 - 3e^{-x}$

40. $dy/dx = -5/x$

41. $y = A (a^{-1} - b^{-1})$

42. $y = A/a$

43. $y = A/a + B/b$

44. $y = (1/A)(a^{-1} - b^{-1})$

45. $y = \ln x^4$

46. $\ln y = \ln y^0 - kt$

47. $y = y^0 + kt$

48. $y = \ln x^{-5}$

49. $y = 40/a - 30/b$

50. $y = 20/a$

51. Area $= (20(e^{-4}/-4) - 15(e^{-0.2}/0.2)) - ((20/-4) - (15/0.2)) \cong 18.55$

52. Area $= 100((e^{-2.5}/-0.5) - (e^{-0.5}/-0.5)) \cong 104.90$

53. Area $= 50((e^{-1.386}/-0.693) + (e^{-12.6}/6.93) + (1/0.693) - (1/6.93)) \cong 46.9$

54. Area $= 0.5((e^6/2) + (e^{-0.6}/0.2) - (1/2) - (1/0.2) \cong 99.477$

55. Area $= (10(e^{-0.4}/-0.1) - 8(e^{-0.2}/0.05)) - ((10/-0.1) - (8/0.05)) \cong 91.973$

56. Area$_{0 \to 5\ h}$ = $(0.05(0.1)) + (0.05(0.35)) + (0.1(1.25)) + (0.1(4.5)) + (0.2(7.25)) =$ 2.047 mg h/L

57. AUC$_{0 \to 350\ min}$ = 1258.60 mg min/L or μg min/mL $\cong$ 21 mg h/L

TABLE A1.1 Data Related to the Answer to Assignment 1.57

$t_{i+1} - t_i$	10	10	20	20	30	30	60	60	110
$(C_{p_{i+1}} + C_p)_2$	0.12	0.42	2.80	6.40	8.00	7.35	5.15	2.85	1.17
Area$_{i \to i+1}$	1.2	4.2	56	128	240	220.5	309	171	128.7

58. Part 1—Using trapezoid rule:

TABLE A1.2 Data Related to Solution to Assignment 1.58

$t_{midpoint}$	0.25	0.75	1.25	1.75	2.25	2.75	3.25	3.75	4.25	4.75
$C_{p_{midpoint}}$	23.30	11.14	6.68	4.52	3.26	2.44	1.88	1.47	1.17	0.94

$$AUC_{0 \to 5\ h} = 0.5(23.30 + 11.14 + 6.68 + 4.52 + 3.26 + 2.44 + 1.88 + 1.47 + 1.17 + 0.94) = 28.4 \text{ mg h/L}$$

Part 2—Using integration:
$$AUC_{0 \to 5\ h} = 0 - 0.025 - 2.03 + 6.5 + 10 + 15 = 29.445 \text{ mg h/L}$$

Part 3—$AUC_{0 \to \infty}$ using trapezoid rule:
$$C_{p_n} = 20e^{-3.2(5)} + 12e^{-1.2(5)} + 6e^{-0.4(5)} = 0.841 \text{ mg/L}$$

Terminal area = $0.812/0.4 = 2.03$ mg h/L
$$AUC_{0 \to \infty} = 28.4 + 2.03 = 30.43 \text{ mg h/L}$$

Part 3—$AUC_{0 \to \infty}$ using integrated equation:
$$AUC = (20/3.2) + (12/1.2) + (6/0.4) = 31.50 \text{ mg h/L}$$

59.

1. $\overline{A} = \dfrac{A_D^0}{s + K}$ $\qquad \to A = A_D^0 e^{-Kt}$

2. $\overline{A}_e = \dfrac{k_{12} A_D^0}{s(s + K)}$ $\qquad \to A_e = \dfrac{k_{12} A_D^0}{K}(1 - e^{-Kt})$

3. $\overline{A} = \dfrac{k_{13} A_D^0}{(s + k_{34})(s + K)}$ $\to A_m = \dfrac{k_{13} A_D^0}{K - k_{34}}(e^{-k_{34}t} - e^{-Kt})$

4. $\overline{A} = \dfrac{k_{34} k_{13} A_D^0}{s(s + k_{34})(s + K)}$ $\to A_{me} = \dfrac{k_{13} A_D^0}{K}\left[1 + \dfrac{1}{k_{34} - K}(Ke^{-k_{34}t} - k_{34}e^{-Kt})\right]$

CHAPTER 4

4.1 Slope = -8636.36
  $K_a = 8636.36$ L/mol
  $n = (23{,}000 + 0.736\,(8636))/8636.36 = 3.4$
4.2 Fraction bound = $(0.8 \times 10^{-3})/(1.4 \times 10^{-3}) = 0.57$
  Free fraction = $1 - 0.57 = 0.43$
  $r = (0.8 \times 10^{-3})/(1 \times 10^{-4}) = 8$
4.3 Slope = $(0.039 - 0.133)/(3.2 - 0.64) = -0.036$
  $K_a = 0.036$
  $n = (0.133 + (0.64 \times 0.036))/0.036 = 4.33$
4.4 $n = 1/0.2 = 5$
  $K_a = (1/0.002)(0.2) = 100$ L/μmol
4.5 $n = 500/250 = 2$
  $K_a = 250$ L/mmol

CHAPTER 5

5.1 Lineweaver–Burk Plot:
  $1/v = 0.0654 + 0.498/[D]$
  $V_{max} = 15.29\ \mu\text{mol L}^{-1}\ \text{min}^{-1}$
  $K_M = 7.61 \mu\text{mol L}^{-1}$
  Hanes plot:
  $[D]/v = 0.492 + 0.0662[D]$
  $V_{max} = 15.10\ \mu\text{mol L}^{-1}\ \text{min}^{-1}$
  $K_M = 7.43 \mu\text{mol L}^{-1}$

Eadie–Hofstee plot:

$v = 15.2 - 7.56\ v/[D]$

$V_{max} = 15.2\ \mu mol\ L^{-1}\ min^{-1}$

$K_M = 7.56\ \mu mol\ L^{-1}$

5.2.1 $V_{max} = 28.57\ \mu mol\ L^{-1}\ min^{-1}$ $K_M = 19.23\ \mu mol\ L^{-1}$

5.2.2 $V_{max} = 54\ \mu mol\ L^{-1}\ min^{-1}$ $K_M = 54\ \mu mol\ L^{-1}$

5.2.3 $V_{max} = 100\ \mu mol\ L^{-1}\ min^{-1}$ $K_M = 20\ \mu mol\ L^{-1}$

5.2.4 $V_{max} = 20\ \mu mol\ L^{-1}\ min^{-1}$ $K_M = 4.6\ \mu mol\ L^{-1}$

5.2.5 $V_{max} = 110\ \mu mol\ L^{-1}\ min^{-1}$ $K_M = 29\ \mu mol\ L^{-1}$

5.2.6 $V_{max} = 13.33\ \mu mol\ L^{-1}\ min^{-1}$ $K_M = 1.28\ \mu mol\ L^{-1}$

CHAPTER 6

6.1

Part One: 6.1.1

Plot of log Cp versus Time (Treatment A) - Assignment 6.1.1

Y = 2.38975 - 0.344304X
R-Sq = 0.997

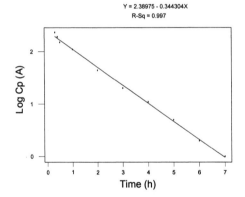

Plot of log Cp versus Time (Treatment B) - Assignment 6.1.1

Y = 2.49909 - 0.337222X
R-Sq = 0.997

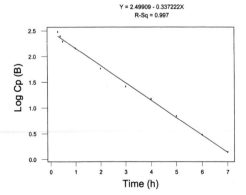

Part One: 6.1.2

TABLE A1.3 Data Related to the Solution to Assignment 6.1—Part Two

Treatment	$T_{1/2}$ (h)	K (h^{-1})	AUC (mg h/L)	Cl_t (L/h)	Cl_t (mL/min)	t_d (h)	$(f_o)_{t=1 h}$
A	0.88	0.79	310.70	6.44	107.34	1.70	0.454
B	0.90	0.77	410.70	4.87	81.16	2.70	0.463

Part One: 6.1.3 Class discussion

Part Two: 6.1.4–6.1.7

TABLE A1.4 Data Related to the Solution to Assignment 6.1—Part Two (6.1.4–6.1.7)

$T_{1/2}$ (h)	K (h^{-1})	C_p^0 (mg/L)	V_d (L)	AUC (mg h/L)	Cl_t (L/h)	Cl_t (mL/min)	$C_{P_{10 h}}$ (mg/L)
2.04	0.34	478.60	4.20	1408	1.42	23.67	16

Part Two: 6.1.8 Class discussion

6.2

6.2.1 50% $(C_p^0)_B = 75$ mg/L; therefore, $(T_{1/2})_B = 4$ h
  $(t_d)_B = 3.3 \times 4$ h $= 13.2$ h
  $(T_{1/2})_A = 2$ h
  $(t_d)_A = 4.3 \times 2$ h $= 8.6$ h
6.2.2 $(t)_{95\%} = 4.3 \times 2$ h $= 8.6$ h
6.2.3 $(t_d)_A = 8.6 + 2 = 10.6$ h
  $(t_d)_B = 13.2 + 4 = 17.2$ h
6.2.4 $(V_d)_A = 7$ L
  Dose $= 7$ L $\times 300$ mg/L $= 2100$ mg
  $(V_d)_B = 2100$ mg/150 mg/L $= 14$ L
  Amount eliminated in $2T_{1/2} = 0.75 \times 2100 = 1575$ mg
6.2.5 $K_A = 0.693/2$ h $= 0.3465$ h^{-1}; therefore, $(AUC)_A = 300/0.3465 = 866$ mg h/L
  $K_B = 0.693/4$ h $= 0.1732$ h^{-1}; therefore, $(AUC)_B = 150/0.1732 = 866$ mg h/L

6.3

6.3.1 $f_b = 10\%$
6.3.2 $f_{el} = 0.75$

6.3.3 $T_{1/2} = 5$ h

6.3.4 $f_b = 0.92$

6.3.5 Initial rate = 240 mg/h

6.3.6 K = 0.1155 h^{-1}

6.3.7 Dose = 2 g

6.3.8 Dose = 100 mg

6.3.9 $T_{1/2} = 2$ h

6.3.10 $T_{1/2} = 10$ h

6.3.11 $Cl_t = 30$ L/h

6.3.12 $t = 9.9$ h

6.4

6.4.1 (A) $\log C_p = 1.76 - 0.0471t$ $K = 0.106$ h^{-1}

(B) $\log C_p = 1.87 - 0.0294t$ $K = 0.067$ h^{-1}

(B$_{dial}$) $\log C_p = 1.72 - 0.0546t$ $K = 0.125$ h^{-1}

6.4.2 $C_{P_A}^0 = 57.54$ mg/L $\quad C_{P_B}^0 = 74.13$ mg/L $\quad C_{P_{Bdial.}}^0 = 52.48$ mg/L

6.4.3 $AUC_A = 542.83$ mg h/L $\quad AUC_B = 1106.40$ mg h/L $\quad AUC_{Bdial.} = 419.84$ mg h/L

6.4.4 $Cl_{tA} = 15.35$ mL/min $\quad Cl_{tB} = 7.53$ml/min $\quad Cl_{tBdial} = 19.84$ mL/min

6.4.5 $(1/K)_A = 9.43$ h $\quad (1/K)_B = 14.92$ h $\quad (1/K)_{Bdial.} = 8$ h

6.4.6 $(f_{el})_A = 0.470$ $\quad (f_{el})_B = 0.331$ $\quad (f_{el})_{Bdial.} = 0.527$

6.4.7 $t_A = 13$ h $\quad t_B = 20.7$ h $\quad t_{bdial.} = 11.09$ h

6.4.8 Class discussion

6.5

6.5.1 $(T_{1/2})_A = 3$ h $\quad (T_{1/2})_B = 6$ h

$(V_d)_A = 15$ L $\quad (V_d)_B = 60$ L

$(Cl_t)_A = 3.465$ L/h $\quad (Cl_t)_B = 6.93$L/h

6.5.2 $(dose)_A = 900$ mg $\quad (dose)_B = 3600$ mg

6.5.3 $(AUC)_A = 259.74$ mg h/L $\quad (AUC)_B = 519.48$ mg h/L

6.5.4 $(A_{el})_A = 675$ mg $\quad (A_{el})_B = 1800$ mg

6.6

$K = 0.46$ h^{-1} $\quad C_p^0 = 1000$ mg

$C_p = 1000(mg)e^{-0.46t}$

6.7

$\log C_p = 1.698 - 0.113t$

$C_p = 50(mg/L)e^{-0.26\,(1/h)\,t}$

6.7.1 $T_{1/2} = 2.66$ h

6.7.2 $V_d = 10$ L
6.7.3 $Cl_t = 2.6$ L/h
6.7.4 $(A_{el})_{2T_{1/2}} = 375$ mg
6.7.5 $t = 3.52$ h

6.8

TABLE A1.5 **Answer to Assignment 6.8**

Parameter/Constant	Drug A	Drug B
Fraction of dose in body at $t = 3$ h	0.50	0.25
AUC (mg h/L)	1302.65	432.90
Mean residence time (h)	4.34	2.16
Total body clearance (mL/min)	51.18	154.32
Rate of elimination at $t = 3$ h (mg/h)	460.62	924.00

6.9

6.9.1 $C_{p_{4h}} = 0.25 \times 25 = 6.25$ mg/L
6.9.2 $Cl_t = (500/25)(0.693/2) = 6.93$ L/h
6.9.3 $f_b = 0.1$
6.9.4 $(A_{el})_{4h} = 0.75 \times 500m = 375$ mg

6.10

$C_p^0 = 250(0.693/2.89) = 60$ mg/L
$C_{p_{MEC}} = 60e^{-0.24 \times 4} = 23$ mg/L

6.11

6.11.1 $C_p^0 = 100$ mg/L, $K = 0.2303$ h^{-1}, $T_{1/2} = 3$ h, $V_d = 20$ L, $t_d = IT_{1/2} = 3$ h
6.11.2 $Cl_t = 20 \times 0.2303 = 4.6$ L/h $= 76.76$ mL/min
6.11.3 6 h $= 2T_{1/2}$; therefore, total amount eliminated $= 1500$ mg
6.11.4 $(\text{rate})_{3h} = (50 \ \mu g/mL) \times (76.76 \ mL/min) = 3838 \ \mu g/min = 230.3$ mg/h
6.11.5 AUC $= 100/0.2303 = 434.21$ mg h/L

6.12

6.12.1 100 mg
6.12.2 2 h
6.12.3 10 h

CHAPTER 7

7.1

7.1.1 $K = 0.594 \text{ h}^{-1} = 0.0099 \text{ min}^{-1}$
$k_0 = 100 \text{ mg/min} = 6 \text{ g/h}$

$$C_{p_{Tic}} = \frac{100 \text{ mg/min}}{100 \text{ mL/min}} (1 - e^{-0.594 \times 0.5}) = 0.257 \text{ mg/mL} = 257 \text{ mg/L}$$

7.1.2 $K = 0.01155 \text{ min}^{-1}$
$k_0 = 200 \text{ mg/h}$

$$C_{p_{CA}} = \frac{200 \text{ mg/h}}{12 \text{ L/h}} (1 - e^{-0.01155 \times 30}) = 4.88 \text{ mg/L}$$

7.1.3 $C_{p_{140 \text{ min}_{Tic}}} = 0.25 \times 257 = 64.25 \text{ mg/L}$
7.1.4 $C_{p_{1 \text{ h}_{CA}}} = 0.5 \times 4.88 = 2.44 \text{ mg/L}$

7.1.5 $V_d = \dfrac{200 \text{ mL/min}}{0.01155 \text{ min}^{-1}} = 17316 \text{ mL} = 17.3 \text{ L}$

7.1.6 $V_d = \dfrac{6 \text{ L/h}}{0.594 \text{ h}^{-1}} = 10.10 \text{ L}$

Amount eliminated $= 3000 \text{ mg} - (257 \times 10.10) = 404.3 \text{ mg}$

7.1.7 $Cl_m = 200 - 100 = 100 \text{ mL/min}$

7.1.8 $C_{p_{ss}} = \dfrac{6 \text{ g/h}}{6 \text{ L/h}} = 1 \text{ g/L} = 1000 \text{ mg/L}$

$$\frac{C_{p_{MEC}}}{C_{p_{ss}}} = \frac{60}{1000} = 0.06$$

$$f_{ss} = 1 - e^{-Kt}$$

Therefore, $t_{onset} = \dfrac{\ln(1 - f_{ss})}{K} = -\dfrac{\ln(1 - 0.06)}{0.594} = 0.104 \text{ h} = 6.24 \text{ min}$

$$t_{dinfusion} = 30 - 6.24 = 23.76 \text{ min} = 0.396 \text{ h}$$

$$t_{dpostinfusion} = \frac{2.303}{0.594} \log \frac{257 \text{ mg/L}}{60 \text{ mg/L}} = 2.45 \text{ h}$$

Therefore, $t_{dtotal} = 0.396 + 2.45 = 2.846 \text{ h}$

7.2

7.2.1 $k_0 = 8.34 \text{ mg/h}$
$K = 0.3465 \text{ h}^{-1}$
$V_d = 150 \text{ L}$

$$Cl_t = 150 \text{ L} \times 0.3465 \text{ h}^{-1} = 52 \text{ L/h}$$

$$C_{p_{ss}} = \frac{8.34 \text{ mg/h}}{52 \text{ L/h}} = 0.16 \text{ mg/L}$$

7.2.2 Flow rate = $(8.34 \text{ mg/h})/(0.4 \text{ mg/mL}) = 20.83 \text{ mL/h}$
   or flow rate = $500/24 = 20.83 \text{ mL/h}$
7.2.3 $C_p = 0.16(1 - e^{-0.3465(6)}) = 0.14 \text{ mg/L}$
7.2.4 $k_0 = KA_{ss} = 8.34 \text{ mg/L}$
7.2.5 $15 \text{ h} > 7T_{1/2}$
   Therefore, $C_p = C_{p_{ss}} = 0.16 \text{ mg/L}$
7.2.6 $D_L = 0.16 \text{ mg/L} \times 150 \text{ L} = 24 \text{ mg}$

7.3

7.3.1 $K = 0.693/6 = 0.1155$
   $Cl_t = 11.55 \text{ L/h}$
   $V_d = 11.55/0.1155 = 100 \text{ L}$
   $D_L = 10 \text{ mg/L} \times 11.55 \text{ L/h} = 115.50 \text{ mg/h}$
7.3.2 Total amount = $115.5 \text{ mg/h} \times 12 = 1386 \text{ mg}$
   Volume of solution = $12 \text{ h} \times 60 \text{ min/h} \times 1 \text{ mL} = 720$
   Concentration = $1387 \text{ mg}/720 \text{ mL} = 1.925 \text{ mg/mL}$
7.3.3 $t = 1T_{1/2} = 6 \text{ h}$
7.3.4 $f_{ss} = 1 - e^{-Kt}$

$$t = \frac{-\ln(1 - f_{ss})}{K} = \frac{-\ln(1 - 0.8)}{0.1155} = 13.9 \text{ h} = 14 \text{ h}$$

7.3.5 $C_{p_{1h}} = 10e^{-0.1155 \times 1} = 8.91 \text{ mg/L}$
   $C_{p_{6h}} = 10 \times 0.5 \text{ 5 mg/L}$
   $C_{p_{12h}} = 10 \times 0.25 = 2.5 \text{ mg/L}$
7.3.6 $Cl_t = 2 + 6.55 = 8.55 \text{ L/h}$
   $K = (8.55 \text{ L/h})/(100 \text{ L}) = 0.0855 \text{ h}^{-1}$
   $T_{1/2} = 8.10 \text{ h}$
   $D_L = 10 \text{ mg/L} \times 100 \text{ L} = 1000 \text{ mg} = 1 \text{ g}$
   $k_0 = 10 \text{ mg/L} \times 8.55 \text{ L/h} = 85.5 \text{ mg/h}$

7.4

7.4.1 $V_d = 0.3 \times 80 \text{ kg} = 24 \text{ L}$
   $K = 0.693 \text{ h}^{-1}$
   $k_0 = 4 \text{ g}/0.5 \text{ h} = 8 \text{ g/h}$

$$C_{p_{6:30}} = \frac{8 \text{ g/L}}{24 \times 0.693} (1 - e^{-0.693 \times 0.5}) = 0.14 \text{ mg/L}$$

7.4.2 $C_{p_{12}} = 0.14e^{-0.693 \times 5.5} = 0.003 \text{ mg/L}$
7.4.3 $A_{12} = 0.003 \times 24 = 0.072 \text{ mg}$
7.4.4 $A_{12:30} = 0.14 \text{ mg/L} \times 24\text{L} + 0.072e^{-0.693 \times 0.5} = 3.41 \text{ mg}$

7.5

250 mg

7.6

0.833 mL/min

7.7

15 mg/L

7.8

75 mg/L

7.9

20 mg/h

7.10

7.10.1 Weight = 176/2.2 = 80 kg

$k_0 = 500$ mg/h, $V_d = 32$ L, $K = 0.007$ min^{-1} = 0.462 h^{-1}

$Cl_t = 14.784$ L/h

$C_{p_{7AM}} = (500/14.784)(1 - e^{-0.462\,(1)}) = 12.5$ mg/L

7.10.2 5 h = $3.3T_{1/2}$

$C_{p_{12noon}} = 0.1 \times 12.51 = 1.25$ mg/L

7.10.3 $(C_{p_{1PM}})_{\text{from 1st dose}} = 1.25e^{-0.462\,(1)} = 0.7875$ mg/L

$(C_{p_{1PM}})_{\text{total}} = 12.51 + 0.7875) = 13.3$ mg/L

7.10.4 $D_L = (15$ mg/L$) \times (32$ L$) = 480$ mg

$k_0 = (15$ mg/L$) \times (14.784$ L/h$) = 221.76$ mg/h = 3.7 mg/min

CHAPTER 8

8.1

8.1.1 The regression equation of the extrapolated line is

$$\log \tilde{C}_p = 1.59 - 0.0054(t)$$

The residuals are 34.00, 29.08, 18.35, and 9.89.

The equation of the residual line is

$$\log(\breve{C}_p - C_p) = 1.66 - 0.0108(t)$$

Treatment A   *Treatment B*

$K = 0.0127$ min^{-1} $K = 0.013$ min^{-1}

$k_a = 0.025$ min^{-1} $k_a = 0.025$ min^{-1}

8.1.2 $F_A = \dfrac{38.9 \times 19(0.025 - 0.0127)}{500 \times 0.025} = 0.727$

$F_B = 0.675$ (no significant difference)

8.1.3 $C_{\text{p max A}} = 10.138$ mg/L $C_{\text{p max B}} = 8.74$ mg/L

8.1.4 $\text{Cl}_{rA} = 132.70$ mL/min $\text{Cl}_{rB} = 212.20$ mL/min

8.2

Treatment A

8.2.1

Extrapolated line: $\breve{C}_p = 91.415(\mu\text{g/L})e^{-0.4(\text{h}^{-1})t}$

Residual line: $\breve{C}_p - C_p = 131.22(\mu\text{g/L})e^{-3.455(\text{h}^{-1})t}$

8.2.2 $T_{\max} = \dfrac{2.303}{3.455 - 0.4} \log \dfrac{3.455}{0.4} = 0.706$ h

8.2.3 $F = \dfrac{91.415 \ \mu\text{g/L} \times 120 \ \text{L} \times (3.455 - 0.4)}{3.455 \ \text{h}^{-1} \times 10 \ \text{mg} \times 1000 \ \mu\text{g/mg}} = 0.97$

8.2.4 $C_{\text{p max}} = \dfrac{0.97 \times 10 \ \text{mg}}{120 \ \text{L}} e^{-0.4 \times 0.7} = 0.061$ mg/L $= 61 \ \mu\text{g/L}$

8.2.5 $\text{AUC} = 91.415 \ \mu\text{g/L}\left(\dfrac{1}{0.4} - \dfrac{1}{3.455}\right) = 202.08 \ \mu\text{gh/L}$

8.2.6 $\text{Cl}_t = \dfrac{0.97 \times 10 \ \text{mg} \times 1000 \ \mu\text{g/mg}}{202 \ \mu\text{gh/L}} = 48.02$ L/h

Treatment B

8.2.1

Extrapolated line: $\breve{C}_p = 67(\mu\text{g/L})e^{-0.389(\text{h}^{-1})t}$

Residual line: $\breve{C}_p - C_p = 97.72(\mu\text{g/L})e^{-2.945(\text{h}^{-1})t}$

8.2.2 $T_{\max} = \dfrac{2.303}{2.945 - 0.389} \log \dfrac{2.945}{0.389} = 0.792$ h

8.2.3 $F = \dfrac{67.95 \times 120 \times (2.945 - 0.389)}{2.945 \times 10,000} = 0.707$

8.2.4 $C_{p_{max}} = \dfrac{0.707 \times 10,000}{120} e^{-0.389 \times 0.792} = 43.30 \ \mu g/L$

8.2.5 $AUC = 67.95\left(\dfrac{1}{0.389} - \dfrac{1}{2.945}\right) = 151.60 \ \mu g \ h/L$

8.2.6 $Cl_t = \dfrac{0.707 \times 10,000}{151.6} = 46.63 \ L/h$

8.2.7

Treatment	T_{max} (h)	F	$C_{p_{max}}$ (mg/L)	AUC (mg h/L)	Cl_t (L/h)
A	0.706	0.970	61	202.08	48.02
B	0.792*	0.707*	43*	151.60*	46.63

*$P < 0.05$

The parameters of Treatment B that are identified by (*) are significantly different from Treatment A. The increase of T_{max} and reduction of AUC are indicative of a slower rate of absorption and a lower availability of the drug given with high fat diet. The decline of F, the fraction of dose absorbed, is consistent with the reduction of AUC. The maximum plasma concentration was also reduced significantly. However, the total body clearance, as it was expected, remained essentially the same. It can be concluded that the high fat diet reduced the bioavailability of the drug and its duration and intensity of action.

8.3

8.3.1 The overall elimination rate constant, $K = 0.5 \ h^{-1}$.
   The following area terms are calculated with the inclusion of the calculated initial plasma concentration:
   $(AUC_0^{7 \ h})_{IV} = 391.38 \ mg \ h/L$
   $(AUC_0^{7 \ h})_{oral} = 241.95 \ mg \ h/L$
   $(\text{Terminal area})_{IV} = 6.039/0.5 = 12.078 \ mg \ h/L$
   $(\text{Terminal area})_{oral} = 4.529/0.5 = 9.058 \ mg \ h/L$
   $(AUC_0^{\infty})_{IV} = 391.38 + 12.078 = 403.46 \ mg \ h/L$
   $(AUC_0^{\infty})_{oral} = 241.95 + 9.058 = 251.00 \ mg \ h/L$
   (Note: AUC_{IV} without the initial plasma concentration is 301.65 mg h/L.)
8.3.2 Krüger–Thiemer method:
   $F = 251/403.46 = 0.622$
   $(C_p^0)_{IV} = 200 \ mg/L$, $(\overleftarrow{C}_p^0)_{p.o.} = 150 \ mg/L$

$$k_a = \frac{K}{1 - \dfrac{FC_p^0}{\bar{C}_p^0}} = \frac{0.5}{1 - \dfrac{0.622 \times 200}{150}} = 2.929 \text{ h}^{-1}$$

Wagner–Nelson method:

TABLE A1.6 Calculations of Wagner–Nelson Method: Solution to Assignment 8.3

K_{AUC}	$C_p + K_{AUC}$	$C_p + K_{AUC}$	$\%(A_D/V_d)$	Time (h)	Log $100-\%A_{D/V_d}$
2.027	49.729	49.729	39.8203	0.17	1.77945
4.212	65.731	65.731	52.6333	0.25	1.67547
6.871	78.318	78.318	62.7125	0.33	1.57156
13.450	96.800	96.800	77.5117	0.50	1.35196
24.114	111.397	111.397	89.2005	0.75	1.03340
34.789	118.300	118.300	94.7277	1.00	0.72200
53.876	123.064				
69.376	124.186				
91.441	124.892				
104.879	125.178				
113.032	125.344				
117.977	125.445				
120.976	125.505				
Average = 124.802					

Average = 124.802
Log $100 - \%AD/V_d = 1.993 - 1.275t$
Therefore, $k_a = 1.275 \times 2.303 = 2.936 \text{ h}^{-1}$
Peeling method:

TABLE A1.7 Calculation of Residuals (Peeling Method): Part of the Answer to Assignment 8.3

$\bar{C}_p$	$\bar{C}_p - C_p$
137.77	90.07
132.37	70.85
128.18	55.73
116.82	33.47

Log $(\overleftarrow{C}_p - C_p) = 2.176 - 1.302t$
Therefore, $k_a = 1.302 \times 2.303 = 2.998 = 3 \text{ h}^{-1}$

8.3.3 Assuming $k_a = 2.9 \text{ h}^{-1}$

$$T_{\text{max}} = \frac{2.303}{2.9 - 0.5} \log \frac{2.9}{0.5} = 0.732 \text{ h}$$

$$V_d = \frac{0.622 \times 2000 \text{ mg}}{0.5 \text{ h}^{-1} \times 251 \text{ mg h/L}} = 9.91 \text{ L}$$

$$C_{\text{Pmax}} = \frac{0.625 \times 2000 \text{ mg}}{9.91 \text{ L}} (e^{-0.5 \times 0.732}) = 87.47 \text{ mg/L}$$

8.4

TABLE A1.8 Answer to Assignment 8.4

Parameter/Constant	Answer
Plasma concentration at $t = 10$ h	25 mg/L
T_{max}	0.968 h
Total amount absorbed	796.54 mg
Area under plasma concentration–time curve	692.64 mg h/L

8.5

$A_D = \text{zero}$

8.6

$t_d = 0$

8.7

$k_a = 2.303 \text{ h}^{-1}$

8.8

$t_1 = 9 \text{ min}$

CHAPTER 9

9.1

9.1.1 $\log \text{ARE} = 2.60 - 0.0603t$
9.1.2 $K = 0.1388 \text{ h}^{-1}$

9.1.3 $T_{1/2} = 5$ h
9.1.4 $f_e = 0.8$
9.1.5 $k_m = 0.0278$ h^{-1}
9.1.6 $\log(\Delta A_e/\Delta t) = 1.74 - 0.098t_{midpoint}$

9.2

9.2.1 $Cl_r = 4$ L/h $= 67.22$ mL/min, $Cl_m = 3.72$ L/h
9.2.2 $f_e = 0.52$
9.2.3 $f_m = 0.48$

9.3

9.3.1 $\log ARE = 2.93 - 0.0904t$, or $ARE = 850e^{-0.208t}$

9.4

9.4.1 $(A_e)_{10\ h} = (A_e)_{2T_{1/2}} = 3$ g $= 75\%$ dose, ie, $A_e^\infty =$ dose
      Therefore, $f_e = 1$ and $k_e = K = 0.138$ h^{-1}
9.4.2 $Cl_r = 3.588$ L/h $= 60$ mL/min
9.4.3 $f_b = 0.5$
9.4.4 $ARE = 4e^{-0.138t}$, or $\log ARE = 0.602 - 0.06t$
      Rate $= 0.552e^{-0.138t_{midpoint}}$, or $\log$ rate $= -0.258 - 0.06t$

9.5

TABLE A1.9 Answer to Assignment 9.5

	A_e^∞ (mg)	k_e (h^{-1})	K_m (h^{-1})	A_m^∞ (mg)	$(f_{el})_{3\ h}$
Rest	60	0.0184	0.211	690	0.5
Exercise	42.4	0.026	0.44	707.6	0.75

9.6

TABLE A1.10 Answer to Assignment 9.6

Parameter/Constant	Drug A	Drug B
Metabolic rate constant (h^{-1})	0.45	0.35
Total amount excreted unchanged (mg)	50	62.5
Total amount eliminated as metabolite(s) (mg)	450	437.5
Metabolic clearance (mL/min)	45	35
Area under plasma concentration–time curve (mg h/L)	166.6	208.3

9.7

The equation of the linear segment of t he curve (last four data points) is

$$Y = 34.93t - 47.90$$

9.7.1 $K = 0.79 \text{ h}^{-1}$
9.7.2 $f_e = 0.58$
9.7.3 $f_m = 0.417$
9.7.4 $T_{1/2} = 0.877 \text{ h}$

9.8

Simulation of the ARE Equation of Assignment 9.8

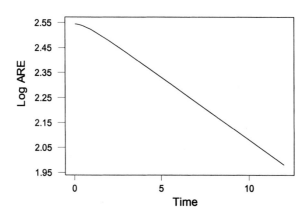

Simulation of the Rate Equation of Assignment 9.8

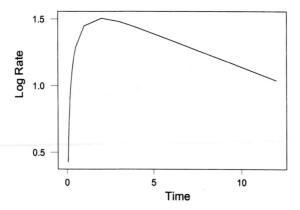

9.9

9.9.1 100 mg
9.9.2 0.1
9.9.3 0.092 h^{-1}
9.9.4 250 mg
9.9.5 1.61 L/h

9.10

9.10.1

TABLE A1.11 Calculations Related to Assignment 9.10

ΔA_e	Δt	$\Delta A_e/\Delta t$	$t_{midpoint}$
160	0.25	640	0.125
140	0.25	560	0.375
200	0.50	400	0.750
250	1.00	250	1.50
188	2.00	94	3.00
46	2.00	23	5.00

Slope $= -0.3$
$K = 0.69$ h^{-1}

9.10.2 $A_e^\infty = 0.6 \times$ dose, dose $= 1.67$ g

9.10.3 $k_e = 0.6 \times 0.69 = 0.414$ h^{-1}

9.10.4 $C_p^0 = (6.25$ mg/L$)/e^{-0.69 \times 4} = 98.75$ mg/L
$V_d = 1670/98.75 = 16.91$ L
$Cl_t = 16.91 \times 0.69 = 11.66$ L/h $= 194.465$ mL/min
$Cl_r = 0.6 \times 194.465 = 116.679$ mL/min $= 6.993$ L/h
$Cl_m = 0.4 \times 194.465 = 77.786$ mL/min $= 4.667$ L/h

9.10.5 ARE $= 1$ (g) $\exp(-0.69$ (h^{-1}) $\times t)$

CHAPTER 10

10.1

10.1.1 $V_d = 17.03$ L, $Cl_t = 6.4$ L/h, $Cl_r = 4.58$ L/h, $K = 0.376$ h^{-1}, $(C_{p_{min}})_1 = 1.29$ mg/L

10.1.2 $(C_{p_{max}})_{ss} = 118.70$ mg/L

10.1.3 $C_{p_{6\,h}} = 12.43$ mg/L, $C_{p_{12\,h}} = (C_{p_{min}})_{ss} = 1.3$ mg/L

10.1.4 $(A_{ave})_{ss} = 0.44$ g

10.1.5 Total amount eliminated $= 2$ g

10.1.6 $A_m^\infty = 0.575$ g

10.1.7 $n\tau = 2.42$ h

10.1.8 $n\tau = 3.68$ h

10.2

10.2.1 Patient A $(C_{p_{min}})_{3rd} = 20.94$ mg/L
          Patient B $(C_{p_{min}})_{3rd} = 43.75$ mg/L
          Patient C $(C_{p_{min}})_{3rd} = 81$ mg/L
10.2.2 Patient A $(C_{p_{max}})_{ss} = 61.92$ mg/L
          $(C_{p_{min}})_{ss} = 21.57$ mg/L
          Patient B $(C_{p_{max}})_{ss} = 100$ mg/L
          $(C_{p_{min}})_{ss} = 50$ mg/L
          Patient C $(C_{p_{max}})_{ss} = 172.84$ mg/L
          $(C_{p_{min}})_{ss} = 102.67$ mg/L
10.2.3 Patient A $C_{p_{t'=4\,h}} = (C_{p_{max}})_{ss}/2 = 30.96$ mg/L
          $C_{p_{t'=8\,h}} = 25\%(C_{p_{max}})_{ss} = 15.48$ mg/L
          Patient B $C_{p_{t'=4\,h}} = 100e^{-0.1155\times4\,h} = 63$ mg/L
          $C_{p_{t'=8\,h}} = 100e^{-0.1155\times8\,h} = 39.7$ mg/L
          Patient C $C_{p_{t'=4\,h}} = 172.84e^{-0.0866\times4\,h} = 122.24$ mg/L
          $C_{p_{t'=8\,h}} = 172.84/2 = 86.42$ mg/L
10.2.4 Patient A $(C_{p_{ave}})_{ss} = 38.54$ mg/L
          Patient B $(C_{p_{ave}})_{ss} = 72.15$ mg/L
          Patient C $(C_{p_{ave}})_{ss} = 134.72$ mg/L
10.2.5 One approach, and obviously not the only one, would be:
          Patient A   Set $\tau = 4$ h. Keep dose the same, ie, $D_M = 500$ mg, $D_L = 1000$ mg.
                          To check:

$$(C_{p_{max}})_{ss} = 1000 \text{ mg}/12.5 \text{ L} = 80 \text{ mg/L}$$

$$(C_{p_{min}})_{ss} = 80/2 = 40 \text{ mg/L}$$

          Patient B   Set $\tau = 6$ h, $D_M = 500$ mg, $D_L = 1000$ mg.

$$(C_{p_{max}})_{ss} = 100 \text{ mg/L}$$

$$(C_{p_{min}})_{ss} = 50 \text{ mg/L}$$

          Patient C   Set $\tau = 8$ h, $D_M = 500$ mg, $D_L = 1000$ mg.

$$(C_{p_{max}})_{ss} = 140 \text{ mg/L}$$

$$(C_{p_{min}})_{ss} = 70 \text{ mg/L}$$

10.3

10.3.1 Patient A $(C_{p_{max}})_{ss} = 6.67$ mg/L, $(C_{p_{min}})_{ss} = 2.67$ mg/L
          Patient B $(C_{p_{max}})_{ss} = 20.65$ mg/L, $(C_{p_{min}})_{ss} = 15.65$ mg/L

10.3.2 Patient A $T_{1/2} = 3$ h, $7T_{1/2} < 24$ h

Therefore, steady-state levels are achieved.

$(C_{p_{max}})_{24\ h} = (C_{p_{max}})_{ss} = 6.67$ mg/L

$(C_{p_{min}})_{24\ h} = (C_{p_{min}})_{ss} = 2.67$ mg/L

Patient B $T_{1/2} = 10$ h, $7T_{1/2} > 24$ h

Therefore, steady-state levels are not achieved.

$(C_{p_{max}})_{n=6} = 16.73$ mg/L

$(C_{p_{min}})_{n=6} = 12.68$ mg/L

10.3.3 Patient A $(C_{p_{ave}})_{ss} = 4.35$ mg/L

Patient B $(C_{p_{ave}})_{ss} = 18.03$ mg/L

10.3.4 Patient A $R = 1.66$

Patient B $R = 4.13$

10.4

$K = 0.1732$ h^{-1}, $k_a = 1.386$ h^{-1}

Half-life of elimination $> 7(T_{1/2})_{ka}$

Set $\tau = 4$ h

$FD_M = 41$ mg/L $\times$ 10 L $\times$ 4 h $\times$ 0.1732 = 284.05

$D_M = 284.05/0.9 = 315.6$ mg $\cong$ 300 mg

$D_L = 315.6/(1 - e^{-0.1732 \times 4}) = 631$ mg $\cong$ 600 mg

Or $D_L = 2D_M$

$$\overleftarrow{C}_p^0 = \frac{0.9 \times 300 \times 1.386}{10(1.386 - 0.1732)} = 30.85 \cong 31 \text{ mg/L}$$

$$(C_{p_{min}})_{ss} = 31 \frac{e^{-0.1732 \times 4}}{1 - e^{-0.1732 \times 4}} = 31 \text{ mg/L}$$

$(T_{max})_{ss} = 1.146$ h

$FD_M/V_d = 28.40$ mg/L

$$(C_{p_{max}})_{ss} = 24 \left(\frac{e^{-0.1732 \times 1.146}}{1 - e^{-0.1732 \times 4}} \right) = 46.63 \text{ mg/L}$$

CHAPTER 11

11.1

Patient A	Patient B
$\overleftarrow{C}_p = 0.6e^{-0.355t}$	$\overleftarrow{C}_p = 0.62e^{-0.16t}$

11.1.1 $b = 0.6\%$ | $b = 0.62\%$

$\beta = 0.355$ h^{-1} | $\beta = 0.16$ h^{-1}

11.1.2 $(T_{1/2})_{biol} = 0.693/0.355 = 1.95$ h | $(T_{1/2}) = 4.4$ h

11.1.3 $(C_p - \overleftarrow{C}_p) = 0.5e^{-3.5}$ | $(C_p - \overleftarrow{C}_p) = 0.48e^{-1.7t}$

11.1.4 $C_p = 0.5e^{-3.5t} + 0.60e^{-0.355t}$ $C_p = 0.48e^{-1.7t} + 0.62e^{-0.16t}$

11.1.5 $C_p^0 = 1.1$ mg% $C_p^0 = 1.1$ mg%

        $V_1 = 1000/1.1$ mg% $= 90.90$ L $V_1 = 90.90$ L

11.1.6   AUC $= 18$ mg h/L   AUC $= 42$ mg h/L

11.1.7 $k_{21} = 2.07$ h^{-1} $k_{21} = 1.00$ h^{-1}

        $k_{10} = 0.60$ h^{-1} $k_{10} = 0.27$ h^{-1}

        $k_{12} = 1.2$ h^{-1} $k_{12} = 0.59$ h^{-1}

11.1.8 $(T_{1/2})_{elim} = 0.693/0.6 = 1.2$ h $(T_{1/2}) = 2.6$ h

11.1.9 $Cl_t = 90.90$ L $\times 0.6 = 55$ L/h $Cl_t = 24$ L/h

        Or $Cl_t = 1000$ mg/18 mg h L$^{-1} = 55$ L/h $Cl_t = 1000/42 = 24$ L/h

11.1.10 Patient A:

$$(AUC_0^\infty)_{peripheral} = \frac{1.2 \times 1000}{3.5 - 0.355}\left(\frac{1}{0.355} = \frac{1}{3.50}\right) = 965.8 \text{ mg h}$$

Patient B:

$$(AUC_0^\infty)_{peripheral} = \frac{0.59 \times 1000}{1.7 - 0.16}\left(\frac{1}{0.16} - \frac{1}{1.7}\right) = 2169.11 \text{ mg h}$$

11.2   **Patient A**   **Patient B**

11.2.1

     $\overleftarrow{C}_p = 26.42e^{-0.608t}$ $\overleftarrow{C}_p = 30.76e^{-0.185t}$

     $(T_{1/2})_{biol} = 0.693/0.608 = 1.14$ h $(T_{1/2})_{biol} = 3.746$ h

11.2.2

     $(C_p - \overleftarrow{C}_p) = 76.03e^{-5t}$ $(C_p - \overleftarrow{C}_p) = 63.97e^{-1.84t}$

     $k_{12} = 5 + 0.608 - 1.74 - \dfrac{0.608 \times 5}{1.74} = 2.12$ h^{-1} $k_{12} = 0.832$ h^{-1}

     $k_{21} = \dfrac{(76.03 \times 0.608) + (26.42 \times 5)}{76.03 + 26.42} = 1.74$ h^{-1} $k_{21} = 0.722$ h^{-1}

11.2.3 $k_{10} = (0.608 \times 5)/1.74 = 1.747$ h^{-1} $k_{10} = 0.471$ h^{-1}

        $(T_{1/2})_{elim} = 0.693/1.747 = 0.4$ h $(T_{1/2})_{elim} = 1.47$ h^{-1}

11.2.4 $A_1 = 670$ mg $A_1 = 750$ mg

        $A_2 = 0$ $A_2 = 0$

11.2.5 $C_p = 76.03e^{-5t} + 26.42e^{-0.608t}$ $C_p = 63.97e^{-1.84t} + 30.76e^{-0.185t}$

11.2.6 $V_1 = 670/(76.03 + 26.42) = 6.53$ L $V_1 = 7.92$ L

11.2.7 $Cl_t = 1.747 \times 6.53 = 11.40$ L/h $Cl_t = 3.73$ L/h

11.2.8 $Cl_m \cong 4.56$ L/h $Cl_m \cong 3.73$ L/h

11.2.9 4 h $> 7(T_{1/2})_\alpha$ 4 h $< 7(T_{1/2})_\alpha$

     $A_2 = \dfrac{670 \times 2.12}{5 - 0.608}e^{-0.608 \times 4} = 28.43$ mg $A_2 = \dfrac{750 \times 0.832}{1.84 - 0.185}$

                                                                   $(e^{-0.185 \times 4} - e^{-1.84 \times t})$

                                                                   $= 179.65$ mg

11.2.10 $A_1 = 6.53\ \text{L}(26.42e^{-0.608\times4}) = 15.16\ \text{mg}$ $A_1 = 117.02\ \text{mg}$

11.2.11 $A_{\text{Total}} = 28.43 + 15.16 = 43.6\ \text{mg}$ $A_{\text{Total}} = 296.65\ \text{mg}$

11.2.12 $6\ \text{h} > 7(T_{1/2})_\alpha$ $6\ \text{h} < 7(T_{1/2})_\alpha$

$\quad C_{p_{6\ \text{h}}} = 26.42e^{-0.608\times6} = 0.7\ \text{mg/L}$ $C_{p_{6\ \text{h}}} = 10.14\ \text{mg/L}$

11.2.13 $(C_{p_{\max}})_2 = 0.7 + (670/6.53) = 103.30\ \text{mg/L}$ $(C_{p_{\max}})_2 = 104.83\ \text{mg/L}$

11.2.14

$$(V_{\text{d}})_{\text{area}} = \frac{670}{0.608 \times \left(\dfrac{76.03}{5} + \dfrac{26.42}{0.608}\right)} = 18.78\ \text{L} \qquad (V_{\text{d}})_{\text{area}} = 20.16\ \text{L}$$

11.2.15

$$T_{\max} = \frac{2.303}{5 - 0.608}\log\frac{5}{0.608} = 2.10\ \text{h} \qquad T_{\max} = 1.39\ \text{h}$$

$$2.10\ \text{h} > 7(T_{1/2})_\alpha \qquad\qquad 1.39\ \text{h} < 7(T_{1/2})_\alpha$$

$$(A_{\max})_{\text{peripheral}} = \frac{2.12 \times 670}{5 - 0.608}e^{-0.608\times2.1} \qquad (A_{\max})_{\text{peripheral}} = 262.33\ \text{mg}$$

$$= 90.24\ \text{mg}$$

11.3 $(T_{1/2})_{\text{biol}} = 0.693/0.533 = 1.30\ \text{h}$

11.4

TABLE A1.12 Answer to Assignment 11.4

Parameter/Constant	Answer	Units
Plasma concentration 6 h after injection	15	μg/mL
Half-life of disposition	6	h
Rate constants of distribution	$k_{21} = 0.01$	min^{-1}
	$k_{12} = 0.015$	
Apparent volume of distribution of central compartment	10	L
Amount of drug in peripheral compartment at $t = 6$ h	282.90	mg
Area under plasma concentration–time curve	300.14	mg h/L
Total body clearance	55.53	mL/min

11.5

$$(T_{1/2})_{\text{biol}} = 0.693 \Big/ \frac{3000\ \text{mg}}{750\ \text{mg h/L} \times 20\ \text{L}} = 3.465\ \text{h}$$

11.6

$$AUC_0^\infty = 500 \text{ mg} \left/ \frac{500 \text{ mg} \times 0.5 \text{ h}^{-1}}{100 \text{ mg/L}} \right. = 200 \text{ mg h/L}$$

CHAPTER 12

12.1

12.1.1 $\beta = \dfrac{0.213}{7.38} = 0.02886 \text{ h}^{-1}$

$(T_{1/2})_{biol} = 0.693/0.02886 = 24 \text{ h}$
72 h $= 2(T_{1/2})_{biol}$ after the steady-state trough level
Therefore, $C_{p_{t'=72 \text{ h}}} = 0.25 \times 1 \ \mu g/mL = 0.25 \ \mu g/mL$

12.1.2 $f_{ss} = 1 - e^{-3 \times 0.029 \times 24} = 0.876$
$(C_{p_{max}})_3 = 0.876 \times 2 \ \mu g/mL = 1.752 \ \mu g/mL$

12.1.3 $n\tau = -3.3 \times 24 \text{ h} \times \log(1 - 0.65) = 36 \text{ h}$

12.1.4 $n\tau = 24 \text{ h}$

12.2

12.2.1 $k_{21} = 0.6 \text{ h}^{-1}$, $k_{10} = 0.6 \text{ h}^{-1}$, $V_1 = 3.3 \text{ L}$
$(C_{p_{ave}})_{ss} = 50/(3.3 \text{ L} \times 0.6 \text{ h}^{-1} \times 6 \text{ h}) = 4.2 \text{ mg/L}$
or
AUC $= 25.25 \text{ mg h/L}$, $(V_d)_{area} = 10 \text{ L}$
$(C_{p_{ave}})_{ss} = 50 \text{ mg}/(10 \text{ L} \times 0.2 \text{ h}^{-1} \times 6 \text{ h}) = 4.2 \text{ mg/L}$

12.2.2 $D_L = 50 \text{ mg}/(1 - e^{-0.2 \times 6}) = 71.55 \text{ mg}$

12.2.3 $(T_{1/2})_\alpha = 0.385 \text{ h}$; therefore, $\tau > 7(T_{1/2})_\alpha$

$$(C_{p_{min}})_{ss} = 3.75\left(\frac{e^{-0.2 \times 6}}{1 - e^{-0.2 \times 6}}\right) = 1.62 \text{ mg/L}$$

12.2.4 $C_{p_{t'=12 \text{ h}}} = 1.6e^{-0.2 \times (12-6)} = 0.488 \text{ mg/L}$

12.2.5 $n\tau = -3.3 \times (0.693/0.2) \times \log(1 - 0.8) = 8 \text{ h}$

12.2.6 $R = 1.43$

12.2.7 $(A_m)_\tau = 23 \text{ mg}$ \qquad $(A_e)_\tau = 27 \text{ mg}$

CHAPTER 14

14.1

14.1.1 $K = 0.693/2.3 \text{ h} = (6 \text{ L/h})/20 \text{ L} = 0.3 \text{ h}^{-1}$
$K_m = (0.4 \text{ L/h})/20 \text{ L} = 0.02 \text{ h}^{-1}$

IBW = 80 kg

$$\overline{C}_{cr} = \frac{(140 - 70)80}{72 \times 4} = 19.44 \text{ mL/min}$$

$$\frac{\overline{K}}{K} = 1 - \left(\frac{0.3 - 0.02}{0.3} \left(1 - \frac{19.44}{120} \right) \right) = 0.212$$

$\overline{D} = (3 \text{ mg kg}^{-1}/\text{d}) \times 0.212 = 0.636 \text{ mg kg}^{-1}/\text{d}$
$\overline{D} = 0.636 \times 80 \text{ kg} = 50.88 \text{ mg/d}$
$\overline{D} = 50.88/3 = 17 \text{ mg t.i.d.}$
Using the accumulation ratio method:
$(A_{ave})_{ss} = (1.44 \times 2.3 \text{ h} \times 1 \text{ mg/kg})/8 \text{ h} = 0.414 \text{ mg/kg}$
$\overline{T}_{1/2} = 0.639/(0.212 \times 0.3) = 10.9 \text{ h}$
$\overline{D} = (0.414 \times 8)/(1.44 \times 10.9) = 17 \text{ mg every 8 h}$
14.1.2 $\overline{D} = (1 \text{ mg/kg}) \times (0.212) \times (12/8) = 0.318 \text{ mg/kg b.i.d.}$
$\qquad\qquad\qquad\qquad\qquad\qquad\quad = 25.44 \text{ mg b.i.d.}$

Using the accumulation ratio method:
$(A_{ave})_{ss} = 0.414 \text{ mg/kg}$
$\overline{D} = (0.414 \times 12)/(1.44 \times 10.9) = 0.316 \text{ mg/kg b.i.d.}$
$\qquad\qquad\qquad\qquad\qquad\qquad\quad = 25.28 \text{ mg b.i.d.}$

14.1.3 $(C_{p_{max}})_{ss} = \dfrac{17 \text{ mg}}{20(1 - e^{-0.0636 \times 8})} = 2.13 \text{ mg/L}$

$\qquad (C_{p_{min}})_{ss} = 2.13 e^{-0.0636 \times 8} = 1.28 \text{ mg/L}$

$\qquad (C_{p_{max}})_{ss} = \dfrac{25 \text{ mg}}{20(1 - e^{-0.0636 \times 12})} = 2.34 \text{ mg/L}$

$\qquad (C_{p_{min}})_{ss} = 1.09 \text{ mg/L}$

14.1.4 $\overline{\tau} = 8 \left(\dfrac{0.3}{0.0636} \right) = 37 \text{ h}$

14.1.5 $\overline{D} = 50.88 \text{ mg/d}$

14.2

$$\overline{K} = 0.12 \left(1 - \left(0.975 \left(1 - \frac{30.3}{120} \right) \right) \right) = 0.0325 \text{ h}^{-1}$$

14.3

14.3.1 $\overline{D} = 260 \text{ mg b.i.d.}$
14.3.2 $\overline{D} = 172 \text{ mg t.i.d.}$

14.4

14.4.1 $\overline{C}_{cr} = 15.93$ mL/min

14.4.2 $\overline{K} = 0.017\left(1 - \left(\dfrac{0.017 - 0.008}{0.017}\left(1 - \dfrac{15.93}{120}\right)\right)\right) = 0.009$ h^{-1}

14.4.3 $\overline{\tau} = 21.7$ h (≈ 24 h)

14.4.4 $\overline{D} = 0.138$ mg

CHAPTER 15

15.1

15.1.1 $\overleftarrow{C}_p^0 = C_p^0 = 21$ mg/L

$$(C_{p_{max}})_{ss} = \frac{250}{12(1 - e^{-0.058 \times 12})} = 41.5 \text{ mg/L}$$

$$(C_{p_{min}})_{ss} = 20.7 \text{ mg/L}$$

15.1.2 $C_{p_{12 \text{ noon}}} = \dfrac{250 e^{-0.058 \times 4}}{12(1 - e^{-0.058 \times 12})} = 32.94$ mg/L

$C_{p_{6 \text{ PM}}} = 32.94 e^{-(0.058 + 0.2) \times 6} = 7.00$ mg/L

15.1.3 $C_{p_{8 \text{ PM}}} = 7 e^{-0.058(2)} = 6.23$ mg/L

$(C_{p_{ave}})_{ss} = 29.93$ mg/L

$D_M = 12(29.93 - 6.23) = 284.40$ mg

CHAPTER 17

17.1

$\text{AUC}_0^{16 \text{ h}} = 11.7$ mg h/L

$\text{AUC}_{terminal} = 2.307$ mg h/L

17.1.1 $\text{AUC}_0^{\infty} = 14$ mg h/L

$\text{AUMC}_0^{16 \text{ h}} = 70.50$ mg h^2/L

$\text{AUMC}_{terminal} = 54.67$ mg h^2/L

$\text{AUMC}_0^{\infty} = 125.17$ mg h^2/L

$\text{MRT} = 8.94$ h

17.1.2 $\text{Cl}_t = \dfrac{0.85 \times 250}{14} = 15.17$ L/h

17.1.3 $f_b = 1 - (6.5/14) = 0.535$

GLOSSARY OF VARIABLES AND CONSTANTS

Symbol	Definition
a	Coefficient of exponential term
A_1	Amount of drug in central compartment
A_2	Amount of drug in peripheral compartment
A_D	Amount of drug at site of absorption
A_e	Total amount excreted unchanged in interval of t
A_e^∞	Total amount excreted unchanged
A_{el}	Total amount eliminated in time t
α	First-order hybrid rate constant
A_{me}^∞	Total amount eliminated as metabolite(s)
a_N	Normalized value of a with respect to the initial concentration
A_{ss}	Amount of drug in body at steady state
A_t	Amount of free drug at time t
AUC	Area under the plasma concentration–time curve
AUMC	Area under first-moment curve
$AUMC_2$	Area under second-moment curve
b	Coefficient of exponential term
b_N	Normalized value of b with respect to initial plasma concentration
β	Disposition rate constant
C	Concentration
C_2	Concentration of drug in peripheral compartment
$C_{arterial}$	Concentration of drug in arterial blood
$(C_{p_{ave}})_{ss}$	Average steady-state plasma concentration
C_{blood}	Concentration of drug in blood
C_{cr}	Creatinine clearance
Cl_l	Lung clearance
Cl_m	Metabolic clearance
Cl_r	Renal clearance
Cl_t	Total body clearance
C_p	Plasma concentration of drug
C_p^0	Initial plasma concentration of drug
$C_{p_{max}}$	Maximum plasma concentration
$(C_{p_{max}})_n$	Maximum plasma concentration before steady state
$(C_{p_{min}})_n$	Minimum plasma concentration before steady state
$(C_{p_{max}})_{ss}$	Steady-state peak level
$(C_{p_{min}})_{ss}$	Steady-state trough level
$C_{p_{MEC}}$	Minimum effective plasma concentration
$(C_{p_t})_n$	Plasma concentration at time t between maximum and minimum
C_{tissue}	Concentration of drug in tissue
D_{coeff}	Diffusion coefficient
D	Dose
dC	Change in concentration

Symbol	Definition
E	Effect (response)
$[E]$	Concentration of enzyme
E_{max}	Maximum effect
ER	Extraction ratio
F	Absolute bioavailability
f_b	Fraction of dose in body
f_e	Fraction of dose excreted unchanged
f_m	Fraction of dose eliminated as metabolite(s)
f_{ss}	Fraction of steady state
GFR	Glomerular filtration rate
J	Flux
K	Overall elimination rate constant
k_0	Zero-order rate of infusion
k_{12}	Distribution rate constant from central to peripheral compartment
k_{21}	Distribution rate constant from peripheral to central compartment
k_a	Absorption rate constant
k_{CE}	Input rate in effect compartment
k_e	Excretion rate constant
k_{EE}	Exit rate from effect compartment
K_{eq}	Equilibrium rate constant
k_m	Metabolic rate constant
K_M	Michaelis–Menten rate constant
k_{me}	Rate constant of elimination of metabolite(s)
MAT	Mean absorption time
MIT	Mean infusion time
MRT	Mean residence time
P	Membrane permeability
Q	Blood flow
R	Accumulation index
τ	Dosing interval
t_d	Duration of action
t_l	Lag time of absorption
$t_{midpoint}$	Midpoint of time interval of sampling
T_{max}	Time to maximum plasma concentration
$(T_{1/2})_\beta$	Biologic half-life
$(T_{1/2})_{k10}$	Elimination half-life
S_{Cr}	Serum creatinine
v	Rate of metabolism
V_1	Volume of central compartment
V_2	Volume of peripheral compartment
V_d	Apparent volume of distribution of one-compartment model
$(V_d)_{area}$	Apparent volume of distribution of two-compartment model
V_{max}	Maximum rate of metabolism
VRT	Variance of residence time

INDEX

*NOTE: A t following a page number indicates tabular material
and an f following a page number indicates a figure.*

NOTES

NOTES